T0332659

Immunology of Sexually Transmitted Diseases

IMMUNOLOGY AND MEDICINE SERIES

Immunology of Endocrine Diseases
Editor: A. M. McGregor

Clinical Transplantation: Current Practice and Future Prospects
Editor: G. R. D. Catto

Complement in Health and Disease
Editor: K. Whaley

Immunological Aspects of Oral Diseases
Editor: L. Ivanyi

Immunoglobulins in Health and Disease
Editor: M. A. H. French

Immunology of Malignant Diseases
Editors: V. S. Byers and R. W. Baldwin

Lymphoproliferative Diseases
Editors: D. B. Jones and D. H. Wright

Phagocytes and Disease
Editors: M. S. Klempner, B. Styrt and J. Ho

HLA and Disease
Authors: B. Bradley, P. T. Klouda, J. Bidwell and G. Laundy

Lymphocytes in Health and Disease
Editors: G. Janossy and P. L. Amlot

Mast Cells, Mediators and Disease
Editor: S. T. Holgate

Immunodeficiency and Disease
Editor: A. D. B. Webster

Immunology of Pregnancy and its Disorders
Editor: C. Stern

Immunotherapy of Disease
Editor: T. J. Hamblin

Immunology of Sexually Transmitted Diseases
Editor: D. J. M. Wright

IMMUNOLOGY
· SERIES · SERIES · SERIES · SERIES · AND SERIES · SERIES · SERIES · SERIES ·
MEDICINE

Immunology of Sexually Transmitted Diseases

Edited by

D. J. M. Wright

Reader/Consultant of Microbiology
Charing Cross Hospital (Fulham)
London

Series Editor: Professor W. G. Reeves

KLUWER ACADEMIC PUBLISHERS
DORDRECHT / BOSTON / LONDON

Distributors

for the United States and Canada: Kluwer Academic Publishers, PO Box 358, Accord Station, Hingham, MA 02018-0358, USA
for all other countries: Kluwer Academic Publishers Group, Distribution Center, PO Box, 322, 3300 AH Dordrecht, The Netherlands

British Library Cataloguing in Publication Data

Immunology of sexually transmitted diseases.
— (Immunology and medicine series).
1. Man. Sexually transmitted diseases.
Immunological aspects
I. Wright, D. J. M.   II. Series
616.9'51079

ISBN 978-0-7462-0087-2

Published in the United Kingdom by Kluwer Academic Publishers, PO Box 55, Lancaster, UK.

Kluwer Academic Publishers BV incorporates the publishing programmes of D. Reidel, Martinus Nijhoff, Dr W. Junk and MTP Press

Typeset by Witwell Ltd, Southport

Contents

Series Editor's Note

The modern clinician is expected to be the fount of all wisdom concerning conventional diagnosis and management relevant to his sphere of practice. In addition, he or she has the daunting task of comprehending and keeping pace with advances in basic science relevant to the pathogenesis of disease and ways in which these processes can be regulated or prevented. Immunology has grown from the era of anti-toxins and serum sickness to a state where the study of many diverse cells and molecules has become integrated into a coherent scientific discipline with major implications for many common and crippling diseases prevalent throughout the world.

Many of today's practitioners received little or no specific training in immunology and what was taught is very likely to have been overtaken by subsequent developments. This series of titles on IMMUNOLOGY AND MEDICINE is designed to rectify this deficiency in the form of distilled packages of information which the busy clinician, pathologist or other health care professional will be able to open and enjoy.

Professor W. G. Reeves, FRCP. FRCPath
Department of Immunology
University Hospital, Queen's Medical Centre
Nottingham

What is the use of immunology.
The results are never what you expect.

Attributed to Oscar Wilde

List of Contributors

J. F. ACKROYD
Department of Medicine
St Mary's Hospital Medical School
London
W2 1PG
UK

S. A. ALLARD
The Kennedy Institute of Rheumatology
6 Bute Gardens
Hammersmith
London, W6 7DW
UK

J. ASHWORTH
Department of Medicine (Dermatology)
Charing Cross Hospital
Fulham Palace Road
London, W6 8RF
UK

S. M. BREATHNACH
Department of Medicine (Dermatology)
Charing Cross Hospital
Fulham Palace Road
London, W6 8RF
UK

G. W. CSONKA
Department of Genito-Urinary Medicine
West London Hospital
Hammersmith Road
London, W6 7QD
UK

P. W. EWAN
MRC Centre
Hills Road
Cambridge, CB2 2QH
UK

M. J. HALL
Research Division, Roche Products Ltd
PO Box 8
Welwyn Garden City
Herts, AL7 3AY
UK

C. A. ISON
Department of Medical Microbiology
St Mary's Hospital Medical School
Paddington
London, W2 1PG
UK

D. J. JEFFRIES
Department of Medical Microbiology
St Mary's Hospital Medical School
Paddington
London, W2 1PG
UK

R. N. MAINI
The Kennedy Institute of Rheumatology
6 Bute Gardens
Hammersmith
London, W6 7DW
UK

M. A. MONNICKENDAM
Section of Virology
Institute of Ophthalmology
Judd Street
London, WC1H 9QS
UK

S. J. NORRIS
Department of Pathology
University of Texas Health Science Center
Medical School
PO Box 20708
Houston, TX 77225
USA

J. D. ORIEL
Department of Genito-urinary Medicine
University College Hospital
London
UK

J. M. PARKIN
Department of Immunology
St Mary's Hospital Medical School
Norfolk Place
London, W2 1PG
UK

A. J. PINCHING
Department of Immunology
St Mary's Hospital Medical School
Norfolk Place
London, W2 1PG
UK

M. A. STANLEY
Department of Pathology
Cambridge Institute
University of Cambridge
Cambridge, CB2 1QP
UK

D. TAYLOR-ROBINSON
Division of Sexually Transmitted Diseases
MRC Clinical Research Centre
Watford Road
Harrow, Middlesex, HA1 3UJ
UK

A. J. ZUCKERMAN
Department of Medical Microbiology
London School of Hygiene and Tropical
Medicine
Keppel Street
London, WC1E 7HT
UK

Introduction: Koch's Last Postulate

D. J. M. WRIGHT

When Koch found the cause of tuberculosis, the criteria he used to identify *Mycobacterium tuberculosis* as the sole agent of the disease, were refined into 'postulates'[1]*. Shortcomings of Koch's postulates and possible modifications have been much discussed[3]. Examples of syndromes where the associated microbe falls short of fulfilling Koch's postulates are spirochaetes in tabes dorsalis or more recently, is acquired immune deficiency syndrome really caused by the human immunodeficiency virus[4]. The problem can be resolved by suggesting that these postulates were not really intended to define a causative agent but to provide methods which can be used to trace the cause of disease[5]. Therefore, new methods which had not been available to Koch, should be incorporated into the catechism. This allows the substitution of 'pure culture' or 're-isolation' in Koch's postulates with the postulates rewritten in terms of substantial DNA hybridization of an unknown DNA. This would embrace both bacterial and viral DNA and even toxin encoding DNA of plasmids.

In addition to the conventional postulates, Wilson and Miles[6] tentatively proposed a further postulate dealing with the immune response to microbes. A proposition particularly useful when investigating sexually transmitted diseases (STD). There is no doubt that multiple infections are more deadly than those caused by a single microbe[7], like the mixed opportunistic infections in acquired immune deficiency syndrome, a subject only understood in terms of the immune response. The causative microbe's relationship to many animal models and analagous natural infections is more relevant to immunity than to Koch's original principles. This is particularly true of chlamydiae and retrovirus animal diseases. In terms of pathogenesis, provided the host survives the initial inflammatory response, specific lymphocyte-mediated immune processes are effectively mobilized in the non-immune host, generally peaking within 3–4 weeks[8]. To disentangle the immune response from the direct action of the microbe is sometimes difficult. In the Jarisch–Herxheimer reaction, immunological phenomena could well

---

*Another consideration which, to some, deserves to be included as a postulate, is *financial support*[2]. This may even be more important now than it was in Koch's day.

be superimposed on what may be an effect of spirochaetal endotoxin-like substances[9,10]. The development of a humoral response is often central to the diagnosis of disease. However, serodiagnosis can be difficult when the antibody response is impaired in the immunocompromized, or misleading because of rare false positive reactions[11]. The cellular response, initially used for diagnosis in sexually transmitted diseases[12,13], is responsible for the effective elimination of intracellular pathogens. Intercurrent infection with such pathogens in those with acquired immune deficiency syndrome, tend to relapse or the patients become carriers, despite standard antimicrobial therapy. Exceptionally, in the few cases reported of Legionnaires disease in patients with acquired immune deficiency syndrome, a carrier state does not occur after adequate treatment[14], presumably because the carrier state is virtually unknown in those with normal immune systems. However, reinfection and asymptomatic carriage are the hallmark of the human STD reservoir. Clinically, in a chronic STD like syphilis, the patient rarely suffers the same disease twice, but has a modified form which corresponds to a progression of the disease from that seen when previously infected[15,16]. This premunition was crystallized in the phrase 'infection immunity'[17]. As a result of further study of the effect of immunization, the development of artificial immunity has been studied and vaccines produced, e.g. for hepatitis B and, experimentally, for herpes. The specific immune response may also be inadvertently damaging. This is particularly true of the antimicrobials used in the treatment of STD, which can act as haptens causing allergic reactions (see Chapter 12). Lastly, inappropriate autoimmune phenomena are encountered often against antigens in organs that could only peripherally be involved in the disease[18]. All these reactions are irrelevant in terms of Koch's original postulates, and can only be understood if immunological aspects are considered. For this reason the clinician, whose work is usually confined to disease and micro-organisms, should take an interest in the immune response induced by microbes which cause sexually transmitted diseases. It is with immunology of the changing pattern of these diseases that the following chapters are concerned.

References

1. Koch, R. (1882). Die aetiologie der tuberculose, *Berl. Klin. Wochenschr.*, **19**, 221–30
2. Huebner, R. J. (1957). The virologist's dilemma. *Ann. NY Acad. Sci.*, **67**, 430–8
3. Evans, A. S. (1976). Causation and Disease: The Henle–Koch postulates revisited. *Yale J. Biol. Med.*, **49**, 175–95
4 Duisberg, P. H. (1987) Retroviruses as carcinogens and pathogens: Expectations and results. *Cancer Res.*, **47**, 1199–220
5 King, L. S. (1952) Dr. Koch's postulates. *J. Hist. Med.*, **7**, 350–61
6 Wilson, G. S. and Miles, A. A. (1975). In Topley and Wilson's (eds.) *Principles of Bacteriology and Immunity.* 5th Edn., Vol. 2 p. 1228. (London: Edward Arnold)
7. Gorbach, S. L. and Bartlett, J. G. (1974). Anaerobic infections. *N. Engl. J. Med.*, **290**, 1174–84, ibid: 1233–45, ibid: 1280–94
8. Isenberg, H. D. and Smith J. K. (1981). The epidemiology and control of nosocomial and opportunistic infection. In Hausler, Wjr and Balows A. (eds.) *Diagnostic procedures for bacterial, mycotic and parasitic infection.* 6th Edn. pp. 119–39. (Washington: Am. Public Health Assoc.)

9. Wright, D. J. M. (1980). Reaction following treatment of murine borreliosis and Shwartzman type reaction with borrelial sonicates. *Parasite Immunol.*, **2**, 201–21
10. Teklu, B., Habte-Michal, A., White, N. J., Warrell, D. A. and Wright, D. J. M. (1983). Meptazinol diminishes the Jarisch–Herxheimer reaction. *Lancet*, **1**, 835–9
11. Wright, D. J. M. (1973). The significance of the fluorescent treponemal antibody (FTA-ABS) test in collagen disorders and leprosy. *J. Clin. Pathol.*, **26**, 968–72
12. Noguchi, H. (1911). A cutaneous reaction in syphilis. *J. Exp. Med.*, **14**, 557–68
13. Frei W. (1925). Eine neue hautreaktion bei 'lymphogranuloma inguinale'. *Klin. Wochenschr.*, **4**, 2148–9
14. Murray, J. F., Felton, C. P., Garay, S. M. *et al.* (1984). Pulmonary complications of the acquired immunodeficiency syndrome. Report of a National Heart, Lung and Blood Institute workshop. *N. Engl. J. Med.*, **310**, 1682–8
15. Ehrmann, S. (1907). Versuche uber autoinfektion bei syphilis. *Verh. Dtsch. Dermatol. Gesel Berl.*, **1**, 265–70
16. Gluck, A., cited by Grin E. I. (1953). *Epidemiology and control of endemic syphilis: report on mass treatment campaign in Bosnia*. Monograph 11, pp. 34–5. (Geneva: WHO)
17. Neisser, A., cited by Chesney, A. (1926). Immunity in syphilis. *Medicine* (Balt.), **5**, 463–87
18. Grimble, A. and Lessof, M. H. (1965). Anti-prostate antibodies in arthritis. *Brit. Med. J.*, **11**, 263–4

1
Syphilis

S. J. NORRIS

Syphilis has long been recognized as one of the most complex infectious diseases, and the immunology of the disease is both a cause and a reflection of this complexity. The human diseases caused by *Treponema pallidum* subspecies *pallidum* and related bacteria (which cause venereal syphilis, endemic syphilis, yaws and pinta) exhibit a similar pattern of pathogenesis involving acute and chronic manifestations, as well as the capacity for long-term acute latent infection. Syphilis represents an ideal host–parasite relationship (from the parasite's point of view): the spirochetes can cause both acute infectious lesions, important in transmission of the disease in the early stages, and also persist in the host for decades despite the presence of demonstrable resistance to infection. The immune response battles valiantly to rid the host of this invader, but usually does not succeed; in many cases its fervour seems to be principally responsible for the pathogenesis of the disease.

During the primary and secondary stages, both antibody and cellular responses develop and recent studies indicate that both arms of the immune response may be important in eradicating most of the organisms present during these fulminant stages of infection. Antibodies specific for numerous *T. pallidum* antigens, lipoidal (cardiolipin) antigens, and in some cases self-antigens, are expressed during all stages of infection, and anti-cardiolipin and anti-treponemal antibodies serve as the basis of serologic diagnosis. Immune complexes are present in variable quantities, and may be responsible in part for the vasculitis seen during secondary syphilis. Based on experimental studies in animal models, the interaction of T-cells and macrophages at the site of infection appears to be involved in the clearance of organisms from early lesions; these same 'protective' cellular reactions also seem to be the primary cause of tissue damage during the late stages of the disease. The mechanisms of latent infection, in which the spirochaetes persist in small numbers despite an immune response capable of preventing reinfection, continues to be the principal mystery of syphilis. During the past decade, there has been much discussion in the literature of 'immunosuppression' during syphilitic infection and its involvement in latency; although certain changes in lymphocyte and macrophage activities have been reported to occur, it is unlikely that these 'aberrations' are responsible for incomplete protection. In any case, syphilis does not cause generalized immunosuppression leading to opportunistic infections, and has no aetiologic link with acquired immunodeficiency disease (AIDS).

In this chapter, no attempt will be made to include all of the vast literature on the immunology of syphilis. Rather, the reader will be directed to the many excellent reviews[1-5] which have accumulated on this subject, along with articles which are either too salient to be excluded or too recent to have been reviewed previously. Much of the information available on the natural course of infection and resistance to re-infection was gathered during the pre-penicillin era, and the textbooks[6] and historical accounts [7-9] of this period chronicle the widespread morbidity and death which this disease once caused. A monograph published by the US Public Health Service in 1968[10] still provides the best brief overview of the clinical aspects of syphilis.

CHARACTERISTICS OF *TREPONEMA PALLIDUM*

The structural and physiologic characteristics of *T. pallidum* are important in understanding some of the unusual features of syphilitic infection. As a result of DNA homology studies, the bacterial species *Treponema pallidum* has recently been expanded to include not only venereal syphilis isolates (subspecies *pallidum*), but also the causative organisms of endemic syphilis (subsp. *endemicum*) and yaws (subsp. *pertenue*)[11]. The causative agent of pinta, *Treponema carateum*, is still considered a separate species due to a lack of genetic information regarding this bacterium. Although these organisms are morphologically identical[4], each exhibits a characteristic pattern of infectivity and pathogenesis in laboratory animals as well as in humans[2]. They also seem to possess antigenic differences as demonstrated in immunologic cross-protection studies[2,12], although the electrophoretic patterns of the antigenic polypeptides of the *pallidum* and *pertenue* subspecies are virtually identical[13-15].

All of the subspecies of *T. pallidum* are obligate parasites, and until recently none had been successfully cultured *in vitro*. In 1981, Fieldsteel *et al.*[16] reported the multiplication of *T. pallidum* subsp. *pallidum* (Nichols strain) in a tissue culture system, and their results have been duplicated by our laboratory[17]. Unfortunately, only a limited degree of multiplication has been obtained in this system (up to 100-fold), and continuous culture has not as yet been achieved[17]. Thus nearly all of the immunologic studies to date have utilized *T. pallidum* propagated *in vivo* in rabbit testes. A maximum of approximately 10^{10} *T. pallidum* cells can be obtained from the infection of a single rabbit, and these organisms must be purified extensively to remove host tissue components[18]. This limitation has greatly hindered research on *T. pallidum* in comparison to what has been achieved with other bacteria, which can be grown easily in culture.

In vivo, *T. pallidum* tends to invade the interstitial spaces of tissue at the site of infection and to disseminate rapidly to other locations. Both of these activities are aided by the active, 'cork-screw' motility of T. pallidum, which allows it to bore its way through tissues. Viable treponemes can be found in the bloodstream in the early stages of infection, and haematogenous spread is important in the transition from local (primary) to disseminated (secondary, latent and late) infection. The organisms multiply at a very slow rate (generation time = 30–33 hours)[19] and accumulate in the interstitial matrix, although a few apparently viable treponemes can be found inside non-phagocytic cells[5]. In vitro, T. pallidum requires the presence of tissue culture cells, a micro-aerobic environment (1–5% oxygen) and serum components for growth[16,17], and its fastidious nature may account for its obligate parasitism and rapid demise outside the host.

Several animal models of T. pallidum infection have been investigated, but except for apes the rabbit appears to offer a pattern of infection and pathogenesis which is most similar to humans[1,2]. In the rabbit model, the primary chancre obtained by intradermal inoculation with T. pallidum subsp. pallidum closely resembles that found in humans, and T. pallidum disseminates and persists at other sites despite an effective clearance of organisms at the primary site, similar to humans. However, secondary lesions can only be generated in young rabbits under special circumstances, and late manifestations have not been documented. Guinea pig and hamster models have also been developed and have been very useful in cell transfer experiments which require inbred animals. However, venereal syphilis isolates do not cause skin lesions in these animals, although systemic infection, lymphadenopathy and both antibody and cellular responses do occur. Thus most studies utilizing guinea pigs or hamsters have used either endemic syphilis or yaws strains (both of which cause dermal lesions) as the source of infection.

The unusual morphology of treponemes is illustrated in Figure 1.1. When viewed by negative staining and electron microscopy, the helical nature of the organism is evident (Figure 1.1a). The periplasmic flagella originate at the ends of the treponemes (Figure 1.1b) and wrap around the body of the organism in between the cytoplasmic membrane and the outer membrane (Figure 1.1, c–f). Thus the outer membrane represents the outer surface of the organism, and the periplasmic flagella are 'internal' antigens. It seems likely, therefore, that those antigens located in the outer membrane are the ones which would be capable of inducing a protective immune response, inasmuch as effector mechanisms (i.e. antibodies, complement and cells) would only be able to interact with the surface constituents of intact organisms. There are indications, however, that anti-flagellar antibodies can inactivate T. pallidum in vitro; this apparent contradiction may be due to the formation of 'transient gaps' in the outer membrane[20], or to breakdown of the structural integrity of the organism during the prolonged in vitro incubation (16–18 hours) required for these assays.

During the past 5–10 years, a tremendous amount of effort has been devoted to the characterization of the structural and antigenic properties of individual T. pallidum proteins, as summarized in Table 1.1. The individual polypeptides are identified by their relative molecular weights (M_r's) as determined by sodium dodecyl sulphate – polyacrylamide gel electrophoresis

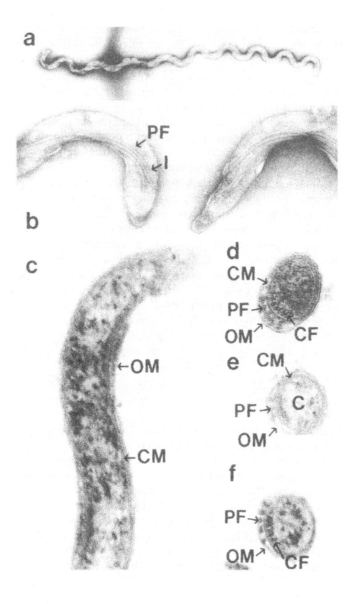

Figure 1.1 Morphologic appearance of *Treponema pallidum*, as demonstrated by electron microscopy. (**a**) Negatively stained preparation of whole *T. pallidum*, showing its helical structure. (**b**) The ends of two negatively stained organisms; the insertion points (I) of the periplasmic flagella (PF) are indicated (I). (**c-f**) Ultrathin longitudinal and cross-sections of *T. pallidum*. The unusual location of the multiple periplasmic flagella (PF) between the outer membrane (OM) and cytoplasmic membrane (CM) is shown in the cross-sections. The function of the cytoplasmic filaments (CF), small tubular structures in the cytoplasm (C) which run parallel to the flagella, is not known, although they may also be involved in motility. A thin peptidoglycan layer is thought to be located in the periplasmic space adjacent to the cytoplasmic membrane, but is not easily visualized by electron microscopy. (**c-f**) are from Reference 18

Table 1.1 Characteristics of some of the major polypeptides of *Treponema pallidum* subp. *pallidum*. The polypeptides are listed according to their relative molecular weight, corresponding to the values given in Figure 1.2. Most references are summarized in ref. 21; sources of more recent information are referenced in the table or footnoted. Several of the major polypeptides are thought to be surface localized and induce a vigorous antibody response, indicating that they may be important in the protective immune response. Cloned recombinant DNA gene products and hybridomas producing specific monoclonal antibodies will be valuable tools in determining the roles of these proteins in immunity

Relative molecular weight (kD)	Other designations	Expressed by recombinant DNA vectors in E. coli	Monoclonal antibodies	Antibodies in normal human serum	Antibodies in syphilitic human serum	Other properties
200	TpF1	Yes				
190	4D	Yes			++	Surface-localized. Ring-like structure. Immunization induces treponemicidal antibodies and partial protection[58]
94					++	
83			Yes[a]	+	++	? Thought to be either a cytadhesin and fibronectin binding protein or an intracellular cytoplasmic filament protein
71			Yes[b]		++	
61	Tp4	Yes[22]	Yes[b]	++	+++	Common Antigen – crossreacts with similar proteins in other bacteria
58	TpA	Yes			+	
47		Yes[23,b]	Yes[23,24]	++	++++	'Immunodominant Antigen' putative outer membrane protein. Anti-47 monoclonal antibody neutralizes viable *T. pallidum*
44.5	TmpA	Yes	Yes[24]		++++	Membrane protein with signal peptide. Gene sequence known

5

Table 1.1 (continued)

Relative molecular weight (kD)	Other designations	Expressed by recombinant DNA vectors in E. coli	Monoclonal antibodies	Antibodies in normal human serum	Antibodies in syphilitic human serum	Other properties
41			Yes	+	+++	
39		Yes				
37	TmpC		Yes[20,25,26]	+	+++	Major flagellar protein[20,25,26,c]
35		Yes	Yes		++++	
34.5			Yes		+++	Flagellar protein[20,25,26,c]
34	TmpB	Yes	Yes			Detectable by SDS–PAGE, but not 2D electrophoresis. Partial gene sequence known
33				++	++	Flagellar protein[20,25,26,c]
30			Yes[26,b]	+	+++	Flagellar protein[20,25,26,c]
29–35	TpD	Yes[27,28]	Yes[27,28,b]		+++	Surface-localized antigen
24–28	TpE	Yes	Yes[b]		+++	
21	TpT	Yes[b]	Yes[b]			
15.5			Yes[a]	+	+++	

[a] A. Cockayne, M. J. Bailey and C. W. Penn, unpublished data
[b] P. Hindersson, R. Agger, L. M. Schouls, N. H. Axelsen and J. D. A. van Embden, submitted
[c] S. J. Norris, N. W. Charon, R. G. Cook, M. D. Fuentes and R. J. Limberger, J. Bacteriol. (In press)

(SDS–PAGE), and further characterization is possible by two-dimensional electrophoresis (see Figure 1.2 and Reference 21). Four approaches have been taken in attempting to determine the relative importance of these proteins in the induction of the immune response during syphilitic infection. First, individual antigens have been identified by electrophoresis combined with either radio-immunoprecipitation (RIP) or immunoblotting techniques. Second, murine hybridomas producing monoclonal antibodies against single polypeptides have been produced by several laboratories. Third, recombinant DNA techniques have successfully led to the expression of a large number of treponemal proteins in *E. coli*. Finally, various approaches have been employed to determine the structural locations and functions of these proteins. Research has been concentrated on those proteins which appear to be surface-localized, including those with M_r's of 190, 47, 44.5 and 28–35 kiloDaltons (kD). These results will be discussed with regard to the antibody responses to treponemal antigens later in this chapter.

HUMORAL RESPONSES

The age of serologic testing in syphilis began in 1906, when August von Wassermann, Albert Neisser and Carl Bruck discovered that sera from syphilitic patients fixed complement when combined with an antigen prepared from syphilitic liver tissue[9]. They reasoned that the tissue extract must contain antigenic components of the recently discovered infectious agent, then called *Spirochaeta pallida*, which reacted with the patient's antibodies. The so-called Wassermann test was a tremendous advance, because it permitted the diagnosis of patients not only during the more easily recognized primary and secondary stages, but also during the sometimes cryptic late manifestations and the 'invisible' period of latency. Gradually over the next few years it was revealed that extracts of normal liver worked just as well as those from syphilitic tissue, and in the 1940s Pangborn identified the antigenic compound as cardiolipin, a normal constituent of mammalian mitochondrial membranes[29]. Serologic tests detecting antibodies against the real culprit were not widely used until the *Treponema pallidum* immobilization (TPI) test was developed in 1949. Thus the pioneering, although technically incorrect, observations of Wassermann led to the fortuitous bifurcation of serologic tests for syphilis into the cardiolipin (or phospholipid) and treponemal types.

The diagnosis of syphilis involves a combination of identification of characteristic lesions, darkfield microscopic examination to detect the presence of spirochetes, history and serologic testing[30–32]. Current serologic diagnosis utilizes a combination of a cardiolipin test for screening and follow-up and a treponemal test for confirmation of diagnosis[33]. The use of both tests in this manner is dictated by their properties[33]. The anti-lipoidal tests, as exemplified by the Venereal Disease Research Laboratory (VDRL) and Rapid Plasma Reagin (RPR) tests, are inexpensive, rapid, and reactive with sera from most patients during every stage of infection. Also, their reactivity titre decreases following effective therapy, enabling their use for verifying the efficacy of treatment. The major disadvantage of the anti-lipoidal tests is the occurrence of false-positive reactions under a number of conditions, including autoimmune diseases, intravenous drug abuse, and pregnancy. Thus the anti-treponemal antibody tests are employed to confirm the diagnosis of syphilis. These include the fluorescent treponemal antibody – absorbed (FTA–ABS) test, haemagglutination tests utilizing erythrocytes coated with *T. pallidum* antigens, (such as the microhaemagglutination – *T. pallidum* (MHA–TP) test and the Haemagglutination Treponemal Test for Syphilis (HATTS)), and recently developed enzyme-linked immunosorbent (ELISA) techniques, such as the Bio–Enza Bead test[34–37]. Although the treponemal tests are highly specific when used in combination with an anti-lipoidal test, their principal disadvantage lies in the retention of reactivity despite effective therapy. Thus a reactive treponemal test is indicative of either present or previous treponemal infection, and the test is not useful for either follow-up of treatment or diagnosis of repeated syphilitic infection. Titre determinations are generally not performed with the treponemal tests, because of the serofast nature of the antibody response and the relative expense and time associated with these tests compared to the cardiolipin tests.

Anti-cardiolipin Antibodies

Both the VDRL and RPR tests are based on the antibody-mediated agglutination of antigen particles consisting of cardiolipin complexed with cholesterol and lecithin. Cardiolipin is the antigenic component, but the presence of the other constituents greatly enhances reactivity with syphilitic sera. The so-called reaginic antibodies of syphilis arise during primary and secondary syphilis, with the incidence of positive tests being approximately 50–70% in the primary stage and approaching 100% during the secondary and early latent stages[38]. Titres tend to decrease during the late latent and tertiary stages, and approximately one-third of untreated patients eventually lose VDRL seropositivity. With the lack of other manifestations, this loss of reactivity is thought to represent a 'biologic cure' of syphilis, in which the host has effectively eradicated infection. As mentioned previously, cardiolipin test reactivity usually dissipates following treatment. Effective therapy is evidenced by a four-fold decrease in titre, but some level of reactivity may be retained for months or years in the later stages of the disease (so-called 'sero-fast' serology).

The source of antigenic exposure giving rise to the anti-lipoidal response remains a mystery. Two possible explanations are that (1) tissue damage occurring during infection results in host cell lysis and release of mitochondrial membranes, thus leading to an autoimmune response to this usually 'hidden' self-antigen, or (2) *T. pallidum* itself contains cardiolipin, which stimulates a response to this 'exogenous' antigen. In support of the first hypothesis, some infectious diseases causing widespread and/or chronic tissue damage (e.g. leprosy) can give rise to anti-cardiolipin antibodies. Preparations of *T. pallidum* have been reported to contain cardiolipin[39], although it is uncertain to what degree it may have represented contamination from rabbit tissue. However, cardiolipin is a common constituent of bacterial membranes, so it is again difficult to discern what particular properties of *T.*

pallidum elicit this response. It may be that the 'antigenic load' and distribution provided by *T. pallidum* dissemination and proliferation is enough to stimulate an anti-lipoidal response, or that the organism may contain a phospholipid which is related to cardiolipin but is sufficiently different to 'break through' self-tolerance (if it exists). Further study of the structure of *T. pallidum* and the nature of the anti-lipoidal response in syphilis is necessary to resolve this question.

An intense area of investigation in recent years has been the nature and specificity of anti-phospholipid antibodies associated with autoimmune disorders[40]. Systemic lupus erythematosus (SLE), thrombosis, intrauterine fetal death and thrombocytopaenia exhibit an unusually high frequency (approximately 30%) of false positive VDRL reactions. Use of more sensitive solid-phase ELISA or radio-immunoassay techniques reveals that many patients with these syndromes possess antibodies that are generally reactive to negatively charged phospholipids, including cardiolipin, phosphatidic acid, phosphatidyl serine, phosphatidyl inositol and phosphatidyl glycerol. Antibodies to phospholipid appear to cross-react to some extent with single-stranded DNA, but the significance of this finding remains to be determined. Harris *et al.*[40] have postulated that the epitopic specificity of syphilitic reaginic (cardiolipin) antibody differs qualitatively from that of autoimmune phospholipid antibodies, in that reaginic antibodies of syphilis have a higher affinity for cardiolipin complexed with cholesterol and lecithin (as in the VDRL and RPR antigens), whereas the autoimmune antibodies tend to have a higher affinity for cardiolipin alone. Indeed, VDRL reactivity and anti-cardiolipin activity as measured by solid-phase immunoassay do not correlate well; patients with high anti-cardiolipin solid phase assay titres often have non-reactive VDRL tests, and *vice versa*. The involvement of antibodies to phospholipid in lupus as a possible mechanism in the pathogenesis of anticoagulant activity and platelet aggregation, are currently under investigation. In the balance, patients exhibiting low-titre VDRL or RPR reactivity in the absence of exposure to or other indications of syphilis should be examined for signs of autoimmune disease.

Treponemal antibodies

All the currently available commercial tests for treponemal antibodies detect immunoglobulins of any isotype which react with whole *T. pallidum* (either acetone-fixed in the case of the FTA–ABS test or sonically disrupted in the microhaemagglutination and ELISA tests). Considerable effort has been directed at the design and evaluation of IgM specific tests[41–43] and assays utilizing purified antigens from *T. pallidum*[44], readily cultivable Treponema[45], or recombinant DNA vectors expressing *T. pallidum* antigens[46,47]. The IgM tests may permit more accurate diagnosis of congenital syphilis through detection of anti-treponemal IgM antibodies in the infant's serum, and might also be helpful in distinguishing between early-phase IgM responses and the later IgG response. The use of individual proteins or purified structures (e.g. the flagella of *T. phagadenis* biotype Reiter) is aimed primarily at increasing the specificity and reducing the cost of the treponemal tests. In all of the present commercial tests for anti-*T. pallidum* antibodies, it is necessary to include a 'sorbent' consisting of Reiter treponeme cultures to reduce false-positive reactions due to the presence of antibodies which react with *T. pallidum* in normal human sera (as discussed later in this section). For example, 20% of normal human sera would be reactive in the FTA–ABS test if sorbent were not used[48]. Use of a purified antigen which exhibits a low background reactivity in normal sera and at the same time elicits a strong Ig response early in syphilis could potentially eliminate the need for absorbtion and increase the sensitivity and specificity of these tests. In addition, identification of 'subspecies-specific' antigens may allow the development of tests which are able to differentiate between venereal syphilis, endemic syphilis and yaws. Thus far, none of the purified antigen tests appear to offer enough of an advantage over the time-tested varieties to warrant their commercial production, although this may change with further developments.

Antigen purification studies in the 1950s and '60s indicated that *T. pallidum* contains both protein and non-protein (presumably carbohydrate) antigens which elicit responses during syphilitic infection[5]. During the past 10 years, there has been an explosion of research directed at the identification of individual protein antigens of *T. pallidum*. The principal questions to be answered by these studies are: (1) what protein antigens elicit an immune response during infection; (2) what are the kinetics of antibody production, i.e. do some antigens produce an antibody response earlier in the course of infection and thus offer an advantage in terms of early diagnosis; and, most importantly, (3) which of these antigens are capable of eliciting a protective immune response?

It has gradually become apparent that nearly all the major proteins present in *T. pallidum* are capable of eliciting an antibody response. Studies utilizing either sodium dodecyl sulphate – polyacrylamide gel electrophoresis (SDS–PAGE) or crossed immunoelectrophoresis (CIE) indicated that antibodies expressed during human or experimental syphilis reacted with 7–23 *T. pallidum* polypeptides (individual protein chains)[15,49–55]. Two-dimensional electrophoresis (2DE), which separates polypeptides on the basis of charge in one dimension and molecular weight in the other[56], resolves a greater number of protein species and thus provides a clearer picture of the antigenic reactivity of individual polypeptides[21,57]. Figure 1.2 shows the protein profile of *T. pallidum* as revealed by 2DE in combination with either silver staining or immunoperoxidase detection of antibody reactivity. Silver staining is a highly sensitive technique for detecting nanogram quantities of proteins, and is thus capable of detecting approximately 100 of the most abundant *T. pallidum* polypeptides (Figure 1.2a). The major polypeptides are identified by their apparent molecular weights (M_r's) in Figure 1.2b.

Antigenic reactivity of electrophoretically separated proteins with antibodies can be detected by incubation of the proteins bound to nitrocellulose with human serum, followed by a peroxidase-conjugated second antibody and a colour reagent for the detection of antibody-associated peroxidase activity[21]. As shown in Figure 1.2c and a number of publications[53–55], normal human serum contains antibodies which bind to several of the major polypeptides of *T. pallidum*, most notably those with

M_r's of 61, 47, 41, 33 and 15.5 kD. This reactivity is thought to arise from exposure to related bacterial antigens; although direct evidence is lacking, treponemes present in the normal gingival flora are favourite candidates as the source of these antigens. These 'natural' treponemal antibodies account for the background reactivity of normal sera with the *T. pallidum* preparations used in the treponemal tests. Naturally occurring treponemal antibodies in normal serum have some treponemicidal activity, as will be discussed in relation to natural immunity later in this chapter.

The pattern of reactivity of sera from human syphilis patients is exemplified in Figure 1.2d. In this case, the *T. pallidum* 2DE pattern was incubated with a pool of syphilitic sera samples which had an RPR titre of $>1:32$; similar results have been obtained with individual sera from patients in the primary, secondary and early latent stages. When the profile of antibody binding is compared to the silver stained pattern in Figure 1.2a, most of the major polypeptides visible by silver staining also bind antibodies from this serum pool, indicating that an antibody response is mounted against most, if not all, of the major proteins of *T. pallidum*. This result is not surprising, in that these bacterial antigens are undoubtedly all recognized by the host as being 'non-self', and the dissemination occurring during the primary and secondary stages assures exposure of the lymphoid system to these antigens. It should be noted that the antibody response to some of these antigens, most notably the 47 kD protein, appears to be more intense than to the other proteins; quantitative and qualitative (e.g. isotype) differences in the immunoglobulin and cellular responses to certain proteins may bear on their relative importance in the immune clearance of infection.

The kinetics of antibody production against individual proteins has been examined by several investigators[4,5,15,49-55]. Although results vary because of the variability in the responses in individuals and differences in the methods employed, the earliest detectable responses are generally against the 'immunodominant' 47 kD antigen and the 37 kD flagellar protein; these proteins would, therefore, be logical candidates for use in antigen-specific serologic tests. As expected, IgM responses are prominent in primary and secondary syphilis, but anti-treponemal IgG is also present as early as the primary stage[53-55].

Monoclonal antibodies and cloned *T. pallidum* proteins have offered a means of studying the importance of individual antigens in the protective immune response. In most cases, monoclonal and monospecific antibodies react only with a single protein species, and have been of value in demonstrating the structural location of proteins and the ability of antibodies directed against certain polypeptides in causing complement-mediated inactivation of *T. pallidum*. The cloning of *T. pallidum* genes into *E. coli* vectors permits the production of relatively large quantities of individual *T. pallidum* proteins; with purification, the cloned proteins can be used as a source of isolated antigens for artificial immunization.

Thus far, over 25 different *T. pallidum* protein genes have been cloned, and at least 40 monoclonal antibodies against 14 different *T. pallidum* antigens have been identified[21-24,26-28]. Of these, the immune responses to three protein antigens have been studied fairly extensively: the 4D antigen (190 kD), the

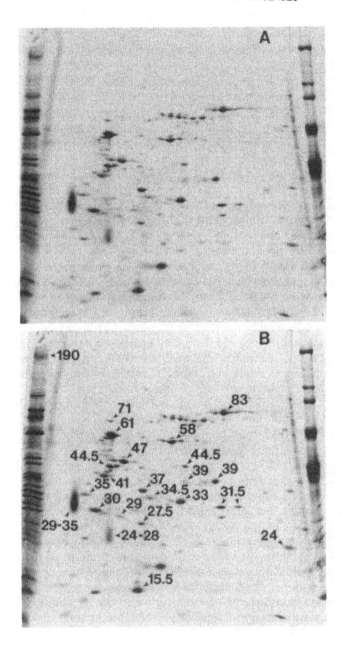

Figure 1.2 Reactivity of normal and syphilitic human sera with *T. pallidum* proteins separated by two dimensional electrophoresis[21,56]. Whole, purified *T. pallidum* were solubilized and subjected to isoelectric focusing followed by sodium dodecyl sulphate – polyacrylamide gel electrophoresis (SDS–PAGE). This procedure separates the proteins on the basis of their net charge (horizontal dimension) and their molecular weight (vertical dimension), thus providing a 'fingerprint' of spots corresponding to the different polypeptides. (**A**) Total protein profile, as revealed by the sensitive silver staining technique[21] (**B**) Same as (**A**), showing the relative

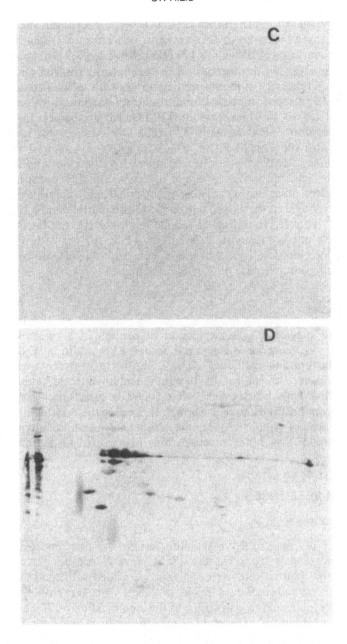

molecular weights (Mrs) of the major polypeptides. (C) Antibody reactivity of a pool of normal human serum with the *T. pallidum* proteins, as demonstrated by immunoperoxidase staining[21] (D) Reaction of pooled sera from syphilis patients (RPR titre $\geq 1:32$) with the *T. pallidum* proteins. the syphilitic sera exhibited reactivity with nearly all of the major polypeptides, indicating the expression of antibodies with many different antigenic specificities. Normal sera reacted less intensely to a smaller group of proteins, corresponding to the presence of naturally-occurring treponemal antibodies. Results are summarized in Table 1.1

47 kD protein and the TpD antigen (28–35 kD). The 4D antigen was isolated and characterized by Lovett and co-workers (see Reference 21) and found to be a protease-resistant oligomer of a 19 kD subunit. The 190 kD oligomer has a characteristic ordered ring structure when examined by electron microscopy and, based on reactivity of monospecific antisera with intact *T. pallidum*, is thought to be surface-localized. Immunization of rabbits with purified 4D antigen has led to the induction of TPI-reactive antibodies and partial protection against challenge with *T. pallidum*[58]. Monoclonal antibodies directed against the 47 kD protein react with intact *T. pallidum* and have treponemicidal activity, supporting structural fractionation studies which suggest that this protein is a major outer membrane constituent[20,21]. Immunoelectron microscopy utilizing monoclonal and monospecific antibodies directed against the cloned antigen TpD also indicate that it is surface-localized[27,28]. Thus far, the effects of vaccination with either the 47 kD or TpD antigens have not been reported. Needless to say, the use of monoclonal antibodies and cloned antigens will continue to yield valuable information on the immunologic importance of *T. pallidum* antigens.

Autoantibodies

As discussed previously, the expression of cardiolipin antibodies during syphilis may represent an autoimmune response. In addition, rheumatoid (anti-IgG) factors and antibodies against fibronectin fragments have been reported to occur in syphilis[59-62]. In experimentally-infected rabbits, antibodies reactive with heart tissue[63] were found to have specific reactivity with the enzyme creatine kinase[64]. The involvement of these autoantibodies in the pathogenesis of syphilis is unknown, although some authors hypothesize that autoimmune 'bystander' reactions may be involved in late manifestations[64].

CELLULAR RESPONSES

Local Responses

The presence of 'round cells' in syphilitic lesions was first reported by von Baerunsprung and Virchow in the 1850s. Several decades later, it was recognized that plasma cells were typically associated with the infiltrate in primary chancres and secondary lesions, and these signs were employed in the diagnosis of syphilis in the years prior to the identification of *T. pallidum* as the causative organism[9]. In recent years, the cellular response has been examined in terms of the involvement of T-cells and macrophages in the local immune clearance of *T. pallidum*, the effects of infection on the systemic activation of T-cells, B-cells and macrophages, and the ability of transferred 'immune' T-cells to protect against infection with *T. pallidum*. It has been shown that T-cells and macrophages play an important role both locally and systemically in the clearance of *T. pallidum*. Many investigators have reported 'aberrant' changes in T-cell proliferation assays, depression of B-cell plaque forming cell responses, and altered phagocytic activity of macrophages. Overall, however, it can be concluded that *T. pallidum* infection leads to an effective cellular response which is, at least in part, responsible for the destruction of the vast majority of organisms in lesions, and that no generalized 'immunosuppression' of the type seen in AIDS occurs during syphilitic infection.

The typical cellular reaction seen in primary and secondary lesions is a perivascular and diffuse monocytic infiltrate with plasma cells (Figure 1.3); at the time of ulceration, the necrotic epidermis is often infiltrated by polymorphonuclear cells. In recent histopathologic studies by Sell and co-workers[65-68] utilizing *T. pallidum*-infected rabbits, T-cells were found to migrate into the site of inoculation within 6 days post-infection, and were the predominant cell type in the nearly confluent lymphocytic infiltrate which accompanied the peak of infection (10-13 days post-infection). Following this 'inductive' phase, macrophages began to accumulate and were shown by electron microscopy to phagocytose and destroy the numerous treponemes that were present (Figure 1.4)[69,70]. This 'reactive' phase in the immune response corresponded to the elimination of the vast majority of organisms within a 4-day period[65,69]. Thus the mechanism of clearance in primary infection in rabbits appears to involve the T-cell mediated recruitment and activation of macrophages. This conclusion is supported by in vitro data demonstrating the expression of macrophage-activating factors by T-cells[5,71] and the phagocytosis and destruction of *T. pallidum* by activated macrophages[72]. The importance of antibodies in this local reaction cannot be excluded, however, since *T. pallidum* antibodies can be detected in extracts from early lesions, and plasma cells are usually present.

The local cellular response in tertiary syphilis (gummata, tabes dorsalis, other forms of neurosyphilis and cardiovascular syphilis) in humans resembles a delayed type hypersensitivity reaction, although characterization of the lymphocyte subsets present has not been reported. Few organisms are present in late lesions in most cases, and almost all of the tissue damage appears to be due to the immunopathologic effects of the cellular infiltrate. Late lesions do not develop in the animal models, making it difficult to study the immunopathologic mechanisms involved in late manifestations.

Systemic Responses

A systemic cellular response is also known to occur. Lymphadenopathy is a common finding in human syphilis, and peripheral blood lymphocytes exhibit *in vitro* proliferation and expression of migration inhibition factors in response to *T. pallidum* antigens[5]. Similar results have been obtained in the rabbit model, as illustrated in Figure 1.5. In the series of studies from which this data was assembled[66-68,73], the proliferative response to treponemal antigens paralleled the antibody response (VDRL reactivity), and increases in the weight of and number of lymphocytes in the spleen and lymph nodes denoted lymphadenopathy. Although other reports indicate a depression of *in vitro* responses to mitogens[74], no change in the response to concanavalin A (a T-cell mitogen) occurred as the result of syphilitic infection of rabbits under the conditions used in these studies (Figure 1.5).

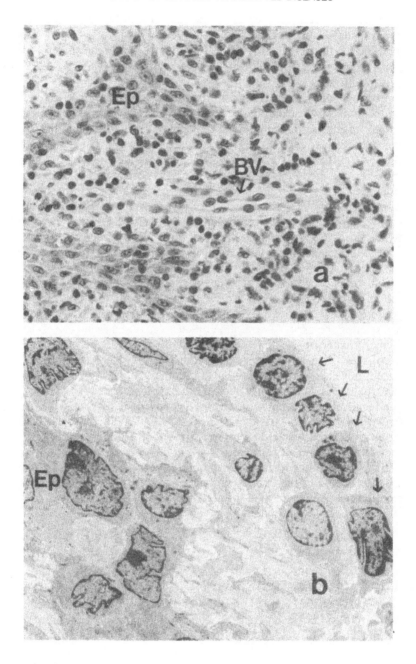

Figure 1.3 Local cellular responses occurring during early syphilitic infection. (a) Low power light micrograph of a skin biopsy from a patient with secondary syphilis, showing the accumulation of mononuclear cells in the dermis underlying the basal layer of the epidermis (Ep). A small blood vessel (BV) in the dermis shows signs of endothelial swelling, a typical feature of syphilitic lesions[10]. (b) An electron micrograph of the tissue in (a), indicating the presence of numerous lymphocytes (L) migrating between collagen bundles in the extracellular matrix

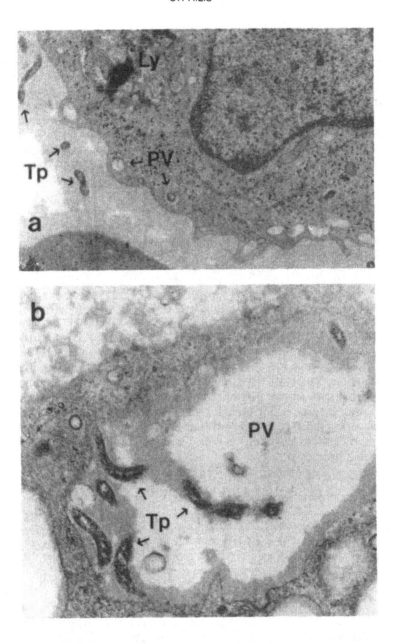

Figure 1.4 Involvement of macrophages in the clearance of *T. pallidum* from syphilitic lesions[70]. Rabbits were infected intratesticularly with *T. pallidum*, and tissue samples were removed and processed for electron microscopy at the time when clearance of treponemes was maximal (day 17 post-infection in this case). (**a**) Electron micrograph of *T. pallidum* (Tp) lying in the extracellular matrix in close proximity to a macrophage. The macrophage contains many phagocytic vesicles (PV) and a large secondary lysosome (Ly) filled with phagocytic debris. (**b**) A higher magnification of a phagocytic vesicle (PV) containing several *T. pallidum*. Electron micrographs graciously provided by Dr S. Sell

Although most evidence indicates that an active immune response occurs during syphilitic infection, some investigators have hypothesized that immunosuppressive mechanisms may inhibit normal responses and thereby delay or prevent the clearance of *T. pallidum* (see Reference 74 and Chapters by Baughn and Folds in Reference 4 for reviews). Findings supporting this theory include: (1) depletion of lymphocytes in the paracortical regions of lymph nodes during infection; (2) depressed responses to mitogens and *T. pallidum* antigens during human and experimental disease; (3) lack of DTH reactions to treponemal antigens during primary and secondary syphilis; (4) inhibition of responses to heterologous antigens (sheep erythrocytes); and (5) T-cell inhibition of the C3b-mediated phagocytosis of sheep erythrocytes by macrophages from infected hamsters[75,76]. Several lines of evidence argue against the overall importance of these observations. First, the evidence for these conclusions is contradictory in many cases[5]. For example, depletion of lymphocytes in lymph nodes is contrary to most historical and recent histopathologic findings. However, lymphocyte traffic studies are required to resolve the point. The changes in lymphocyte proliferation assays have also differed greatly from study to study. Second, most of the findings supporting immunosuppression have used *indirect* measures of the immune response, rather than *functional* and *antigen-specific* activities involved in the clearance of *T. pallidum*. Schell *et al.*[77] showed that transfer of 'immune' spleen cells in hamsters conferred resistance to the recipients, despite the fact that the response to mitogens was depressed in these same cell populations. Many of the changes in activity observed may represent changes in the immunoregulatory 'circuits' which are part of the normal immune response, but the end result is that the vast majority of *T. pallidum* are destroyed by the host with an efficiency similar to or greater than that seen with other disseminated bacterial infections invoking cell-mediated immunity (e.g. tuberculosis, leprosy and listeriosis).

THE IMMUNE RESPONSE AND THE COURSE OF INFECTION

Bacterial pathogenesis is generally characterized as being either toxic (caused by the elaboration of toxins) or invasive (involving widespread proliferation of the organism in the host). Despite recent reports of mammalian cell cytotoxicity caused by high concentrations of *T. pallidum in vitro* (see Fitzgerald and Repesh in Reference 4), syphilis has the properties of an invasive disease. In the early stages, large numbers of organisms accumulate at the sites of infection, and millions of treponemes disseminate throughout the body. Most of the tissue damage which occurs appears to be due primarily to the ensuing immune response. Other mechanisms and cellular reactions are undoubtedly involved, however, since characteristic lesions occur in congenital syphilis and in immunocompromised individuals.

Primary and secondary syphilis

The primary chancre of syphilis heals spontaneously within 4–6 weeks, accompanied by a local mononuclear infiltrate, lymphadenopathy and the

SYSTEMIC EFFECTS OF T. PALLIDUM INFECTION IN RABBITS

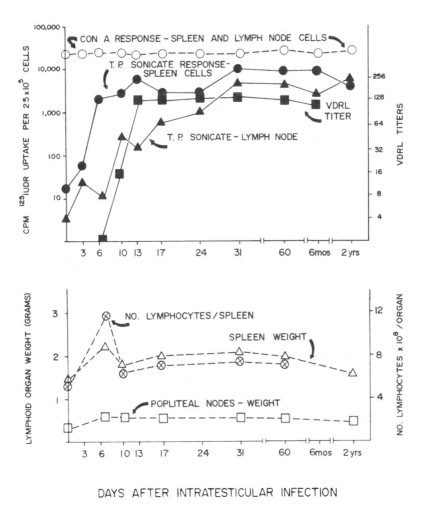

STAGES: INDUCTIVE|REACTIVE| LATENT

DAYS AFTER INTRATESTICULAR INFECTION

Figure 1.5 Systemic cellular responses to syphilitic infection in the rabbit model. Six to ten days following intratesticular infection with *T. pallidum*, spleen and lymph node cells developed a proliferative response to sonically disrupted *T. pallidum* as detected by incorporation of ^{125}I-labelled 2′-deoxyuridine in an *in vitro* assay[73]. Antibody responses developed at the same time, as indicated by the rise in VDRL titre. Proliferative responses to concanavalin A (Con A), a T-cell mitogen, were unaffected by syphilitic infection, although others have reported decreased mitogenic responses in infected patients and animals[74]. Lymphadenopathy is indicated by an increase in the weight of the spleen and draining lymph nodes and by a doubling of the total number of lymphocytes in the spleen, due primarily to T-cell hyperplasia[68]. Adapted from Reference 5

beginning of a systemic humoral response. The clearance of *T. pallidum* from the local nidus of infection indicates that the local immune response is effective in eradicating the organisms. It is somewhat of a paradox, therefore, that this local victory is followed by rampant disseminated (secondary) infection in approximately 25% of untreated cases[76]. The inability of the host to prevent widespread multiplication of *T. pallidum* in these cases is apparently due to a delay in the transition from local to systemic immunity, whereas the balance may be tipped in favour of systemic resistance in those patients who do not exhibit secondary lesions.

Obstructive vasculitis of small vessels is a common finding in most stages of syphilis, and is accompanied by perivascular cuffing with round cells and plasma cells as well as endothelial cell proliferation[6,10]. The resulting breakdown in the vasculature and effective blood flow to lesions may be in part responsible for tissue changes (such as ulceration in primary lesions). Antigen–antibody complexes have been detected in the sera of secondary syphilis patients, and may be involved in dermal neutrophilic vascular reactions and glomerulonephritis seen at this stage of infection[62,79]. Baughn *et al.*[62] found that these immune complexes contained treponemal antigens (most notably an 87 kD polypeptide), but fibronectin–antifibronectin complexes were also present. Skin biopsies exhibited a neutrophil infiltrate, endothelial swelling, and deposition of *T. pallidum* antigens, IgG and complement components in the media of blood vessels in three of nine secondary syphilitic patients[79].

Latent infection

Latent infection appears to be an universal phenomenon in untreated syphilis cases, based on persistent seroreactivity in the absence of other clinical manifestations. Viable *T. pallidum* are scattered throughout the body at an extremely low concentration, and are generally not detectable by any means other than infectivity of tissue samples, most notably lymph nodes. In approximately a third of all untreated syphilis cases, the cardiolipin tests eventually become non-reactive over a period of years; this change is thought to represent a 'biological cure' of infection (i.e. eventual elimination of all *T. pallidum* by the immune response). Another third of the patients appear to maintain a lifelong latent infection, whereas the remainder go on to develop tertiary symptoms[78].

Several mechanisms of latency have been proposed, including (1) residence of *T. pallidum* in sites where they are protected from the immune response ('immunoprotective niches')[80]; (2) intracellular localization[4,5]; (3) suppression of normal lymphoid cell activity[74]; and (4) coating of the organisms with host proteins and glycosaminoglycans so as to conceal treponemal antigens (as reviewed by Baseman and Alderete in Reference 4). It is unlikely that any of the mechanisms of latency will be proven conclusively because of the difficulty posed in studying these low level infections. However, recent studies have shown that intradermal reinfection of 'immune' rabbits with *T. pallidum* results in prolonged survival of treponemes in nerves, dense connective tissue and arrector pili muscles at the site of injection[81]. The ability of *T. pallidum* to burrow through tissue may allow it to localize in such privileged sites and thus avoid contact with lymphoid cells and antibodies. In this model, the organisms would continue to multiply and exit the protective site at random, thus continuing to stimulate the immune response (and maintain seroreactivity). The dynamic balance between continued proliferation of the organisms and the activities of the immune response would determine whether the patient underwent spontaneous cure, continued latent infection, or experienced tertiary symptoms.

Late manifestations

The late manifestations of syphilis appear to be caused either by a delayed type hypersensitivity reaction to 'smouldering' infections of *T. pallidum* or, in some cases, to a local, intense treponemal infection. Gummata, which are essentially a DTH reaction with few *T. pallidum*, can be located in any organ, with the manifestations reflecting the effects of compression, 'bystander' reactions and other pathologic changes on the surrounding tissue. Cases of aortitis have revealed the presence of large numbers of treponemes in the media, with concomitant infiltration by lymphocytes and plasma cells around the vasa vasorum and replacement of the elastic fibres with fibrotic scar tissue[6].

Neurosyphilis exhibits multiple forms. Meningovascular syphilis is most commonly associated with secondary syphilis and is typified by monocytic infiltration and concomitant vascular changes in the meninges and associated vessels. Paresis represents a sometimes rampant infection of the brain parenchyma, with neuronal necrosis, microglial proliferation and endarteritis. The demyelination and dorsal root degeneration characteristic of tabes dorsalis are accompanied by a diffuse lymphocytic infiltrate. Cerebrospinal fluid (CSF) changes in neurosyphilis include a mononuclear infiltrate and a positive VDRL reaction in most cases. Intrathecal production of antibodies has been demonstrated by identification of specific clonotypes of anti-*T. pallidum* antibodies in CSF by isoelectric focusing[82], as well as by comparing CSF VDRL and anti-*T. pallidum* antibody titres (relative to albumin levels) with those found in paired serum samples[83,84].

Congenital syphilis

Congenital syphilis continues to be a significant health problem[85]. As an example, 6% of perinatal mortalities were attributable to congenital syphilis in a recent study in Addis Ababa, Ethiopia[86]. Screening pregnant women for cardiolipin antibodies during the first trimester and then close to the time of birth provides an effective means of detecting this preventable disease.

The severity of congenital syphilis tends to be related to the time of maternal infection, which affects both the number of organisms infecting the fetus and the efficacy of the mother's immune response. If the mother is infected in the third trimester, the relatively high number of *T. pallidum* present in the bloodstream cross the placenta easily. The humoral response of the mother is still developing, so that relatively little treponemicidal IgG crosses the placenta. Thus these infants tend to have a rampant disseminated infection, resulting in severe early congenital syphilis. If the mother is infected prior to conception or early in pregnancy, the maternal immune response becomes partially protective, resulting in clearance of most of the organisms. Infants infected in this manner will generally have a less fulminant infection at birth; they will also be resistant to re-infection from the mother or other sources, due to the presence of maternal IgG. These children will still have early signs of congenital syphilis (such as bone deformities), but will not have severe, life-threatening perinatal infections. Both forms of congenital syphilis can lead to late manifestations, including bone and tooth deformities, rhagades (facial scars), interstitial keratitis and deafness[6,10,85,87].

Early congenital syphilis may represent a circumstance where much of the pathogenesis seems to be evoked by non-immunologic mechanisms. For example, osteochondritis and delayed liver development are difficult to attribute to the immune response, and most likely are direct effects of treponemal infection. However, the presence of lymphocytic infiltrates in many of the affected tissues, along with IgM anti-*T. pallidum* antibodies produced by the fetus or infant, demonstrate an active, if ineffectual, perinatal immune response. Two recently developed animal models of congenital syphilis may shed some light on the pathogenic mechanisms involved[88,89].

AIDS and syphilis

Despite some dubious and dangerously misleading reports linking syphilis and AIDS[90], there is no evidence that syphilis in any way causes the manifestations of AIDS. There is a growing number of cases, however, which indicate that Human Immunodeficiency Virus (HIV) infection may exacerbate the symptoms of syphilis. Neurosyphilis[91-93], syphilitic retinitis[94,95] and cutaneous secondary syphilis[96] have all been reported to exhibit an accelerated course or more severe symptoms in HIV-infected patients. The hypothesis that immunosuppression of T-cell responses can lead to poor clearance of *T. pallidum* and more severe infection is supported by results obtained with immunosuppressive agents in animal models[2], as well as in unusual presentations of syphilis in immunosuppressed transplant patients[97,118]. It is, therefore, recommended that individuals diagnosed as having HIV infection be screened and monitored for serologic and clinical signs of syphilis, particularly since HIV-infected homosexual and bisexual males have an extremely high incidence of past or present syphilis (56% in one study)[99,100].

Jarisch-Herxheimer reaction

The Jarisch–Herxheimer reaction or JHR (as reviewed recently by Young in Reference 4) results from the treatment of syphilis, and is characterized by an exacerbation of dermal lesions, fever, and other physiologic effects, including hypertension and hyperventilation. Immunologic manifestations resulting from the rapid release of treponemal antigens, such as immune complex formation and allergic reactions, have been postulated as possible mechanisms for this syndrome. Endotoxin-mediated toxicity as an alternative explanation is possibly discounted by the lack of detectable endotoxin in purified *T. pallidum*. Young *et al.*[100] found no consistent correlation between the JHR and the presence of circulating immune complexes; they also found no evidence of immunoglobulin or complement deposition in lesions. The strongest evidence for the involvement of antibodies in this syndrome is the ability to induce JHR by injection of hyperimmune serum into infected rabbits. Elucidation of the mechanism of JHR will require further study.

RESISTANCE TO INFECTION

Natural immunity

Only about half the individuals exposed through sexual contact to infectious primary or secondary syphilis lesions develop the disease themselves[101,102]. This observation and the detection of treponemicidal antibodies in normal human serum (see Bishop and Miller, Reference 4) have led some authors to conclude that natural immunity to *T. pallidum* infection exists in humans. However, carefully controlled inoculation studies by Magnuson *et al.*[103] demonstrated that humans previously unexposed to syphilis had a high susceptibility to the disease. All eight volunteers with no evidence of prior exposure developed darkfield-positive lesions following the intradermal injection of *T. pallidum* (Nichols strain), with the median infectious dose being 57 bacteria. This ID_{50} compared favourably with that obtained in the same experiment for intradermal inoculation of rabbits (23 organisms)[103], and intratesticular infection of rabbits can result from inoculation with as few as 1–2 *T. pallidum*[2,104]. Thus it seems likely that the 50% attack rate is due to physical parameters, including the apparent inability of *T. pallidum* to penetrate intact epithelia and its extreme sensitivity to oxygen, dessication and other physical conditions, rather than to the existence of innate immunity.

Acquired immunity

The occurrence of resistance to re-infection (so-called chancre immunity) has long been recognized by physicians, and was confirmed in the rabbit model in the early part of this century[1]. It is generally accepted that significant immunity develops 3–6 months post-infection both in humans and experimentally infected animals[1,2,103,104]. However, it is important to recognize that this immunity is partial, inasmuch as the immune response is incapable of eradicating *T. pallidum* infection in most individuals, yielding a persistent latent infection and, in approximately a third of untreated patients, late manifestations. In addition, immunity to re-infection is incomplete, and re-exposure to syphilis can bring about an asymptomatic infection[103,104]. Finally, resistance subsides following treatment and is extremely difficult to induce by artificial immunization. The incomplete nature of syphilitic immunity has important implications in the prospects of artificial immunization against syphilis, as discussed below.

In the aforementioned human inoculation study by Magnuson et al.[103], 54 volunteers with a history of syphilis were inoculated with 10^5 virulent T. pallidum at a single intradermal site to determine their resistance to re-infection. Five patients with untreated latent syphilis exhibited no skin reaction or serologic changes following infection, indicating resistance to superinfection. In contrast, all 11 patients with a previous history of treated early syphilis ($<$ 2 years duration) developed lesions (9 darkfield positive) and increased cardiolipin and treponemal (TPI) test reactivity. Of the 26 subjects which had been previously treated for late latent syphilis, 50% did not develop lesions or increased serologic reactivity; most of the others developed atypical (darkfield negative) lesions and increased serologic test titres. Thus resistance to symptomatic infection apparently arises after the primary and secondary stages of infection, but dissipates after effective therapy.

Mechanisms of immunity

Adoptive transfer studies conducted in rabbits, hamsters and guinea pigs have indicated that both the humoral and cellular components of the immune response are active in limiting infection. A large number of studies have shown that transfer of serum or purified immunoglobulins from 'immune' donors to normal recipient animals delays the onset of lesion development following injection with T. pallidum[4,5,105-109], as reviewed by Bishop and Miller in Reference 4. In most cases, lesions appear at the site of infection 2–3 weeks after antibody injections have been discontinued. A possible explanation of this phenomenon is that a small number of the injected organisms are able to persist in 'protective niches' at the inoculation site, but are held in check by the presence of treponemicidal antibodies in the surrounding tissue. When the administration of antibodies is stopped and titres decline, these organisms are then capable of proliferating, causing lesions, and disseminating to other sites. This pattern thus reinforces the 'protective niche' theory of latent infection. Complement activity appears to be important in the antibody-mediated clearance of T. pallidum, in that depletion of C3 by administration of cobra venom factor to hamsters abolishes the ability of immune serum transfer to protect against infection[110,111].

Although partial protection of rabbits from T. pallidum infection has been achieved through cell transfer[112], most of the successful lymphocyte transfer studies have utilized inbred strains of hamsters or guinea pigs. Using endemic syphilis and yaws treponemal strains, Schell and co-workers have demonstrated that enriched populations of T-cells from previously infected hamsters conferred resistance to recipients, as assessed by the lack of dermal lesion development and lymph node infection[105,113]. Similar results have been reported by Pavia and Neiderbuhl[114] in the guinea pig model. The anti-treponemal activity of T-cell populations was present at the same time that responses to T-cell mitogens were depressed[77]. Therefore, decreased T-cell proliferative responses do not indicate a decreased ability of the cellular component to respond effectively to *T. pallidum* infection. *In vivo* and *in vitro* evidence suggests that T-cells promote the clearance of *T. pallidum* through the recruitment and activation of macrophages (see Sell review in Reference 4).

Vaccination

In contemplating the potential usefulness of vaccination against syphilis, four basic issues must be considered. First, conditions must be avoided which prevent primary or secondary lesions but permit the establishment of latent infection. If vaccination permits the occurrence of asymptomatic infection, vaccinated individuals exposed to syphilis could eventually develop tertiary manifestations, by far the most dangerous stage of the disease. Second, vaccination would under most circumstances lead to serologic reactivity in the treponemal tests, presenting a diagnostic problem similar to that posed by BCG vaccination for tuberculosis. Third, resistance to re-infection fades in syphilis patients following treatment; by inference, resistance due to vaccination may also be transient. Fourth, syphilis has a low incidence in the general population in most countries, and vaccination would have to be targeted at high risk populations.

Although at least partial resistance develops during syphilitic infection, it has been difficult to induce protective immunity through artificial immunization. Despite numerous attempts utilizing either inactivated *T. pallidum, T. phagedenis*, or other non-pathogenic treponemes[5], there are only two reports of successful vaccination. In 1969, Metzger and Smogor[115] immunized rabbits with up to 1.2×10^{10} *T. pallidum* rendered avirulent by storage at 4°C for 7–10 days. Five of ten rabbits immunized with the highest dose were resistant to infection with 3×10^5 virulent *T. pallidum*, as demonstrated by lack of lesion development, absence of virulent organisms in the draining lymph nodes, and the lack of a post-infection serologic response. The remainder of the rabbits exhibited either symptomatic infection (lesions) or asymptomatic infection (lymph nodes containing virulent organisms). In 1979, Miller[116] reported complete protection of rabbits against *T. pallidum* subsp. *pallidum* infection by intravenous injection of treponemes inactivated by gamma irradiation. The immunized rabbits were resistant to challenge with 10^3 and 10^5 *T. pallidum* and were shown to be protected one year after the completion of vaccination. Unfortunately, the immunization regimen involved 60 injections given over 37 weeks, a procedure unlikely to appeal to humans. Similar injections given over a 12-week-period were not protective. Interestingly, the 37-week immunization regimen did not protect against infection with *T. pallidum* subsp. *pertenue* (Haiti B strain), providing further evidence that venereal syphilis, yaws and endemic syphilis strains possess significant antigenic differences despite morphologic identity, > 90% DNA homology and nearly identical protein profiles[13-15]. Based on the above evidence, vaccination against syphilis, although possible, is not practical at the present time.

Recently, attempts have been made to use purified antigens from other organisms or cloned *T. pallidum* gene products for vaccination, to circumvent our inability to produce large quantities of *T. pallidum* inexpensively. Hindersson *et al.*[117] reported recently that immunization of rabbits with purified flagella from *T. phagedenis* biotype Reiter failed to protect against *T. pallidum* infection. Borenstein *et al.*[58] recently reported acceleration and reduced severity of lesion development resulting from *T. pallidum* infection following immunization of rbabits with the 4D (190 kD) recombinant DNA antigen; this result may reflect heightened cell-mediated immunity. The use of cloned *T. pallidum* antigens for immunization will undoubtedly be an area of intense investigation over the next several years.

ACKNOWLEDGMENTS

I thank D. G. Edmondson and M. Fuentes for superb technical assistance and Dr Stewart Sell for his advice and support. This work was supported by US Public Health Service grant number P01-21290 and World Health Organization agreement number V3/181/73.

References

1. Chesney, A. M. (1927). *Medicine Monographs. XII. Immunity in Syphilis.* (Baltimore: Williams and Wilkins)
2. Turner, T. B. and Hollander, D. H. (1957). *Biology of the Treponematoses.* (Geneva: World Health Organization)
3. Cannefax, G. R., Norins, L. C. and Gillespie, E. J. (1967). Immunology of syphilis. *Annu. Rev. Med.*, **18**, 471–82
4. Schell, R. F. and Musher, D. M. (eds.) (1983). *Pathogenesis and Immunology of Treponemal Infection.* (New York: Marcel Dekker)
5. Sell, S. and Norris, S. J. (1983). The biology, pathology and immunology of syphilis. *Int. Rev. Exp. Pathol.*, **24**, 203–76
6. Stokes, J. H., Beerman, H. and Ingraham, N. R., Jr. (1944). *Modern Clinical Syphilology: Diagnosis, Treatment, Case Study.* (Philadelphia: W. B. Saunders)
7. Pusey, W. A. (1933). *The History and Epidemiology of Syphilis.* (Springfield, IL: C. C. Thomas)
8. Dennie, C. C. (1962). *A History of Syphilis.* (Springfield, IL: C. C. Thomas)
9. Crissey, J. T. and Parish, L. C. (1981). *The Dermatology and Syphilology of the Nineteenth Century.* (New York: Praeger)
10. U. S. Public Health Service (1968). *Syphilis: a Synopsis.* Publication No. 1660 (Washington: US Government Printing Office)
11. Krieg, N. R. and Holt, J. G. (eds.). (1984). *Bergey's Manual of Systematic Bacteriology. The genus* Treponema, Vol. I, p. 49. (Baltimore: Williams and Wilkins)
12. Schell, R. F., Azadegan, A. A., Nitskansky, S. G. and LeFrock, J. L. (1982). Acquired resistance of hamsters to challenge with homologous and heterologous virulent treponemes. *Infect. Immun.*, **37**, 617–21
13. Thornburg, R. W. and Baseman, J. B. (1983). Comparison of major protein antigens and protein profiles of *Treponema pallidum* and *Treponema pertenue. Infect. Immun.*, **42**, 623–7
14. Baker-Zander, S. A. and Lukehart, S. A. (1983). Molecular basis of immunological cross-reactivity between *Treponema pallidum* and *Treponema pertenue. Infect. Immun.*, **42**, 634–8
15. Stamm, L. V. and Bassford, P. J., Jr. (1985). Cellular and extracellular protein antigens of *Treponema pallidum* synthesized during *in vitro* incubation of freshly extracted organisms. *Infect. Immun.*, **47**, 799–807

16. Fieldsteel, A. H., Cox, D. L. and Moeckli, R. A. (1981). Cultivation of virulent *Treponema pallidum* in tissue culture. *Infect. Immun.*, **32**, 908-15
17. Norris, S. J. and Edmondson, D. G. (1986). Factors affecting the multiplication and subculture of *Treponema pallidum* subsp. *pallidum* in a tissue culture system. *Infect. Immun.*, **53**, 534-9
18. Hanff, P. A., Norris, S. J., Lovett, M. A. and Miller, J. N. (1984). Purification of *Treponema pallidum*, Nichols strain, by Percoll density gradient centrifugation. *Sex. Transm. Dis.*, **11**, 275-86
19. Magnuson, H. J., Eagle, H. and Fleischman, R. (1948). The minimal infectious inoculum of *Spirochaeta pallida* (Nichols strain) and a consideration of its rate of multiplication *in vivo*. *Am. J. Syph.*, **32**, 1-18
20. Blanco, D. R., Radolf, J. D., Lovett, M. A. and Miller, J. N. (1986). The antigenic interrelationship between the endoflagella of *Treponema phagedenis* biotype Reiter and *Treponema pallidum* Nichols strain. I. Treponemicidal activity of cross-reactive endoflagellar antibodies against *T. pallidum*. *J. Immunol.*, **137**, 2973-9
21. Norris, S. J., Alderete, J. F., Axelsen, N. H., Bailey, M. J., Baker-Zander, S. A., Baseman, J. B., Bassford, P. J., Baughn, R. E., Cockayne, A., Hanff, P. A., Hindersson, P., Larsen, S. A., Lovett, M. A., Luckehart, S. A., Miller, J. N., Moskophidis, M. A., Müller, F., Norgard, M. V., Penn, C. W., Stamm, L. V., van Embden, J. D. and Wicher, K. (1987). Identity of *Treponema pallidum* subsp. *pallidum* polypeptides: Correlation of sodium dodecyl sulfate-polyacrylamide gel electrophoresis results from different laboratories. *Electrophoresis*, **8**, 77-92.
22. Hindersson, P., Knudsen, J. D. and Axelsen, N. H. (1987). Cloning and expression of *Treponema pallidum* common antigen (Tp-4) in *Escherichia coli* K12. *J. Gen. Microbiol.*, **133**, 587-96
23. Norgard, M. V., Chamberlain, N. R., Swancutt, M. A. and Goldberg, M. S. (1986). Cloning and expression of the major 47-kilodalton surface immunogen of *Treponema pallidum* in *Escherichia coli*. *Infect. Immun.*, **54**, 500-6
24. Bailey, M. J., Cockayne, A. and Penn, C. W. (1987). Monoclonal antibodies directed against surface-associated polypeptides of *Treponema pallidum* define a biologically active antigen. *J. Gen. Microbiol.*, **133**, 1793-803
25. Radolf, J. D., Blanco, D. R., Miller, J. N. and Lovett, M. A. (1986). Antigenic interrelationship between endoflagella of *Treponema phagedenis* biotype Reiter and *Treponema pallidum* (Nichols): molecular characterization of endoflagellar proteins. *Infect. Immun.*, **54**, 626-34
26. Cockayne, A., Bailey, M. J. and Penn, C. W. (1987). Analysis of sheath and core structures of the axial filament of *Treponema pallidum*. *J. Gen. Microbiol.*, **133**, 1397-407
27. Swancutt, M. A., Twehous, D. A. and Norgard, M. V. (1986). Monoclonal antibody selection and analysis of a recombinant DNA-derived surface immunogen of *Treponema pallidum* expressed in *Escherichia coli*. *Infect. Immun.*, **52**, 110-19
28. Hindersson, P., Cockayne, A., Schouls, L. M. and van Embden, J. D. A. (1986). Immunochemical characterization and purification of *Treponema pallidum* antigen TpD expressed by *Escherichia coli* K12. *Sex. Transm. Dis.*, **13**, 237-44
29. Pangborn, M. C. (1951). *Cardiolipin antigens: preparation and chemical and serological control*. Monograph Series No. 6 (Geneva: World Health Organization)
30. Sparling, P. F. (1971). Diagnosis and treatment of syphilis. *N. Engl. J. Med.*, **284**, 642-53
31. Lee, T. J. and Sparling, P. F. (1979). Syphilis: an algorithm. *J. Am. Med. Assoc.*, **242**, 1187-9
32. Luger, A. (1981). Diagnosis of syphilis. *Bull. WHO*, **59**, 647-54
33. Miller, J. N. (1975). Value and limitations of nontreponemal and treponemal tests in the laboratory diagnosis of syphilis. *Clin. Obst. Gynecol.*, **18**, 191-202
34. Chen, J., Lin, T. M., Schubert, C. M. and Halbert, S. P. (1986). Treponemal antibody-absorbent enzyme immunoassay for syphilis. *J. Clin. Microbiol.*, **23**, 876-80
35. Stevens, R. W. and Schmitt, M. E. (1985). Evaluation of an enzyme-linked immunosorbent assay for treponemal antibody. *J. Clin. Microbiol.*, **21**, 399-402
36. Moyer, N. P., Hudson, J. D. and Hausler, W. J., Jr. (1987). Evaluation of the Bio-EnzaBead Test for syphilis. *J. Clin. Microbiol.*, **25**, 619-23
37. Burdash, N. M., Hinds, K. K., Finnerty, F. A. and Manos, J. P. (1987). Evaluation of the

syphilis Bio-EnzaBead assay for detection of treponemal antibody. *J. Clin. Microbiol.*, **25**, 808-11

38. Matthews, H. M., Yang, T.-K. and Jenkin, H. M. (1979). Unique lipid composition of *Treponema pallidum* (Nichols virulent strain). *Infect. Immun.*, **24**, 713-19

39. Huber, T. W., Storms, S., Young, P., Phillips, L. E., Rogers, T. E., Moore, D. G. and Williams, R. P. (1983). Reactivity of microhemagglutination, fluorescent treponemal antibody absorbtion, venereal disease research laboratory, and rapid plasma reagin tests in primary syphilis. *J. Clin. Microbiol.*, **17**, 405-9

40. Harris, E. N., Hughes, G.R. V. and Gharavi, A. E. (1987). Antiphospholipid antibodies: an elderly statesman dons new garments. *J. Rheumatol.*, **14**, 208-13

41. Lindenschmidt, E.-G., Laufs, R. and Muller, F. (1983). Microenzyme-linked immunosorbent assay for the detection of specific IgM antibodies in human syphilis. *Br. J. Vener. Dis.*, **59**, 151-6

42. Farshy, C. E., Hunter, E. F., Larsen, S. A. and Cerny, E. H. (1984). Double-conjugate enzyme-linked immunosorbent assay for immunoglobulins G and M against *Treponema pallidum*. *J. Clin. Microbiol.*, **20**, 1109-13

43. Farshy, C. E., Hunter, E. F., Helsel, L. O. and Larsen, S. A. (1985). Four-step enzyme-linked immunosorbent assay for detection of *Treponema pallidum* antibody. *J. Clin. Microbiol.*, **21**, 387-9

44. Morrison-Plummer, J., Alderete, J. F. and Baseman, J. B. (1983). Enzyme-linked immunosorbent assay for the detection of serum antibody to outer membrane proteins of *Treponema pallidum*. *Br. J. Vener. Dis.*, **59**, 75-9

45. Pedersen, N. S., Petersen, C. S. and Axelsen, N. H. (1982). Enzyme-linked immunosorbent assay for detection of immunoglobulin M antibody against the Reiter treponeme flagellum in syphilis. *J. Clin. Microbiol.*, **16**, 608-14

46. Rodgers, G. C., Laird, W. J., Coates, S. R., Mack, D. H., Huston, M. and Sninsky, J. J. (1986). Serological characterization and gene localization of an *Escherichia coli*-expressed 37 kilodalton *Treponema pallidum* antigen. *Infect. Immun.*, **53**, 16-25

47. Radolf, J. D., Lernhardt, E. B., Fehniger, T. E. and Lovett, M. A. (1986). Serodiagnosis of syphilis by enzyme-linked immunosorbent assay with purified recombinant *Treponema pallidum* antigen 4D. *J. Infect. Dis.*, **153**, 1023-7

48. Hunter, E. F., Deacon, W. E. and Meyer, P. E. (1964). An improved FTA test for syphilis, the absorbtion procedure (FTA-ABS). *Pub. Hlth. Rep.*, **79**, 410-12

49. Baseman, J. B. and Hayes, E. C. (1980). Molecular characterization of receptor binding proteins and immunogens of virulent *Treponema pallidum*. *J. Exp. Med.*, **151**, 573-86

50. Alderete, J. F. and Baseman, J. B. (1981). Analysis of serum IgG against *Treponema pallidum* protein antigens in experimentally infected rabbits. *Br. J. Vener. Dis.*, **57**, 302-8

51. van Eijk, R. V. W. and van Embden, J. D. A. (1982). Molecular characterization of *Treponema pallidum* proteins responsible for the human immune response to syphilis. *Antonie van Leeuwehoek*, **48**, 486-7

52. Lukehart, S. A., Baker-Zander, S. A. and Gubish, E. R., Jr. (1982). Identification of *Treponema pallidum* antigens: comparison with a nonpathogenic treponeme. *J. Immunol.*, **129**, 833-8

53. Hanff, P. A., Fehniger, T. E., Miller, J. N. and Lovett, M. A. (1982). Humoral immune response in human syphilis to polypeptides of *Treponema pallidum*. *J. Immunol.*, **129**, 1287-91

54. Moskophidis, M. and Müller, F. (1984). Molecular analysis of immunoglobulins M and G immune response to protein antigen of *Treponema pallidum* in human syphilis. *Infect. Immun.*, **43**, 127-32

55. Baker-Zander, S. A., Hook, E. W., III, Bonin, P., Handsfield, H. H. and Lukehart, S. A. (1985). Antigens of *Treponema pallidum* recognized by IgG and IgM antibodies during syphilis in humans. *J. Infect. Dis.*, **151**, 264-72

56. O'Farrell, P. (1975). High resolution two-dimensional electrophoresis of proteins. *J. Biol. Chem.*, **250**, 4007-21

57. Norris, S. J. and Sell, S. (1984). Antigenic complexity of *Treponema pallidum*: antigenicity and surface localization of major polypeptides. *J. Immunol.*, **133**, 2686-92

58. Borenstein, L. A., Fehninger, T. E., Radolf, J. D., Blanco, D. R., Miller, J. N. and Lovett, M. A. (1988). Immunization of rabbits with a recombinant *Treponema pallidum* surface

antigen (4D) alters the course of experimental syphilis. *J. Immunol.*, **140**, 2415-21

59. Peltier, A. and Christian, C. L. (1959). The presence of the 'rheumatoid factor' in sera from patients with syphilis. *Arthritis Rheum.*, **2**, 1-7

60. Bloomfield, N. (1960). Reactions in the latex-fixation test for rheumatoid arthritis with serum of syphilitic individuals. *J. Lab. Clin. Med.*, **55**, 73-6

61. Mustakallio, K. K., Lassus, A. and Wager, O. (1967). Autoimmune phenomena in syphilitic infection: rheumatoid factor and cryoglobulins in different stages of syphilis. *Int. Arch. Allergy Appl. Immunol.*, **31**, 417-26

62. Baughn, R. E., McNeely, M. C., Jorizzo, J. L. and Musher, D. M. (1986). Characterization of the antigenic determinants and host components in immune complexes from patients with secondary syphilis. *J. Immunol.*, **136**, 1406-14

63. Casavant, C. H., Wicher, V. and Wicher, K. (1978). Host response to *Treponema pallidum* infections. III. Demonstration of autoantibodies to heart in sera from infected rabbits. *Int. Arch. Allergy Appl. Immunol.*, **56**, 171-8

64. Strugnell, R. A., Williams, W. F., Raines, G., Pedersen, J. S., Drummond, L. P., Toh, B. H. and Faine, S. (1986). Autoantibodies to creatine kinase in rabbits infected with *Treponema pallidum*. *J. Immunol.*, **136**, 667-71

65. Lukehart, S. A., Baker-Zander, S. A., Lloyd, R. M. C. and Sell, S. (1980). Characterization of lymphocyte responsiveness in early experimental syphilis. II. Nature of cellular infiltration and *Treponema pallidum* distribution in testicular lesions. *J. Immunol.*, **124**, 461-7

66. Sell, S., Gamboa, D., Baker-Zander, S. A., Lukehart, S. A. and Miller, J. N. (1980). Host response to *Treponema pallidum* in intradermally-infected rabbits: evidence for persistence of infection at local and distant sites. *J. Immunol.*, **75**, 470-5

67. Baker-Zander, S. A. and Sell, S. (1980). A histopathologic and immunologic study of the course of syphilis in the experimentally infected rabbit: demonstration of long-lasting cellular immunity. *Am. J. Pathol.*, **101**, 387-414

68. Sell, S., Baker-Zander, S. A. and Lloyd, R. M. C. (1980). T-cell hyperplasia of lymphoid tissues of rabbits infected with *Treponema pallidum*. *Sex. Transm. Dis.*, **7**, 74-84

69. Ovcinnikov, N. M. and Delektorskij, V. V. (1972). Electron microscopy of phagocytosis in syphilis and yaws. *Br. J. Vener. Dis.*, **48**, 227-48

70. Sell, S., Baker-Zander, S. and Powell, H. C. (1982). Experimental syphilitic orchitis in rabbits: ultrastructural appearance of *Treponema pallidum* during phagocytosis and destruction by macrophages *in vivo*. *Lab. Invest.*, **46**, 355-64

71. Lukehart, S. A. (1982). Activation of macrophages by products of lymphocytes from normal and syphilitic rabbits. *Infect. Immun.*, **37**, 64-9

72. Lukehart, S. A. and Miller, J. N. (1978). Demonstration of the *in vitro* phagocytosis of *Treponema pallidum* by rabbit peritoneal macrophages. *J. Immunol.*, **121**, 2014-24

73. Lukehart, S. A., Baker-Zander, S. A. and Sell, S. (1980). Characterization of lymphocyte responsiveness in early experimental syphilis. I. *In vitro* response to mitogens and *Treponema pallidum* antigens. *J. Immunol.*, **124**, 454-60

74. Pavia, C. S., Folds, J. D. and Baseman, J. B. (1978). Cell-mediated immunity during syphilis: a review. *Br. J. Vener. Dis.*, **54**, 144-50

75. Tabor, D. R., Azadegan, A. A., Schell, R. F. and LeFrock, J. L. (1984). Inhibition of macrophage C3b-mediated ingestion by syphilitic hamster T-cell-enriched fractions. *J. Immunol.*, **135**, 2698-705

76. Tabor, D. R., Bagasra, O. and Jacobs, R. F. (1986). Treponemal infection specifically enhances node T-cell regulation of macrophage activity. *Infect. Immun.*, **54**, 21-7

77. Schell, R. F., Le Frock, J. L. and Chan, J. K. (1982). Transfer of resistance with syphilitic immune cells: lack of correlation with mitogenic activity. *Infect. Immun.*, **35**, 187-92

78. Gjestland, T. (1955). The Oslo study of untreated syphilis. An epidemiologic investigation of the natural course of syphilitic infection based upon a re-study of the Boeck-Bruusgaard material. *Acta Dermatol. Vener.*, **35** (Suppl. 34) 1-365

79. Jorizzo, J. L., McNeely, M. C., Baughn, R. E., Solomon, A. R., Cavallo, T. and Smith E. B. (1986). Role of circulating immune complexes in human secondary syphilis. *J. Infect. Dis.*, **153**, 1014-22

80. Medici, M. A. (1972). The immunoprotective niche – A new pathogenic mechanism for syphilis, the systemic mycoses and other infectious diseases. *J. Theor. Biol.*, **36**, 617-25

81. Sell, S., Salman, J. and Norris, S. J. (1985). Reinfection of chancre-immune rabbits with *Treponema pallidum*: I. Light and immunofluorescence studies. *Am. J. Pathol.*, **118**, 248-55

82. Vartdal, F., Vanvik, B., Micaelsen, T. E., Loe, K. and Norrby, E. (1981). Neurosyphilis: intrathecal synthesis of oligoclonal antibodies to *Treponema pallidum*. *Ann. Neurol.*, **11**, 35-40

83. Lowhagen, G.-B., Andersson, M., Blomstrand, C. and Roupe, G. (1983). Central nervous system involvement in early syphilis. I. Intrathecal immunoglobulin production. *Acta Derm. Venereol. (Stockholm)*, **63**, 409-17

84. Muller, F., Moskophidis, M. and Prange, H. W. (1984). Demonstration of locally synthesized immunoglobulin M antibodies to *Treponema pallidum* in the central nervous system of patients with untreated neurosyphilis. *J. Neuroimmunol.*, **7**, 43-54

85. Mascola, L., Pelosi, R., Blount, J. H., Alexander, C. E. and Cates, W., Jr. (1985). Congenital syphilis revisited. *Am. J. Dis. Child.*, **139**, 575-80

86. Judge, D. M., Tafari, N., Naeye, R. L. and Marboe, C. (1986). Congenital syphilis and perinatal mortality. *Pediatr. Pathol.*, **5**, 411-20

87. Fiumara, N. J. and Lessell, S. (1983). The stigmata of late congenital syphilis: an analysis of 100 patients. *Sex. Transm. Dis.*, **10**, 126-9

88. Fitzgerald, T. J. (1985). Experimental congenital syphilis in rabbits. *Can. J. Microbiol.*, **31**, 757-62

89. Kajdacsy-Balla, A., Howeedy, A. and Bagasra, O. (1987). Syphilis in the Syrian hamster. A model of human venereal and congenital syphilis. *Am. J. Pathol.*, **126**, 599-601

90. McKenna, J. J., Miles, R., Lemen, D., Dunford, S. A. and Renirie, R. (1986). Unmasking AIDS: chemical immunosuppression and seronegative syphilis. *Med. Hypotheses*, **21**, 421-30

91. Zaidman, G. W. (1986). Neurosyphilis and retrobulbar neuritis in a patient with AIDS. *Ann. Ophthalmol.*, **18**, 260-1

92. Berry, C. D., Hooton, T. M., Collier, A. C. and Lukehart, S. A. (1987). Neurologic relapse after benzathine penicillin therapy for secondary syphilis in a patient with HIV infection. *N. Engl. J. Med.*, **316**, 1587-9

93. Johns, D. R., Tierney, M. and Felsenstein, D. (1987). Alteration in the natural history of neurosyphilis by concurrent infection with the human immunodeficiency virus. *N. Engl. J. Med.*, **316**, 1569-72

94. Stoumbos, V. D. and Klein, M. L. (1987). Syphilitic retinitis in a patient with acquired immunodeficiency syndrome-related complex. (letter) *Am. J. Ophthalmol.*, **103**, 103-4

95. Zambrano, W., Perez, G. M., and Smith, J. L. (1987). Acute syphilitic blindness in AIDS. *J. Clin. Neurol. Ophthalmol.*, **7**, 1-5

96. Rosenheim, M., Brucker, G., Leibowitch, M. Niel, G., Bournerias, I., Duflo, B. and Gentilini, M. (1987). Syphilis maligne chez un malade porteur d'anticorps anti-VIH. *N. Presse Med.*, **16**, 777

97. Petersen, L. R., Mead, R. H. and Perlroth, M. G. (1983). Unusual manifestations of secondary syphilis occurring after orthotopic liver transplantation. *Am. J. Med.*, **75**, 166-70

98. Guinan, M. E., Thomas, P. A., Pinsky, P. F., Goodrich, J. T., Selik, R. M., Jaffe, H. W., Haverkos, H. W., Noble, G. and Curran, J. W. (1984). Heterosexual and homosexual patients with the acquired immunodeficiency syndrome. A comparison of surveillance, interview, and laboratory data. *Ann. Intern. Med.*, **100**, 213-18

99. Moss, A. R., Osmond, D., Bacchetti, P., Chermann, J.-C., Barre-Sinoussi, F. and Carlson, J. (1987). Risk factors for AIDS and HIV seropositivity in homosexual men. *Am. J. Epidemiol.*, **125**, 1035-47

100. Young, E. J., Weingarten, N. M., Baughn, R. E. and Duncan, W. C. (1982). Studies on the pathogenesis of the Jarisch-Herxheimer reaction: development of an animal model and evidence against a role for classical endotoxin. *J. Infect. Dis.*, **146**, 606-15

101. Moore, M. B., Price, E. V., Knox, J. M. and Elgin, L. W. (1963). Epidemiologic treatment of contacts to infectious syphilis. *Pub. Hlth. Rep.*, **78**, 966-70

102. Schroeter, A. L., Turner, R. H., Lucas, J. B. and Brown, W. J. (1971). Therapy for incubating syphilis. Effectiveness of gonorrhea treatment. *J. Am. Med. Assoc.*, **218**, 711-13

103. Magnuson, H. J., Thomas, E.W., Olansky, S., Kaplan, B. I., De Mello, L. and Cutler, J. C. (1956). Inoculation syphilis in human volunteers. *Medicine*, **35**, 33-82

104. Magnuson, H. J. and Rosenau, B. J. (1948). The rate of development and degree of

acquired immunity in experimental syphilis. *Am. J. Syph.*, **32**, 418–36

105. Schell, R. F., Chan, J. K. and Le Frock, J. L. (1979). Endemic syphilis: passive transfer of resistance with serum and cells in hamsters. *J. Infect. Dis.*, **140**, 378–83

106. Azadegan, A. A., Schell, R. F. and Le Frock, J. L. (1983). Immune serum confers protection against syphilitic infection on hamsters. *Infect. Immun.*, **42**, 42–7

107. Azadegan, A. A., Schell, R. F., Steiner, B. M., Coe, J. E. and Chan, J. K. (1986). Effect of immune serum and its immunoglobulin fractions on hamsters challenged with *Treponema pallidum* subsp. *pertenue*. *J. Infect. Dis.*, **153**, 1007–13

108. Pavia, C. S. and Niederbuhl, C. J. (1985). Acquired resistance and expression of a protective humoral immune response in guinea pigs infected with *Treponema pallidum* Nichols. *Infect, Immun.*, **50**, 66–72

109. Pavia, C. S., Niederbuhl, C. J. and Saunders, J. (1985). Antibody-mediated protection of guinea pigs against infection with *Treponema pallidum*. *Immunology*, **56**, 195–202

110. Azadegan, A. A., Tabor, D. R., Schell, R. F. and LeFrock, J. L. (1984). Cobra venom factor abrogates passive humoral resistance to syphilitic infection in hamsters. *Infect. Immun.*, **44**, 740–2

111. Steiner, B. M., Schell, R. F., Liu, H. and Harris, O. N. (1986). The effect of C3 depletion on resistance of hamsters to infection with the yaws spirochete. *Sex. Transm. Dis.*, **13**, 245–50

112. Metzger, M. and Smogor, W. (1975). Passive transfer of immunity to experimental syphilis in rabbits by immune lymphocytes. *Arch. Immunol. Ther. Exp.*, **23**, 625–30

113. Chan, J. K., Schell, R. F. and Le Frock, J. L. (1979). Ability of enriched immune T cells to confer resistance in hamsters to infection with *Treponema pertenue*. *Infect. Immun.*, **26**, 448–52

114. Pavia, C. S. and Niederbuhl, C. J. (1985). Adoptive transfer of anti-syphilis immunity with lymphocytes from *Treponema pallidum*-infected guinea pigs. *J. Immunol.*, **135**, 2829–34

115. Metzger, M. and Smogor, W. (1969). Artificial immunization of rabbits against syphilis. *Br. J. Vener. Dis.*, **45**, 308–12

116. Miller, J. N. (1973). Immunity in experimental syphilis. VI. Successful vaccination of rabbits with *Treponema pallidum*, Nichols strain, attenuated by gamma-irradiation. *J. Immunol.*, **110**, 1206–15

117. Hindersson, P., Petersen, C. S. and Axelsen, N. H. (1985). Purified flagella from *Treponema phagedenis* biotype Reiter does not induce protective immunity against experimental syphilis in rabbits. *Sex. Transm. Dis.*, **12**, 124–7

118. Johnson, P. C., Norris, S. J., Miller, G. P. G., Scott, L. D., Sell, S., Kahan, B. D. and van Buren, C. T. (1988). Early syphilitic hepatitis following renal transplantation. *J. Infect. Dis.* (In press)

2
Reiter's Syndrome and Reactive Arthritis

S. A. ALLARD AND R. N. MAINI

The association of gastrointestinal and lower genital tract infections and the subsequent development of arthritis has been recognized for many years. As long ago as 1818 Sir Benjamin Brodie[1] described a series of patients with the condition that a century later became eponymously linked with Hans Reiter[2]. However, it was only in 1942 that it was suggested that the characteristic triad of non-gonococcal urethritis, poly- or monarthritis and conjunctivitis, should be regarded as a distinct clinical syndrome[3]. It is now well recognized that often the whole triad is not present, and patients may only display evidence of urethral discharge and arthritis; the term 'incomplete Reiter's syndrome' has been used to describe such patients[4] (Figure 2.1). In addition, the term 'reactive arthritis' is being used more frequently to describe the rheumatological features of Reiter's syndrome, and other arthropathies associated with infections at sites distant from joints. The consideration of a diagnosis of reactive arthritis has the added advantage of alerting the physician to the possibility of an infective trigger, which in many instances may give rise to unremarkable symptoms and may antedate the joint symptoms by some weeks[5].

The concept of a reactive arthritis links the presence of a recent infection at a distant site with an absence of viable organisms in the affected joint(s)[6]. When the infection is in the genital tract, epidemiological evidence suggests that it is acquired by sexual contact; hence the term 'sexually acquired reactive arthritis' (SARA) has been used as a description of this form of Reiter's syndrome[7]. It serves to distinguish it from reactive arthritis following an acute gastrointestinal infection. Circumstantial evidence implies that a host reaction provoked by the micro-organism is somehow involved in the pathogenesis of the disease. The concept may be broadened to include a range of infections which are associated with an arthritis, but with no evidence of a live organism within the joints (Table 2.1). Little is known about the mechanisms of disease in such conditions, and at the present time it is uncertain whether distinct pathogenetic processes are involved in the arthritis observed in the context of Reiter's syndrome.

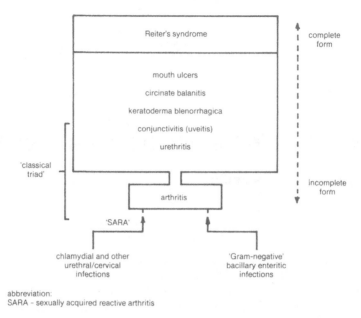

Figure 2.1 'Incomplete Reiter's syndrome' refers to the presence of arthritis plus another feature(s), but not including the full 'classical triad'

In patients with reactive arthritis, the associated infection is of a type that is known to affect many more individuals than ever show joint symptoms. Genetic factors are believed to play a part, although it has been suggested that this is at the level of disease expression rather than susceptibility to infection.

In Reiter's syndrome, the association with the histocompatibility antigen HLA–B27 is well established,[8,9] HLA–B27 is also strongly associated with conditions in which the role of infection is less clear, such as ankylosing spondylitis, and with sacroiliitis and/or spondylitis seen in psoriatic arthritis and inflammatory bowel disease[10]. The mode of interaction between HLA–B27 and an infecting organism is unknown at present, and neither is it understood why inflammation localizes to sites such as the enthesis (the site of insertion of ligament or tendon into bone), synarthrodial joints, synovium and the uveal tract.

REITER'S SYNDROME: CLINICAL FEATURES

The spectrum of clinical features in Reiter's syndrome ranges from a disabling multisystem disease to transient painless joint effusion or arthralgia with trivial or no symptoms. Since the original descriptions many other characteristic clinical features have been noted. These features are largely common to all the B27-associated reactive arthropathies, and have been reviewed extensively elsewhere[5–11] – a brief overview will be given here.

Table 2.1 Reactive arthritis: different types and postulated mechanisms

Clinical disorder	Micro-organism	Site of infection	Postulated disease mechanism
Rheumatic fever	β-haemolytic streptococcus	pharynx	cross-reactive antibody
Reiter's syndrome	– chlamydia	genital	antigen in synovium; local immune response
	– shigella	enteric	epitope sharing with HLA–B27
	– salmonella	,,	
	– yersinia	,,	
	– campylobacter	,,	
Meningococcal fever	meningococcus	systemic	vasculitis associated with circulating antigen–antibody complexes; complement fixation
Hepatitis	hepatitis B virus	liver	circulating HBsAg–Ab complexes
Rubella	rubella virus	systemic	virus/antigen in joints
Parvovirus arthritis	parvovirus	systemic	circulating antigen (viral) – antibody complexes

HLA–B27 – human leukocyte antigen B27
HBsAg – hepatitis B surface antigen
Ab – antibody

Musculoskeletal symptoms

In the majority of patients the arthritic symptoms usually develop within 30 days of the urogenital or enteric symptoms. However, both can arise simultaneously. The joint disease predominantly affects knees, ankles, feet and wrists in an oligoarticular, asymmetrical pattern. Ten per cent of patients may have just a monarthritis, which most commonly affects the knee. X-ray changes in synovial joints are rare, although juxta-articular osteoporosis and cartilage loss do occur and bone erosions, fibrous ankylosis and subluxation are features of chronic disease.

Enthesopathies affecting the Achilles' tendon and plantar fascia insertions at the calcaneum are not uncommon, and reactive arthritis should be considered as the most likely diagnosis in a young man presenting with heel pain. Similar inflammatory lesions may occur at other junctional zones between tendon or fascia and bone. Characteristic bony spurs will develop at these sites, and are visible on X-rays, although the early radiographic features are those of local osteoporosis or erosions.

Low back pain is common during the acute episode, and studies using bone scanning have suggested that this is associated with sacroiliitis[12]. The prevalence of sacroiliitis and spondylitis in patients with reactive arthritis has been difficult to estimate because of the similarities between severe, chronic or recurrent reactive disease and the other spondyloarthropathies. This has contributed to the considerable debate as to the relationship between these diseases. Radiographically, changes seen at the sacro–iliac joints and spine may be identical. Non-marginal syndesmophytes or bony bridges that were at one time thought to be characteristic of reactive disease have also been described in psoriatic spondylitis and some asymptomatic, normal individuals[13].

Ocular symptoms

Although a feature of the characteristic triad, symptomatic ocular inflammation occurs in less than one-third of patients with reactive arthritis. Unilateral or bilateral conjunctivitis which is usually mild and resolves without complication is the typical lesion. Rarely, symptoms may be severe with secondary infection. Although acute anterior uveitis is rare in the acute stage, a patient with a red eye and arthritis should be seen urgently by a specialist for slit-lamp examination in view of the risk of rapid deterioration in vision in patients with acute anterior uveitis. A past history of uveitis may be obtained in patients with Reiter's disease.

Skin and mucous membrane lesions

Characteristic cutaneous lesions include keratoderma blenorrhagica, which presents as a scaling pustular rash on the soles of the feet and palms. Psoriaform lesions of circinate balanitis occur on the glans or shaft of the penis, and similar skin lesions have been reported on the external female genitalia. It is of great interest that histologically these lesions resemble those of pustular psoriasis[14]. These lesions may be less common in enteric forms of reactive arthritis than in SARA[5]. In contrast, erythema nodosum has been well described in yersinial arthritis but appears to be rare in sexually acquired disease.

Shallow painless ulcers on the buccal mucosa, tongue and palate may be present. Inflammation of the urethral mucosa occurs not only in patients with local infection, but also in patients with Reiter's syndrome following an enteric infection.

Other lesions

Electrocardiographic abnormalities, including complete heart block and pericarditis may occur. Aortic valve disease and other chronic myocardial abnormalities have been described[15]. Numerous other disorders have also been described, including pulmonary infiltrates, neurological defects, thrombophlebitis and thyroid disorders, but these are extremely rare, and their significance uncertain.

PATHOLOGY AND IMMUNOPATHOLOGY

Histological studies on the joint tissue from patients with Reiter's syndrome have suggested that there are distinct changes in the synovial membrane during the early acute stage which were not seen in early rheumatoid arthritis (RA) or pyogenic septic arthritis[14,16]. These changes include a subacute inflammatory infiltrate localized to the superficial vascular regions of the involved membranes, intense hyperaemia, the presence of many neutrophils and minimal synovial lining layer hyperplasia. At this stage the predominent cell type in the synovial fluid is also the neutrophil. Characteristic inclusions have been described within large mononuclear cells both in synovial fluid[17] and synovial membrane[18]. Abnormalities of mitochondrial morphology in Type B synovial-lining cells have also been described in acute Reiter's syndrome[19]. The specificity of these findings for Reiter's syndrome is unknown. It is more usual to observe changes of chronic synovial inflammation, irrespective of the stage of the disease, resembling that seen in rheumatoid synovitis, including the appearance of perivascular lymphoid aggregates, plasma cells, and synovial-lining layer hyperplasia.[16]

Immunopathological studies of synovial fluid and tissues have been less numerous than those investigating rheumatoid arthritis. Deposits of immunoglobulin and complement have been noted in synovial membrane, and evidence for local complement activation and deposition of immune complexes within the joint have been shown to occur in a few patients[20,21], although this does not appear to be as marked a feature as observed in rheumatoid synovitis.

Recent studies using monoclonal antibodies to characterize the phenotype of mononuclear cells in the peripheral blood of patients with Reiter's disease have demonstrated that the ratio of helper/inducer (CD4) positive cells to suppressor/cytotoxic (CD8) cells did not differ between patients with reactive synovitis and normal controls[22]. In contrast, in the synovial fluid, CD4-positive cells occur in excess of CD8 cells[23]. The same group have studied the mononuclear cell populations of synovial fluid, following depletion of polymorphonuclear leukocytes[24]. In this study the percentage of monocytes was found to be far greater in the reactive arthritis group compared with RA. Although MHC Class II positive cells formed about 60% of the monoculear cells seen in both conditions, other activation markers detected by antibodies to the interleukin-2 receptor (anti-Tac), the transferrin receptor (OKT9) and a marker of activated cytotoxic T-cells and natural killer cells (4F2) were markedly increased in reactive arthritis compared with RA. These results were thought to demonstrate an active cell-mediated immune response in reactive synovitis. Similar detailed studies on synovial membrane have not yet been performed.

It should be noted, however, that samples of synovial fluid and tissue are often obtained early in the course of disease in patients with reactive arthritis, whereas in a chronic disorder such as rheumatoid arthritis, the patient population is often more heterogeneous, with many patients having had a long disease duration and a wide spectrum of disease-modifying drugs. Therefore caution must prevail in drawing far-reaching conclusions by comparison of such disparate groups. A recent study may exemplify this point, it showed significantly increased levels of the proteoglycan keratan sulphate in the synovial fluid of patients with Reiter's syndrome, but not in patients with rheumatoid or osteoarthritis.[25]

Chlamydial inclusion bodies have been reported in the synovial membranes of some patients with acute joint disease[26-29], and using an antibody against chlamydia, specific antigen has been detected[28-29]. Ultrastructural studies using antisera identified chlamydial antigen in the vacuoles of synovial macrophages in two of these joints[29]. In another study, using a fluorescein-conjugated monoclonal antibody to *C. trachomatis* ('MicroTrak'; Syva), the presence of chlamydial antigen was demonstrated in synovial material from patients with SARA following recent chlamydial infection[30]. Control material from the joints of 13 patients with other rheumatic diseases were negative using this test. The same group have also claimed the presence of chlamydial antigen in synovial tissue from four women with unexplained oligo- or monarthritis[31]. These promising findings require better proof of the chlamydial origin of antigen, since cross-reactions with other micro-organisms have been recorded[32]. In addition, a true cause-and-effect relationship would be strengthened by negative findings in relevant controls, such as synovium from patients with reactive arthritis following enteric infections and in synovium from an age-matched sexually active group without arthritis.

INITIATING INFECTIONS

Genital infections

Genital tract infection is thought to be the commonest initiator of reactive arthritis in some parts of Europe and in the USA. Arthritis develops in approximately 1% of men presenting with non-gonococcal urethritis (NGU) at hospital clinics[33], however this figure is only an approximation as many individuals with mild joint disease may not seek medical attention. In addition, the incidence of SARA in women is unknown largely because of the underdiagnosis of genital tract infection[34].

Chlamydial infections

Approximately 50% of cases of NGU in men are caused by *Chlamydia trachomatis*, and it is also thought to be a common pathogen of the female genital tract[35]. Its role in the pathogenesis of Reiter's syndrome derives from (1) clinical studies, (2) identification of the organism or antigen originating from it, and (3) the immune response of the host.

Clinical studies – have shown a close association between the development of arthritis and sexually transmitted genital tract infection. Several studies have shown that the intervals between the development of urethritis and arthritis were relatively constant[9,36,37]. In addition, the onset of this disease pattern is often associated with multiple or new sexual contacts. However, inflammation of the genital tract has been described in association with gastrointestinal infection, and, therefore, the presence of urethritis alone is not sufficient evidence to indicate sexually transmitted disease[38].

In identifying the organism or antigen originating from C. trachomatis – since the development of sensitive cell-culture techniques for isolation, major studies have shown that chlamydiae can be recovered from the urethra of approximately 35% of men with non-diarrhoeal Reiter's syndrome[34]. There have been great variations between isolation rates from the genital tract in the different studies, varying between 0-69%[39,40]. This presumably reflects differences in patient selection, prior antibiotic therapy, differences in isolation methods and variations in aetiology in different regions. It is reasonable to assume that other sexually-transmitted micro-organisms are implicated in chlamydia-negative SARA.

The question of whether viable organisms reach the joint in Reiter's syndrome associated with NGU is central to the concept of this disorder being truly 'reactive'. In some early studies, positive isolations from both synovial membrane and fluid were described[41]. However, this has not been substantiated by other studies, and it is an exceptional patient in whom isolation of the organism appears to have been reported[42-43] However, the high titres of neutralizing chlamydial antibody in the synovial fluids of patients with SARA, could contribute to the difficulty of culturing organisms.

The failure to detect viable organisms in the joint does not, however, exclude the possibility that antigenic material derived from chlamydiae does not reach and persist in the joint. Recent studies [28-31] using monoclonal antibodies to chlamydiae suggest that this might occur. Further experimental evidence derives from animals with a septic chlamydial arthritis, in which joint cultures become negative after 3 or 4 weeks despite the persistence of synovitis[44]. The fact that bacterial cell wall constituents can induce synovitis in experimental animals in a variety of situations[45-47], and the finding of raised levels of antibody to bacterial peptidoglycan in patients with Reiter's syndrome[48] also supports this concept.

Isolation of organisms from the conjunctivae of patients with Reiter's syndrome has similarly produced largely negative results, and it has likewise been assumed that this lesion also has a 'reactive' basis.

The immune responses of the host to C. trachomatis – appear to be enhanced in patients with SARA when compared to individuals with uncomplicated chlamydial urethritis or other forms of arthritis. The complement-fixation test for chlamydial group-specific antibody, which has been used successfully in the diagnosis of lymphogranuloma venereum (LGV) and psittacosis, has produced conflicting results when applied to Reiter's syndrome. Using this test, chlamydial serum antibody was found in only 21-31% of patients, the prevalence and titre being similar to patients with uncomplicated NGU[34].

The more sensitive micro-immunofluorescence test, which also allows identification of immunoglobulin class has resulted in more convincing evidence implicating *C. trachomatis* in SARA. Several studies have now shown that patients with SARA produce significantly higher titres of IgG serum antibody to chlamydia than controls. In one study, these controls included some patients with reactive arthritis associated with diarrhoea[36]. Only 6% of these controls had antibody present, compared to 58% of the patients with Reiter's syndrome. Keat *et al.*[9] found that 22/30 (73%) men with SARA had serum chlamydial IgG antibody titres of > 64 at presentation. These included nine who had positive urethral chlamydia isolates. These patients had antibody titres that were significantly greater than those in 50 men with uncomplicated NGU. In a few patients who were studied serially, more than half (8/15) showed the typical changes in IgM and IgG antibody levels that are associated with a primary immune response to infection. The titre of IgM antibody was usually maximal at presentation and then fell, while maximal titres of IgG antibody were seen about 6 weeks after the onset of the arthritis. A subsequent study from Finland included seven women all of whom had high chlamydial IgG antibody titres[43]. These high levels of chlamydial antibody are rarely found in patients with uncomplicated chlamydial genital tract infection, even in those who have had a recurrent infection[34]. Therefore, this is likely to be a real difference and not an anamnestic response, and is compatible with the systemic spread of the organism from the urethra in patients with SARA.

In investigations to further study any differences between the humoral response of patients with chlamydially-induced Reiter's syndrome and uncomplicated chlamydial NGU, a study using immunoblotting of antigens of *C. trachomatis* did not reveal an antibody response unique to Reiter's syndrome[50]. However, IgA antibodies to a 59 kD antigen were present in all the Reiter's syndrome patients examined (11/11), but in only 2/6 patients with uncomplicated NGU.

An exaggerated proliferative response to chlamydial antigens in a lymphocyte transformation test has been recorded in some patients with Reiter's syndrome. This appeared to be specific for chlamydial antigens, since similar responses were not observed against measles, rubella or influenza viruses, nor against *Candida albicans*[36]. Other studies, however, could not find any difference between patients with Reiter's syndrome and uncomplicated NGU[51].

A recent report of Reiter's syndrome occurring in patients with the acquired immunodeficiency syndrome (AIDS) who are deficient in the number of helper–inducer CD4+ T-lymphocytes has suggested that lymphocytes of this phenotype may not play an important part in the mediation of inflammation at the effector level[52]. The nature of the arthritis was particularly aggressive in these patients, and it may be that non-compromised cell populations – such as the CD8+ (cytotoxic) lymphocytes or B-lymphocytes play a more critical role in Reiter's syndrome. However, a lack of CD4+ lymphocytes may depress the evolution of a normal anti-bacterial immune response, for example, as a result of lack of interleukin-2, which is essential for the generation of antibody and T-cell cytotoxicity. Thus the elimination of the putative organism and its antigens may be impaired and favour a persistent reactive arthritis.

Gonococcal infections

Genital infection with *Neisseria gonorrhoeae* may be associated with a blood-borne pyogenic arthritis in which invasion of the synovium by the bacterium can be proven in about half of the patients. The low isolation rate may reflect the microbiological techniques used for isolation of the gonococcus. In the majority of patients, the genital infection and arthritis resolves quickly after antibiotic therapy. However, there are some patients in whom the symptoms of urethritis and arthritis persist despite therapy, and in these patients a second clinical diagnosis of Reiter's syndrome seems appropriate. Whether arthritis in these patients is initiated by a co-existent chlamydial infection, which may be present in 20–30% of patients[34] and set in train a reactive arthritis, or whether the gonococcus may trigger an 'aseptic arthritis' in its own right is unclear. Rosenthal et al.[53] favour the possibility of the arthritis being initiated by the gonococcus, and suggest that cell-mediated immune mechanisms play a part, since lymphocyte stimulation induced by gonococcal antigen in these patients is significantly greater than in patients with non-gonococcal reactive arthritis or in controls. Goldenberg[54] is of the opinion that in patients in whom blood and joint fluid cultures do not yield gonococci, the arthralgias and tenosynovitis resemble a circulating immune complex disorder. More direct evidence is required to substantiate the role of the different organisms and mechanisms of disease in patients apparently infected with more than one organism, or when growth characteristics require special attention.

Other non-gonococcal genital infections

Urethritis is known to be associated with infections with ureaplasma and mycoplasma strains[55]. Mycoplasmas have occasionally been isolated from joints of patients with Reiter's syndrome[16], although recent attempts have not confirmed their presence. Synovial lymphocyte proliferative responses to ureaplasma antigens were noted in approximately 25% of sexually transmitted Reiter's syndrome cases, whilst the remainder of the cohort showed responses to chlamydial antigens[56]. Unlike the exaggerated antibody response to chlamydia in reactive arthritis, the antibody levels to mycoplasma in reactive arthritis and patients with non-specific urethritis are similar[57]. Eradication of these organisms from the genital tract does not influence the course or development of the arthritis[37]. Although inconclusive, the overall evidence suggests that reactive arthritis may sometimes be associated with mycoplasma or ureaplasma infection of the genital tract.

Enteric infections

Reiter's syndrome and its incomplete variants has been described in 2–3% of individuals following acute enteric infections with *Salmonella enteritidis* and *S. typhimurium, Shigella flexneri* and *Sh. dysenteriae, Yersinia enterocolitica* and *Y. pseudotuberculosis* and *Campylobacter jejuni*[5]. This association has been clearly demonstrated following outbreaks of bacterial diarrhoea, during which the incidence of reactive arthritis has often been higher, particularly with Yersinia infection[58]. Unlike SARA, males and females are equally affected.

A great deal of recent work on immunological changes in reactive arthritis associated with enteric infections comes from studies of Yersinia infection. Increased polyclonal immunoglobulin levels and antigen non-specific circulating immune complexes, occur in patients both with and without arthritis who have active infection[59]. However, as with chlamydiae, titres of antibodies against yersiniae have been reported to be higher and to persist for longer in patients with arthritis than in patients with uncomplicated bowel infection[60].

Studies on patients with yersiniae infection have shown the expected MHC Class II restriction in antigen presentation in an *in vitro* T-cell proliferation assay[61]. In one study, the lymphocyte proliferation assay was found to be significantly lower in patients with arthritis than in patients with only bowel infection[62], although in another study increased lymphocyte responses were found in the arthritic group[63]. Previous work by Ford *et al.*, [56,64] had shown an expansion of T-cells responsive to a variety of Gram-negative organisms in the joints of patients with Reiter's syndrome, however, responses in peripheral blood lymphocytes have been inconsistent. More specific responses of circulating lymphocytes have been demonstrated to a formalin-killed strain of Yersinia (serum strain 3), known to be associated with reactive arthritis but not to a strain (serum type 8) not associated with arthritis[65]. The antigen specificity was explained on the basis that heat-killed bacteria in other studies led to a loss of antigenic determinants not susceptible to formalin treatment. The prevalence of circulating sensitized lymphocytes following enteric infections does not of course explain why the immune response localizes to joints in only some patients, and also why only some micro-organisms appear to be arthritogenic. Specific properties of organisms, as well as the host, would appear to be important in the induction of arthritis, and the apparent lack of Reiter's syndrome in infections with *Shigella sonnei* emphasizes the role of a microbial factor[66].

Yersinia has not been isolated from the joints of patients with reactive arthritis, however, recent studies from Finland have demonstrated Yersinia-specific immune complexes in the synovial fluid of three out of 12 patients with Yersinia-triggered reactive arthritis, and in none of 16 control patients[67]. Circulating Yersinia-specific IgA immune complexes were previously found in arthritic but not non-arthritic patients, and antigen-specific IgM immune complexes were found in higher titre in the first 2 months of disease in the former group[68].

Infections in idiopathic forms of seronegative arthritis and spondylitis

There are many case reports of various organisms being associated with peripheral arthritis or sacroiliitis, but an aetiological role is difficult to establish. Chronic prostatitis has been found in a high proportion of men with sacroiliitis and spondylitis[69]. In addition, a high percentage of women with acute salpingitis developed sacroiliitis in Scandinavian studies[70]. However, more detailed microbiological analyses are needed to demonstrate these causal relationships.

Recent work examining the small and large bowel of patients with various forms of HLA–B27 arthritis have shown subclinical inflammation in the bowel mucosa[71]. Microscopic signs of gut inflammation were also observed in 67 out of 87 patients suffering from idiopathic arthritis not obviously due to a known trigger[72]. In contrast, only two of 18 patients with SARA presented histological abnormalities. Similar abnormalities in the bowel were found more often in ankylosing spondylitis patients with peripheral joint involvement than those with axial involvement alone. These studies have led to the supposition that repetitive bouts of subclinical bowel inflammation may result in abnormal gut permeability and permit entry of various antigens into the circulation, leading to inflammatory reactions in distant tissues in genetically predisposed individuals.

GENETIC SUSCEPTIBILITY

The original association of HLA-B27 was described in relation to ankylosing spondylitis[73,74], and has been found in more than 90% of patients in Caucasians and some American Indian groups. However, this is not true for all racial groups; for example, there is only a 50% association with American blacks. Other antigens that cross-react with B27 have been found with increased frequency in B27-negative patients[75]. This cross-reactive group (termed CREG), which include B7, Bw22 and B40, are also frequently found in the general population, and, therefore, their relevance in the pathogenesis of the disease is uncertain. The basis for this cross-reactivity is a common public antigenic determinent located on the heavy chain of these molecules[76].

The existence of inherited factors predisposing to reactive arthritis initiated by genital or gut infections has been confirmed by the finding of the genetic marker HLA-B27 in 60-90% of patients, but in less than 10% of healthy controls[5]. However, as in ankylosing spondylitis, there are racial differences, and in a recent study, only 29% of Israeli patients have been found to be HLA-B27 positive[77]. In contrast, HLA-B27 is not found more frequently in association with arthritis secondary to various bacterial and viral infections [78-80]. A recent family study of patients with Reiter's syndrome showed that the degree of familial aggregation approaches that seen in ankylosing spondylitis[81]. However, in this study, none of the relatives of Reiter's disease patients had ankylosing spondylitis, and vice versa, suggesting that in addition to HLA-B27 shared by both, other susceptibility factors distinct to each condition were involved. In addition, clinical differences between ankylosing spondylitis and Reiter's syndrome, in particular in relation to prognosis and chronicity, imply that findings related to one disease should not automatically be applied to the other syndrome. Despite several similarities reactive arthritis only rarely progresses to ankylosing spondylitis. However, patients with reactive arthritis who are HLA-B27 positive tend to have disease that is both more severe and of longer duration[9,82]. Similar disease mechanisms may occur in ankylosing spondylitis and some patients with HLA-B27 positive reactive arthritis.

How do HLA molecules affect the pathogenesis of these diseases? There has been some debate as to whether the B27 antigen interacts alone with the putative infecting organism or whether B27 is just an innocent marker for a separate disease susceptibility or immune response gene in linkage disequilibrium with the B27 gene. It may be that HLA molecules act as specific receptors for micro-organisms. However, in studies using adherence to epithelial cells[83] and binding of radiolabelled HLA molecules to bacteria[84], no specific receptor-interaction of B27 and arthritogenic organisms could be identified. HLA–dependent abnormalities in the immune response, such as an exaggerated or aberrant response to inflammatory mediators, are a possibility but still have little experimental support.

The postulated cross-reactivity of HLA antigens and microbial antigens has received the most widespread attention in the literature, and in particular the studies of the Ebringers[85] and Geczy and his co-workers[86-89] have examined the relationship of *Klebsiella pneumoniae* with ankylosing spondylitis. A detailed discussion of these controversial studies has been reviewed extensively elsewhere[87,90-91]. The original observation by Geczy drew attention to a rabbit antiserum directed against a certain strain of *K. pneumoniae* which proved cytotoxic for lymphocytes from B27 patients with ankylosing spondylitis, but not of B27-positive cells of normal individuals or B27 negative patients[86]. Later it was claimed that the supernatant from the klebsiella culture could modify 'normal' B27 cells so that they too were lysed by klebsiella antibodies[87]. Preliminary evidence suggested that this factor might be a plasmid[88]. In fact these studies have proved difficult to reproduce, although recent confirmation is reported from the Netherlands[92]. Further work from the Geczy group has shown that bacteria with cross-reactive antigenic determinents are found in the bowel flora of B27-positive spondylitic patients, but almost never in B27 positive controls[89]. This cross-reactivity was shared by many organisms and were not confined to a particular genus or species.

A similar cross-reactivity has recently been described between antibodies raised in rabbits against *C. trachomatis* and mononuclear cells of B27 positive patients with ankylosing spondylitis[93]. This cross-reactivity was observed in a serotype (D) known to be associated with urethritis, but not in one (L2) that causes lymphogranuloma venereum but not urethritis. Binding of the antibody was not blocked by monoclonal HLA–B27 antiserum, and it was, therefore, thought unlikely that B27 itself was responsible for this cross-reactivity. However, similar studies in patients with post-yersinial reactive arthritis and post-chlamydial reactive arthritis have failed to show any cross-reactivity with B27[94]. More recently monoclonal antibodies have been made that show cross-reactivity, for example, between HLA–B27 lymphoblastoid cell lines and *Yersinia enterocolitica*[95]. These varying results demonstrate the need for some standardization of the antigens used and some unification in the test systems employed to be able to make any relevant comparisons or conclusions.

Two monoclonal antibodies to HLA–B27 have recently been described[96]. These, designated M1 and M2, are thought to define separate determinants on the B27 molecule. Although M1 has been shown to bind to serotypes of Yersinia and Klebsiella and M2 to *Shigella flexneri*[97], no clearcut association between either variant and disease has been shown. Similarly, studies using cytotoxic T-cell clones, which have also defined B27 subsets, have so far failed to demonstrate any differences between the B27 of patients with arthritis and the B27 in normals[98]. A sequence homology of six amino acids between *K. pneumoniae* nitrogenase and HLA-B27 has recently been shown[99]. Antibodies to the peptide were found in patients with ankylosing spondylitis and Reiter's syndrome, and suggest a mechanism for the induction of auto-antibodies to HLA-B27. The pathogenic role, if any, of the antibody is less obvious, but the data does open new areas of investigation on host-parasite relationships in these disorders.

CONCLUSIONS

Although much has been learned over recent years regarding infectious agents, the response of the host and the genetic factors predisposing to the development of Reiter's disease, the exact mechanisms of how these factors interact remain elusive. Further studies particularly at the molecular level will, it is hoped, answer whether specific organisms are particularly arthritogenic or whether it is a predetermined or induced factor in the host which enables many organisms to have this potential. In addition, the concept of this disease being truly reactive will depend on future studies being unable to demonstrate specific antigenic components within the joints themselves.

References

1. Brodie, B. C. (1818). *Pathological and surgical observations on diseases of the joints.* pp. 51-63 (London: Longman).
2. Reiter, H. (1916). Uber einer bisher Unerkannte Spirochaeteninfektion (Spirochaetosis arthritica). *Dtsch. Med. Wochenschr.*, **42**, 1535-6
3. Bauer, W. and Engleman, E. P. (1942). A syndrome of unknown etiology characterized by urethritis, conjunctivitis and arthritis (so-called Reiter's disease). *Trans. Assoc. Am. Phys.*, **57**, 307-13
4. Arnett, F. C. (1979). Incomplete Reiter's syndrome: Clinical comparisons with classical triad. *Ann. Rheum. Dis.*, **38** (Suppl.), 73-7
5. Keat, A. (1983). Reiter's syndrome and reactive arthritis in perspective. *N. Engl. J. Med.*, **309**, 1606-15
6. Aho, K. (1984). Pathogenesis of Reiter's syndrome and reactive arthritis. *Scand. J. Rheumatol.*, **52** (Suppl.), 30-6
7. Keat, A. C., Maini, R. N., Nkwazi, G. C., Pegrum, G. D., Ridgway, G. L. and Scott, J. T. (1978). Role of *Chlamydia trachomatis* and HLA-B27 in sexually acquired reactive arthritis. *Br. Med. J.*, **1**, 605-7
8. Brewerton, D. A., Caffrey, M., Nicolls, A., Walters, D. and James, D. C. O. (1973). Reiter's disease and HLA-B27. *Lancet*, **2**, 996-8
9. Keat, A. C., Maini, R. N., Pegrum, G. D. and Scott, J. T. (1979). The clinical features and HLA associations of reactive arthritis associated with non-gonococcal arthritis. *Q J. Med.*, **48**, 323-42
10. Wright, V. (1978). Seronegative polyarthritis. A unified concept. *Arthritis. Rheum.*, **21**, 619-33
11. Calin, A. (1985). Reiter's syndrome. In Kelley, W. N., Harris, E., Ruddy, S. and Sledge, C. (eds.) *Textbook of Rheumatology*, pp. 1007-20. (Philadelphia: W. B. Saunders)
12. Russell, A. S., Davis, P., Percy, J. S. and Lentle, B. C. (1977). The sacroiliitis of acute Reiter's syndrome. *J. Rheumatol.*, **4**, 293-6
13. Sundaram, M. and Patton, J. T. (1975). Paravertebral ossification in psoriasis and Reiter's disease. *Br. J. Radiol.*, **48**, 628-33
14. Kulka, J. P. (1962). The lesions of Reiter's disease. *Br. J. Vener. Dis.*, **53**, 260-2
15. Ribeiro, K., Morley, K. D., Shapiro, L. M., Garnett, R. A. F., Hughes, G. R. V. and Goodwin, J. F. (1984). Left ventricular function in patients with ankylosing spondylitis and Reiter's disease. *Eur. Heart J.*, **5**, 419-22
16. Weinberger, H. W., Ropes, M. W., Kulka, J. P. and Bauer, W. (1962). Reiter's syndrome, clinical and pathologic observations. *Medicine (Baltimore)*, **41**, 35-91

17. Pekin, T. J., Malinin, T. I. and Zvaifler, N. J. (1965). Leucocyte-containing macrophages in Reiter's syndrome. Presented at the *11th International Congress on Rheumatology*, December, Mar del Plata, Argentina
18. Norton, W. L., Lewis, D. and Ziff, M. (1966). Light and electron microscopic observations on the synovitis of Reiter's disease. *Arthritis Rheum.*, **9**, 747–57
19. Morris, C. J., Farr, M., Hollywell, C. A., Hawkins, C. F., Scott, D. L. and Walton, K. W. (1983). Ultrastructure of the synovial membrane in seronegative inflammatory arthropathies. *J. R. Soc. Med.*, **76**, 27–31
20. Yates, D. B., Maini, R. N., Scott, J. T. and Sloper, J. C. (1975). Complement activation in Reiter's syndrome. *Ann. Rheum. Dis.*, **34**, 468
21. Baldassare, A. R., Weiss, T. D., Tsai, C. C., Arthur, R. E., Moore, T. L. and Zuckner, J. (1981). Immunoprotein deposition in synovial tissue in Reiter's syndrome. *Ann. Rheum. Dis.*, **40**, 281–5
22. Veys, E. M., Verbruggen, G., Hermanns, P., Mielants, H., van Bruwaene, P., de Brabanter, G., de Landsheere, D. and Immesoete, C. (1983). Peripheral blood T lymphocytes subpopulations in HLA–B27 related rheumatic diseases: ankylosing spondylitis and reactive synovitis. *J. Rheumatol.*, **10**, 140–3
23. Nordstrom, D., Konttinen, Y. T., Bergroth, V. and Leirisalo-Repo, M. (1985). Synovial fluid cells in Reiter's syndrome. *Ann. Rheum. Dis.*, **44**, 852–6
24. Konttinen, Y. T., Nordstrom, D., Bergroth, V., Leirisalo-Repo, M. and Skrifvars, B. (1986). Cell-mediated immune response in the diseased joints in patients with reactive arthritis. *Scand. J. Immunol.*, **23**, 685–91
25. Ratcliffe, A., Maini, R. N., Docherty, M. and Hardingham, T. (1987). The determination of the raised level of keratan sulphate in the synovial fluids of patients with reactive arthritis. *Br. J. Rheumatol.*, **26** (Suppl. 1), 66
26. Coste, F., Amor, B. and Delbarre, F. (1965). Sur l'etiologie virale du syndrome oculo-urethro-synoviale. Presented at the *11th International Congress of Rheumatology*, December, Mar del Plata, Argentina
27. Levy, J. P., Ryckewaert, A., Silvestre, D., Kahn, M-F. and Mitrovic, D. (1966). Etude par microscopie electronique des inclusions des cellules synoviales dans un cas de syndrome oculo-urethro synovial (Fiessinger–Leroy–Reiter). *Pathol. Biol.*, **14**, 216–23
28. Ishikawa, H., Ohno, O., Yamasaki, K., Ikuta, S. and Hirohata, K. (1986). Arthritis presumably caused by Chlamydia in Reiter's syndrome. *J. Bone Jnt. Surg.*, **68A**, 777–9
29. Schumacher, H. R., Cherian, P. V., Sieck, M. and Clayburne, G. (1986). Ultrastructural identification of chlamydial antigens in synovial membrane in acute Reiter's syndrome. *Arthritis Rheum.*, **29**, S31
30. Keat, A., Thomas, B., Dixey, J., Osborn, M., Sonnex, C. and Taylor-Robinson, D. (1987). *Chlamydia trachomatis* and reactive arthritis: the missing link. *Lancet*, **1**, 72–4
31. Dixey, J., Thomas, B., Taylor-Robinson, D., Osborn, M. and Keat, A. (1987). *Chlamydia trachomatis* and unexplained knee arthritis in women. *Arthritis Rheum.*, **30**, S42
32. Krech, T., Gerhard-Fsandi, D., Hofmann, N. and Miller, S. M. (1985). Interference of *Staphylococcus aureus* in the detection of *Chlamydia trachomatis* by monoclonal antibodies. *Lancet*, **1**, 1161–2
33. Csonka, G. W. (1958). The course of Reiter's syndrome. *Br. Med. J.*, **1**, 1088–90
34. Keat, A., Thomas, B, J. and Taylor-Robinson, D. (1983). Chlamydial infection in the aetiology of arthritis. *Br. Med. Bull.*, **39**, 168–74
35. Taylor-Robinson, D. and Thomas, B. J. (1980). The role of *Chlamydia trachomatis* in genital tract and associated diseases. *J. Clin. Pathol.*, **33**, 205–33
36. Martin, D. H., Pollock, S., Kuo, C-C., Wang, S-P., Brunham, R. C. and Holmes, K. K. (1984). *C. trachomatis* infections in men with Reiter's syndrome. *Ann. Intern. Med.*, **100**, 207–13
37. Ford, D. K. and Rasmussen, G. (1964). Relationships between genitourinary infection and complicating arthritis. *Arthritis Rheum.*, **7**, 220–7
38. Editorial. (1985). Is Reiter's syndrome caused by Chlamydia? *Lancet*, **1**, 317–19
39. Ford, D. K. and McCandlish, L. (1971). Isolation of human genital TRIC agents in nongonococcal urethritis and Reiter's disease by an irradiated cell culture method. *Br. J. Vener. Dis.*, **47**, 196–7
40. Koussa, M., Saikku, P., Richmond, S. and Lassus, A. (1978). Frequent association of

chlamydial infection with Reiter's syndrome. *Sex. Transm. Dis.*, **5**, 57–61

41. Schachter, J. (1976). Can chlamydial infections cause rheumatic disease? In Dumonde, D. C. (ed.). *Infection and Immunology in the Rheumatic Diseases*, pp. 151–7. (Oxford: Blackwell)

42. Shatkin, A. A., Popov, N. L. and Scherbakova, N. I. (1976). Morphology of Halprowia (chlamydia) isolated in Reiter's syndrome. *Zh. Mikrobiol. Epidemiol. Immunobiol.*, **4**, 60–4

43. Vippula, A. II., Yli-Kertulla, U. I., Ahlroos, A. K. and Terho, P. E. (1981). Chlamydia isolation and serology in Reiter's syndrome. *Scand. J. Rheumatol.*, **10**, 181–5

44. Storz, J. (1971). Chlamydial polyarthritis. In   (ed.) *Chlamydia and chlamydia-induced diseases*, pp. 216–32. (Springfield, Il: C. C. Thomas)

45. Cromartie, W. J., Craddock, J. G., Schwab, J. H., Anderle, S. K. and Yang, C. H. (1977). Arthritis in rats after systemic injection of streptococcal cells or cell walls. *J. Exp. Med.*, **146**, 1585–602

46. Wilder, R. L., Allen, J. B., Wahl, L. M., Calandra, G. B. and Wahl, S. M. (1983). The pathogenesis of group A streptococcal cell wall-induced polyarthritis in the rat. *Arthritis Rheum.*, **26**, 1442–51

47. Goldenberg, D. L., Reed, J. I. and Rice, P. A. (1984). Arthritis in rabbits induced by killed *Neisseria gonorrhoeae* and gonococcal polysaccharide. *J. Rheumatol.*, **11**, 3–8

48. Park, H., Schumacher, H. R., Zeiger, A. R. and Rosenbaum, J. T. (1984). Antibodies to peptidoglycan in patients with spondylarthritis: a clue to disease aetiology? *Ann. Rheum. Dis.*, **43**, 725–8

49. Keat, A. C., Thomas, B. J., Taylor-Robinson, D., Pegrum, G. D., Maini, R. N. and Scott, J. T. (1980). Evidence of *Chlamydia trachomatis* infection in sexually acquired reactive arthritis. *Ann. Rheum. Dis.*, **39**, 431–7

50. Inman, R. D., Johnston, M. E. A., Chiu, B., Falk, J. and Petric, M. (1987). Immunochemical analysis of immune response to *Chlamydia trachomatis* in Reiter's syndrome and nonspecific urethritis. *Clin. Exp. Immunol.*, **69**, 246–54

51. Amor, B., Kahan, A., Lecoq, F. and Delbarre, F. (1972). Le test de transformation lymphoblastique par des antigenes bedsoniens (TTL Bedsonien). *Rev. Rhum.*, **39**, 671–6

52. Winchester, R., Bernstein, D. H., Fischer, H. D., Enlow, R. and Solomon, G. (1987). The co-occurrence of Reiter's syndrome and acquired immunodeficiency. *Ann. Intern. Med.*, **106**, 19–26

53. Rosenthal, L., Olhagen, B. and Ek, S. (1980). Aseptic arthritis after gonorrhoea. *Ann. Rheum. Dis.*, **39**, 141–6

54. Goldenberg, D. L. (1983). 'Postinfectious arthritis'. *Am. J. Med.*, **74**, 925–8

55. Csonka, G. W., Williams, R. E. O. and Corse, J. (1967). T-strain mycoplasmas in non-gonococcal urethritis. *Ann. NY Acad. Sci.*, **143**, 794–8

56. Ford, D. K., da Roza, D. M. and Shah, P. (1981). Cell-mediated immune responses of synovial mononuclear cells to sexually transmitted, enteric and mumps antigens in patient's with Reiter's syndrome, rheumatoid arthritis and ankylosing spondylitis. *J. Rheumatol.*, **8**, 220–32

57. Taylor-Robinson, D., Thomas, B. J., Furr, P. M. and Keat, A. C. (1983). The association of *Mycoplasma hominis* with arthritis. *Sex. Transm. Dis.*, **101** (Suppl.), 341–4

58. Tertti, R., Granfors, K., Lehtonen, O-P., Mertsola, J., Makela, A.-L., Valimaki, T., Hanninen, P. and Toivanen, A. (1984). An outbreak of *Yersinia pseudotuberculosis* infection. *J. Infect. Dis.*, **149**, 245–50

59. Leirisalo, M., Gripenberg, M., Julkunen, I. and Repo, H. (1984). Circulating immune complexes in yersinia infection. *J. Rheumatol.*, **11**, 365–8

60. Granfors, K., Viljanen, M. K., Tiilikanen, A. and Toivanen, A. (1980). Persistence of IgM, IgG and IgA antibodies to yersinia and yersinia arthritis. *J. Infect. Dis.*, **141**, 424–9

61. Vuento, R., Eskola, J., Leino, R., Viander, M. and Toivanen, A. (1984). Role of Ia-positive cells in the lymphocyte responses to Yersinia. *Scand. J. Rheumatol.*, **20**, 141–7

62. Toivanen, A., Granfors, K., Lahesmaa-Rantala, R., Leino, R., Stahlberg, T. and Vuento, R. (1985). Pathogenesis of yersinia-triggered reactive arthritis: immunological, microbiological and clinical aspects. *Immunol. Rev.*, **86**, 47–70

63. Brenner, M. B., Kobayashi, S., Wiesenhutter, C., Huberman, A. K., Bales, P. and Yu, D. T. Y. (1984). *In vitro* T lymphocyte proliferative response to *Yersinia enterocolitica* in Reiter's syndrome. Lack of response in other HLA–B27 positive individuals. *Arthritis. Rheum.*, **27**, 250–7

64. Ford, D. K., da Roza, D. M. and Schulzer, M. (1982). The specificity of synovial mononuclear cell responses to microbial antigens in Reiter's syndrome. *J. Rheumatol.*, **9**, 561-7
65. Yu, D. T. Y., Ogasawara, M., Hill, J. L. and Kono, D. H. (1985). Study of Reiter's syndrome with special emphasis on *Yersinia enterocolitica*. *Immunol. Rev.*, **86**, 27-45
66. Kaslow, R. A., Ryder, R. P. and Calin, A. (1979). Search for Reiter's syndrome after an outbreak of *Shigella sonnei* dysentery. *J. Rheumatol.*, **6**, 562-6
67. Lahesmaa-Rantala, R., Granfors, K., Isomaki, H. and Toivanen, A. (1987). Yersinia specific immune complexes in the synovial fluid of patients with yersinia triggered reactive arthritis. *Ann. Rheum. Dis.*, **46**, 510-14
68. Lahesmaa-Rantala, R., Granfors, K., Kekomaki, R. and Toivanen, A. (1987). Circulating yersinia specific immune complexes after acute yersiniosis: a follow up study of patients with and without reactive arthritis. *Ann. Rheum. Dis.*, **46**, 121-6
69. Grainger, R. G. and Nicol, C. S. (1959). Pelvic infection as a cause of bilateral sacroiliac arthritis and ankylosing spondylitis. *Br. J. Vener. Dis.*, **35**, 92-8
70. Szanto, E. and Hagenfeldt, K. (1979). Sacroiliitis and salpingitis: quantitative 99m Tc pertechnate scanning in the study of sacroiliitis in women. *Scand. J. Rheumatol.*, **8**, 129-35
71. Mielants, H., Veys, E. M., Cuvelier, C., Vos, M. de and Botelberghe, L. (1985). HLA-B27 related arthritis and bowel inflammation. *J. Rheumatol.*, **12**, 294-8
72. Mielants, H. and Veys, E. M. (1987). Ileocolonoscopic findings in seronegative spondylarthropathies. In Andrianakos, A., Kappou, I., Mavrikakis, M. and Moutsopoulos, H. (eds.), *Eurorheumatology* (Suppl.), pp. 52-4. (Athens: Tagas)
73. Brewerton, D. A., Caffrey, M., Hart, F. D., James, D. C. O., Nicholls, A. and Sturrock, R. D. (1973). Ankylosing spondylitis and HL-A27. *Lancet*, **1**, 904-7
74. Schlosstein, L., Terasaki, P. I., Bluestone, R. and Pearson, C. M. (1973). High association of an HL-A antigen, W27, with ankylosing spondylitis. *N. Engl. J. Med.*, **288**, 704-6
75. Arnett, F. C., Jr., Hochberg, M. C. and Bias, W. B. (1977). Cross-reactive HLA antigens in B27-negative Reiter's syndrome and sacroiliitis. *Johns Hopkins Med. J.*, **141**, 193-7
76. Schwartz, B. D., Luehrman, L. K. and Rodey, G. E. (1979). Public antigenic determinant on a family of HLA-B molecules. *J. Clin. Invest.*, **64**, 938-94
77. Ben-Chetrit, E., Brautbar, C. and Rubinow, A. (1985). HLA antigens in Reiter's syndrome in Israeli patients. *J. Rheumatol.*, **12**, 964-6
78. Caughey, D. E., Douglas, R., Wilson, W. and Hassall, I. B. (1975). HL-A antigens in Europeans and Maoris with rheumatic fever and rheumatic heart disease. *J. Rheumatol.*, **2**, 319-22
79. Robitaille, A., Cockburn, C., James, D. C. O. and Ansell, B. M. (1976). HLA frequencies in less common arthropathies. *Ann. Rheum. Dis.*, 271-3
80. Friis, J. (1975). HL-A27 in neisseria infected patients with arthritis. *Scand. J. Rheumatol.* (Suppl.), **8**, Abstr. No. 30-12
81. Calin, A., Marder, A., Marks, S. and Burns, T. (1984). Familial aggregation of Reiter's syndrome and ankylosing spondylitis: a comparative study. *J. Rheumatol.*, **11**, 672-7
82. Leirisalo, M., Skylv, G., Kousa, M., Voipio-Pulkki, L-M., Suoranta, H., Nissila, M., Hvidman, L., Nielson, E. D., Svejgaard, A., Tiilikainen, A. and Laitinen, O. (1982). Follow-up study on patients with Reiter's disease and reactive arthritis, with special reference to HLA-B27. *Arthritis Rheum.*, **25**, 249-59
83. Robinson, S., Panayi, G. S., Marshal, L. and Wolheim, F. A. (1985). Attachment of certain gram-negative bacteria to buccal epithelial cells from patients with Yersinia arthritis. In Ziff, M. and Cohen, S. B. (eds.). *Advances in Inflammation Research*. Vol. 9. pp. 217-24. (New York: Raven)
84. Maeda, K., Kono, D., Kobayashi, S., Brenner, M. B. and Yu, D. T. Y. (1984). A study of the specificity of the direct binding between bacteria and HLA antigens. *Clin. Exp. Immunol.*, **57**, 694-702
85. Ebringer, A. (1983). The cross-tolerance hypothesis, HLA-B27 and ankylosing spondylitis. *Br. J. Rheumatol.*, **22**, (Suppl. 2), 53-66
86. Seager, K., Bashir, H. V., Geczy, A. F., Edmonds, J. and Tyndall, A. (1979). Evidence for a specific B27 associated cell surface marker on lymphocytes of patients with ankylosing spondylitis. *Nature*, **277**, 68-70
87. McGuigan, L. E., Geczy, A. F. and Edmonds, J. P. (1985). The immunopathology of

ankylosing spondylitis – a review. *Semin. Arthritis, Rheum.*, **15**, 81–105
88. Cameron, F. H., Russell, P. J., Sullivan, J. and Geczy, A. F. (1983). Is a Klebsiella plasmid involved in the aetiology of ankylosing spondylitis in HLA-B27-positive individuals? *Mol. Immunol.*, **20**, 563–6
89. McGuigan, L. E., Prendergast, J. K., Geczy, A. F., Edmonds, J. P. and Bashi, H. V. (1986). Significance of non-pathogenic bowel flora in patients with ankylosing spondylitis. *Ann. Rheum. Dis.*, **45**, 566–571
90. Kinsella, T. D. (1985). Review on research on the role of Klebsiella antigens in the spondyloarthropathies. In Ziff, M. and Cohen, S. B. (eds.). *Advances in Inflammation Research*. Vol. 9, pp. 139–49. (New York: Raven)
91. Keat, A. (1986). Is spondylitis caused by Klebsiella? *Immunol. Today*, **7**, 144–9
92. Van Rood, J. J., Van Leeuwen, A., Ivanyi, P., Cats, A., Breur-Vriesendorp, B. S., Dekker-Saeys, A. J., Kijlstra, A. and Van Kregten, E. (1985). Blind confirmation of Geczy factor in ankylosing spondylitis. *Lancet*, **2**, 943–4
93. Wakefield, D., Easter, J., Robinson, P., Graham, D. and Penny, R. (1986). Chlamydial antibody cross-reactivity with peripheral blood mononuclear cells of patients with ankylosing spondylitis. *Clin. Exp. Immunol.*, **63**, 49–57
94. Inman, R. D., Chiu, B., Johnston, M. E. A. and Falk, J. (1986). Molecular mimicry in Reiter's syndrome: cytotoxicity and ELISA studies of HLA-microbial relationships. *Immunology*, **58**, 501–6
95. Kono, D. H., Ogasawara, M., Effros, R. B., Park, M. S., Waldord, R. L. and Yu, D. T. Y. (1985). Ye-1, a monoclonal antibody that cross-reacts with HLA-B27 lymphoblastoid cell lines and an arthritis causing bacteria. *Clin. Exp. Immunol.*, **61**, 503–8
96. Grumet, F. C., Calin, A., Engleman, E. G., Fish, L. and Young, S. K. H. (1985). Studies of HLA-B27 using monoclonal antibodies: ethnic- and disease-associated variants. In Ziff, M. and Cohen, S. B. (eds.). *Advances in Inflammation Research*, Vol. 9, pp. 41–53. (New York: Raven)
97. Van Bohemen, C. G., Grumet, F. C. and Zanen, H. C. (1984). Identification of HLA-B27M1 and -M2 cross-reactive antigens in Klebsiella, Shigella and Yersinia. *Immunology*, **52**, 607–10
98. Turek, P. J., Grumet, F. C. and Engleman, E. G. (1985). Molecular variants of the HLA-B27 antigen in healthy individuals and patients with spondylarthropathies. *Immunol. Rev.*, **86**, 71–91
99. Schwimmbeck, P. L., Yu, D. T. Y. and Oldstone, M. B. A. (1987). Autoantibodies to HLA B27 in the sera of HLA B27 patients with ankylosing spondylitis and Reiter's syndrome. *J. Exp. Med.*, **166**, 173–81

3
Viral Hepatitis

A. J. ZUCKERMAN

INTRODUCTION

Many viruses may infect the liver of animals and man and produce severe inflammation. In man, the general term viral hepatitis refers to infections caused by at least five different viruses, hepatitis A (infectious or epidemic hepatitis), hepatitis B (serum hepatitis), hepatitis D virus (the delta agent), non-A, non-B hepatitis, which appears to be caused by more than one virus, and an epidemic form of non-A hepatitis. Viral hepatitis is recognized as a major public health problem occurring in all parts of the world.

Acute viral hepatitis is a generalized infection with emphasis on inflammation of the liver. The clinical picture of the infection varies in its presentation from asymptomatic or subclinical infection, mild gastro-intestinal symptoms and the anicteric form of the disease, acute illness with jaundice, severe prolonged jaundice to acute fulminant hepatitis. Hepatitis B and co-infection with the delta form, and the parenterally transmitted non-A, non-B hepatitis may be associated with a persistent carrier state, and these forms of infection may progress to chronic liver disease, which may be severe. There is now compelling evidence of an aetiological association between hepatitis B virus and hepatocellular carcinoma, one of the ten most common malignant tumours worldwide. Hepatitis A, hepatitis B and hepatitis D viruses have been characterized, and these infections can now be differentiated by sensitive and specific laboratory tests. Non-A, non-B hepatitis is at present the most common form of post-transfusion hepatitis occurring in some areas and an important cause of sporadic hepatitis in adults, although virological criteria and specific laboratory tests are not yet available.

HEPATITIS A

Hepatitis A occurs endemically in all parts of the world, but the exact incidence is difficult to estimate because of the high proportion of asymptomatic and anicteric infections, differences in surveillance and differing patterns of disease. The degree of under-reporting is very high. Serological surveys have shown that while the prevalence of hepatitis A in industrialized countries is in the order of 30–50% of the population by middle age, the infection is almost universal in the less developed countries.

Incubation period

The incubation period of hepatitis A is between 3–5 weeks with a mean of 28 days. Subclinical and anicteric infections are common, and although the disease has, in general, a low mortality, adult patients may be incapacitated for many weeks. There is no evidence of persistence of the infection and progression to chronic liver damage does not occur.

Mode of spread

Hepatitis A virus (HAV) is spread by the faecal–oral route, most commonly by person to person contact, and infection is particularly common in conditions of poor sanitation and overcrowding. Common source outbreaks result most frequently from faecal contamination of drinking water and food, but waterborne transmission is not a major factor in the industrialized communities. On the other hand, many, and an increasing number, of food-borne outbreaks have been reported in developed countries. This can be attributed to the shedding of large amounts of virus in the faeces during the incubation period of the illness in infected food handlers, and the source of the outbreak can often be traced to uncooked food or food which has been handled after cooking. The consumption of raw or inadequately cooked shellfish cultivated in polluted water is associated with a high risk of hepatitis A infection. However, although hepatitis A is common in the developed countries, the infection occurs mainly in small clusters and often with only few identified cases. Hepatitis A is highly endemic in many tropical and subtropical areas with the occasional occurrence of large epidemics. This infection is common in male homosexuals. Hepatitis A is frequently acquired by travellers from areas of low to areas of high endemicity.

Outbreaks of hepatitis A have also been described among handlers of newly captured non-human primates, particularly chimpanzees and other great apes. As a general rule, hepatitis A is not transmitted by blood and blood products, and very rarely is transmitted by the parenteral route, although this has been achieved experimentally in volunteers and in susceptible non-human primates.

Age incidence

All age groups are susceptible to hepatitis A. The highest incidence in the civilian population is observed in children of school age, but in many countries in northern Europe and in North America most cases occur in adults. This shift in age incidence is similar to the change in age incidence which occurred with poliomyelitis during and after the Second World War, reflecting improvement in socio-economic and hygienic conditions. Nevertheless, as noted above, serological surveys have shown that approximately 50% of adults in the United Kingdom have antibody to hepatitis A.

Pathological changes in the liver

The constant histological features in acute viral hepatitis are parenchymal cell necrosis and histiocytic periportal inflammation. Usually the reticulin framework of the liver is well preserved except in some cases of massive and submassive necrosis. The pattern of changes in the liver is essentially similar in hepatitis types A and B and consists of marked focal activation of sinusoidal lining cells; accumulations of lymphocytes in histiocytes within the parenchyma, often replacing hepatocytes lost by necrosis; mild diffuse hepatocytic changes with occasional coagulative necrosis in the form of acidophilic bodies; and focal regeneration and portal inflammatory reaction with alteration of bile ductules. The lesions in hepatitis A develop earlier and the duration of morphological changes is shorter, while the lesions in hepatitis B linger on, fluctuate and regress slowly. There is some difference in the distribution of the lesions: in hepatitis A, the localization of parenchymal changes is predominantly periportal, whereas in hepatitis B the lesions are diffuse and tend to be accentuated around the hepatic vein tributaries, and streaks of focal necrosis may extend from portal tracts to hepatic vein tributaries.

The nature of hepatitis A virus and laboratory tests

In 1973, small cubic virus particles measuring 27 nm in diameter, were identified by immune electron microscopy in faecal extracts obtained during the early acute phase of illness of adult volunteers infected orally or by the parenteral route with the MS-1 strain of hepatitis A virus. The availability of viral antigen permitted the identification of specific antibody and the development of serological tests for hepatitis A. Human hepatitis A has been transmitted experimentally to certain species of marmosets and to chimpanzees free of hepatitis A antibody. The infection in non-human primates is mild, often subclinical and always anicteric.

Large numbers of virus particles are found during the incubation period of the infection, beginning as early as nine days after exposure, and shedding of the virus usually continues until peak elevation of serum aminotransferases. The virus is also detected during the acute phase of illness, but the number of infectious virus particles decreases rapidly after the onset of clinical jaundice. Prolonged virus excretion and a persistent carrier state have not been demonstrated. Antibody to hepatitis A virus is found in the serum during the late incubation period of the infection coinciding approximately with the onset of rising serum aminotransferase levels.

Hepatitis A virus is unenveloped containing a linear genome of single-stranded RNA with a molecular weight of 1.9×10^6, and polypeptides with similar molecular weights to the four major polypeptides of the *Enterovirus* genus within the Picornaviridae, and it has been classified as Enterovirus type 72. The virus is ether resistant, stable at pH 3.0 and relatively resistant to inactivation by heat. Hepatitis A virus is partially inactivated by heat at 56°C for 1 hour, mostly inactivated at 56°C for 10 hours and inactivated at 100°C for 5 minutes. The virus is inactivated by ultraviolet irradiation and by treatment with 1:4000 concentration of formaldehyde solution at 37°C for 72 hours. There is also evidence that hepatitis A virus is inactivated by chlorine at a concentration of 1 mg/litre for 30 minutes.

The successful propagation of hepatitis A virus in 1979 in primary monolayer and explant cell cultures and in continuous cell strains of primate origin has led to the development of live attenuated and killed hepatitis A vaccines, which are undergoing phase I clinical trials.

Specific serological tests for hepatitis A antigen and antibodies include radio-immunoassay and enzyme-linked immunosorbent assay (ELISA). Hepatitis A antibody (anti-HAV) is always demonstrable by radio-immunoassay or enzyme immunoassay during the early phase of the illness and titres increase rapidly. The antibody usually persists for many years and its presence indicates immunity. Serological diagnosis of recent infection can be established conveniently by the demonstration of hepatitis A antibody of the IgM class. Hepatitis A IgM is detectable in serum for 45–60 days after the onset of symptoms.

Control

Control of the infection is difficult. Since faecal shedding of the virus is highest during the late incubation period and prodomal phase of the illness, strict isolation of cases is not a useful control measure. Spread of hepatitis A is reduced by simple hygienic measures and the sanitary disposal of excreta.

Normal human immunoglobulin, containing at least 100 international units/ml of anti-HAV, given intramuscularly before exposure to the virus or early during the incubation period will prevent or attenuate a clinical illness. The dosage should be at least 2 i.u. of anti-HAV/kg body weight, but in special cases such as pregnancy or in patients with liver disease the dose may be doubled. Immunoglobulin does not always prevent infection and excretion of hepatitis A virus, and inapparent or subclinical hepatitis may develop. Immunoglobulin is used most commonly for close personal contacts of patients with hepatitis A and for those exposed to contaminated food. Immunoglobulin has also been used effectively for controlling outbreaks in institutions such as homes for the mentally-handicapped and in nursery schools. Prophylaxis with immunoglobulin is recommended for persons without hepatitis A antibody visiting highly endemic areas. After a period of 6 months the administration of immunoglobulin for travellers should be repeated, unless it has been demonstrated that the recipient has developed his own hepatitis A antibodies.

Live attenuated and killed hepatitis A vaccines are under clinical evaluation. Vaccines produced by recombinant DNA techniques are under development.

HEPATITIS B

The discovery, in 1965, of Australia antigen in the circulation and subsequently its association with hepatitis B led to rapid advances in the understanding of this infection.

Serological markers of hepatitis B

Infection with hepatitis B virus leads to the appearance in the plasma during the incubation period of a specific antigen, hepatitis B surface antigen (HBsAg, originally referred to as Australia antigen), about 2–8 weeks before biochemical evidence of liver damage or the onset of jaundice. The antigen persists during the acute illness, and it is usually cleared from the circulation during convalescence. Next to appear in the circulation is specific DNA polymerase associated with the core or nucleocapsid of the virus, and at about the same time another antigen, the e antigen, becomes detectable, again preceding serum aminotransferase elevations. The e antigen (HBeAg) is a distinct soluble antigen which is located within the core of the virus particle. The e antigen correlates closely with the number of virus particles, free hepatitis B DNA in the serum and the relative infectivity of the plasma or serum. Antibody to the core is found 2–4 weeks after the appearance of the surface antigen, and it is usually detectable during the early phase of the illness, persisting after recovery. The next antibody to appear in the circulation is directed against the e antigen, and there is evidence that, in general terms, anti-e (anti-HBe) indicates a relatively low infectivity of serum. Antibody to the surface antigen component, hepatitis B surface antibody (anti-HBs), is the last to appear late during convalescence. Precipitating antibodies reacting with specificities on the complete virus particle have also been described. Other antibodies include those reacting with proteins expressed by the pre-S1, pre-S2 and under certain circumstances the X region of the genome of the virus. Cell-mediated immunity is important in terminating hepatitis B infection.

Hepatitis B serological markers can now be detected by sensitive laboratory techniques, and these have proved extremely useful for unravelling the epidemiology of hepatitis B, establishing the global dissemination and public health importance of this infection.

Structure of Hepatitis B virus (HBV)

Examination of serum specimens containing hepatitis B surface antigen by electron microscopy and immune electron microscopy reveals a remarkable pleomorphism of virus-like particles consisting of small roughly spherical particles measuring about 22 nm in diameter, tubular forms of varying length but with a diameter close to 22 nm and large double-shelled particles about

42 nm in diameter. The 42 nm particle consists of a core about 28 nm in diameter with a 2 nm shell and an outer coat approximately 7 nm in thickness. The 42 nm particle is the hepatitis B virus, whereas the small particles and the tubular forms are non-infectious surplus virus coat protein (Figure 3.1).

The core of the virus (HBcAg) has a subunit structure organized according to the principles of icosahedral symmetry and an endogenous core antigen-associated DNA-dependent DNA polymerase in close association with a DNA template. Double-stranded DNA has been isolated from circulating virus and also from cores extracted from the nuclei of infected hepatocytes. The DNA consists of circular nucleic acid molecules with a mean contour

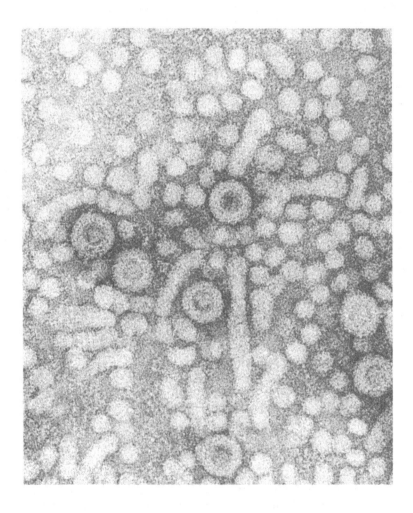

Figure 3.1 Electron micrograph showing the complex morphology of hepatitis B virus in serum: large double shelled complete virus particles, small 22 nm spherical surface antigen particles and tubular forms. × 200,000

length of $0.79 \pm 0.09\,\mu$m, with a molecular weight of about 2.3×10^6. The DNA has been characterized by gel electrophoresis and restriction enzyme cleavage, and shown to be a structure approximately 3200 nucleotides in length containing a single-stranded gap of 600–2100 nucleotides. The endogenous DNA polymerase reaction repairs the gap. The entire DNA of hepatitis B virus has been cloned in *Escherichia coli*, in yeast (*Saccharomyces cerevisiae*) and also in several strains of mammalian cells.

Mode of replication of hepatitis B virus

The inability to cultivate hepatitis B virus *in vitro*, the difficulties of obtaining suitable liver tissue, and, until recently, the lack of suitable experimental systems and techniques, hindered the investigation of the mode of replication of this virus. On the basis of studies of the duck hepatitis B virus, it has been proposed that the replication cycle of hepatitis B-like viruses is strikingly different from other DNA viruses in that RNA-directed DNA synthesis plays an essential role in the life cycle of these viruses, suggesting a close similarity to the RNA retroviruses. The principal unusual feature is the use of an RNA copy of the genome as an intermediate for the replication of the DNA genome. Infecting DNA genomes are converted to the double-stranded form, which serve as a template for transcription of RNA. Multiple RNA transcripts are then synthesized from each infecting genome, and these transcripts have either messenger function or DNA replicative function. The term pre-genomes has been used for the transcripts with DNA replicative function since these are precursors of the progeny DNA genomes, they are assembled into nucleocapsid and reverse-transcribed before coating and release from the cell. Each mature virus particle contains, therefore, a DNA copy of the RNA pre-genome and a DNA polymerase.

The pre-genome appears to be a single polyadenylated viral specific plus strand RNA of approximately one genome in length (3 kb). The first DNA to be synthesized is a minus strand, and it is initiated at a unique site on the viral genome. Very small nascent DNA minus strands, as short as 30 nucleotides in length, are covalently attached at the 5' end of the minus strand to a protein, and the protein probably serves as a primer for the synthesis of the minus strand DNA. Growth of the minus strand is accompanied by degradation of the pre-genome so that a full length single stranded DNA is produced (although hybrid DNA–RNA molecules have also been reported more recently). Plus strand DNA synthesis has been found after completion of the minus strand, and it is initiated at a unique site a few hundred nucleotides from the 5' end of the minus strand. However, complete elongation of the plus strand is not required for coating and release of the nucleocapsid cores, so that most extracellular virions contain incomplete plus strand, and a single-stranded gap in the genome. Based on this mode of replication, the ability of an infected cell to produce virus will depend on the continuous presence of a transcriptionally active form of viral DNA or 'proviral' DNA. The 'proviral' DNA must be present continuously since each pre-genomic RNA molecule can give rise to only one virus particle.

The major forms of intracellular virus-specific DNA in the livers of experimentally infected ground squirrels have been characterized. A variety of DNA structures have been found, covalently closed circular molecules, relaxed circular molecules and a heterogeneous collection of molecules associated with protein and containing minus strands in eight to ten-fold mass excess of plus strands. These results are in agreement with the analysis of intracellular forms of the duck hepatitis B virus.

The DNA replicative intermediates of hepatitis B virus present in the liver of human and chimpanzee carriers were studied in another laboratory. The viral DNA forms consisted of a full length 3.2 kb double-stranded hepatitis B viral DNA in both linear and relaxed circles, partially double-stranded DNA species of heterogeneous length and with mobility in the range of 2.8–2.0 kb, and single-stranded DNA of heterogeneous length with mobilities relative to double-stranded DNA of 1.6 kb and less, exclusively in the form of minus strand DNA. The 3.2 kb double-stranded and single-stranded DNA species are considered to be replicative intermediates since, unlike the partially double-stranded species, they are not found in hepatitis B DNA obtained from plasma. This pattern of single-stranded replicative intermediates exclusively in the form of DNA minus strands is inconsistent with a semiconservative mechanism of DNA replication and is more like the mechanism of asymmeric replication using reverse transcription of an RNA pre-genome, as described above.

Distinct hybrid DNA–RNA molecules have also been found in virus particles obtained from the plasma and liver of persistently infected patients and the liver of infected ducks. Examination of the hybrid molecules revealed the presence of viral minus strand DNA hydrogen bonded to plus strand RNA. The localization of hepatitis B viral DNA predominantly in the cytoplasm of liver cells by an *in situ* hybridization technique, and the presence in the liver of a patient with chronic active hepatitis B of mainly minus stranded viral DNA in the cytoplasm of hepatocytes using *in situ* hydridization and by Southern blot analysis are in agreement with the view of replication of the human hepatitis B virus through an RNA intermediate. Thus, the mode of replication of four of the hepadna viruses reported to date (the human hepatitis B virus, the woodchuck hepatitis B virus, the ground squirrel hepatitis virus and the duck hepatitis B virus) is remarkably similar and differs from that known for all other DNA viruses.

Hepatitis B subtypes

Careful serological analysis of the reactivities of the surface antigen has shown that the hepatitis B surface antigen particles share a common group-specific antigen *a*, and generally carry at least two mutually exclusive subdeterminants, *d* or *y* and *w* or *r*. The subtypes are the phenotypic expressions of distinct genotype variants of hepatitis B virus. Four principal phenotypes are recognized, *adw, adr, ayw* and *ayr*, but other complex permutations of these subdeterminants and new variants have been described, all apparently on the surface of the same physical particles. The major subtypes have differing geographical distribution. For example, in northern

Europe, the Americas and Australia subtype *adw* predominates. Subtype *ayw* occurs in a broad zone which includes northern and western Africa, the eastern Mediterranean, eastern Europe, northern and central Asia and the Indian subcontinent. Both *adw* and *adr* are found in Malaysia, Thailand, Indonesia and Papua New Guinea, while subtype *adr* predominates in other parts of south-east Asia including China, Japan and Pacific Islands.

Epidemiology of hepatitis B

Hepatitis B had been defined on the basis of infection occurring about 60–180 days after the injection of human blood or plasma fractions or the use of inadequately sterilized syringes and needles. The availability of specific laboratory tests for hepatitis B confirmed the importance of the parenteral routes of transmission, and infectivity appears to be especially related to blood. However, a number of factors have altered the epidemiological concepts that hepatitis B is spread exclusively by blood and blood products. These include the findings that under certain circumstances the virus is infective by mouth, that it is endemic in closed institutions and institutions for the mentally-handicapped, that is more prevalent in adults in urban communities and in poor socio-economic conditions, that there is a huge reservoir of carriers of markers of hepatitis B virus in the human population exceeding 280 million worldwide, and that the carrier rate and age distribution of the surface antigen varies in different regions.

There is much evidence for transmission of hepatitis B by intimate personal contact and by the sexual route. At very high risk are male homosexuals and others who change sexual partners frequently, for example, prostitutes. Hepatitis B surface antigen has been found repeatedly in blood and in various body fluids such as saliva, menstrual and vaginal discharges, seminal fluid and serous exudates, and these have been implicated in the spread of infection. Transmission of the infection may result from accidental inoculation of minute amounts of blood or fluids contaminated with blood such as may occur during medical, surgical and dental procedures, immunization with inadequately sterilized syringes and needles, intravenous and percutaneous drug abuse, tattooing, ear piercing and nose piercing, acupuncture, laboratory accidents and accidental inculation with razors, toothbrushes and similar objects which have been contaminated with blood.

The modes of transmission of hepatitis B in the tropics are similar to those in other parts of the world, but additional factors may be of importance. These include traditional tattooing and scarification, blood letting, ritual circumcision with unsterile instruments and perhaps as a result of repeated biting by blood-sucking arthropod vectors. Results of investigations into the role which biting insects may play in the spread of hepatitis B are conflicting. Hepatitis B surface antigen has been detected in several species of mosquitoes and in bed-bugs which have either been trapped in the wild or fed experimentally on infected blood, but no convincing evidence of replication of the virus in insects has been obtained. Mechanical transmission of the infection is a possibility, particularly as a result of interrupted feeding in high prevalence areas, but this remains unproven.

It is clear, therefore, that there are different possible ways of transmission of hepatitis B from person to person including spread by parenteral, inapparent parenteral and non-percutaneous routes. There is also evidence of clustering of hepatitis B within family groups. On the whole, the frequency of serological markers of hepatitis B in family contacts is not in accord with the hypothesis of autosomal recessive inheritance and does not reflect maternal or venereal transmission, and the mechanisms of intrafamilial spread of the infection have not been elucidated.

Transmission of hepatitis B virus from carrier mothers to their babies can occur during the perinatal period, and this is an important factor in determining the prevalence of the infection particularly in south-east Asia. The risk of infection may reach 50–60% or more, although it varies from country to country and appears to be related to ethnic groups. The risk is greatest if the mother has a history of transmission to previous children, has a high titre of hepatitis B surface antigen and/or e antigen. There is also a substantial risk of perinatal infection if the mother has acute hepatitis B in the second or third trimester of pregnancy or within 2 months after delivery. Although hepatitis B virus can infect the fetus *in utero*, this is uncommon and appears to occur in less than 5%. Most children infected during the perinatal period become persistent carriers.

The carrier state

On the basis of longitudinal studies of patients with hepatitis B, the carrier state is defined as persisitence of hepatitis B surface antigen in the circulation for more than 6 months. The carrier state, which may be lifelong, may be associated with liver damage ranging from minor changes in the nuclei of hepatocytes to chronic active hepatitis and cirrhosis. A number of risk factors have been identified in relation to the development of the carrier state. It is commonest in males, more likely to follow infections acquired in childhood than those acquired in adult life, and more likely to occur in patients with natural or acquired immune deficiencies. A carrier state becomes established in approximately 5–10% of infected adults. In countries in which hepatitis B infection is common, the highest prevalence of the surface antigen is found in children aged 4–8 years with steadily declining rates amongst older age groups. Hepatitis B e antigen has been reported to be commoner in young than in adult carriers, while the prevalence of e antibody appears to increase with age.

Survival of hepatitis B virus is ensured by the reservoir of carriers, estimated to number at least 280 million. the prevalence of carriers, particularly among blood donors in northern Europe, North America and Australia is 0.1% or less; in central and eastern Europe up to 5%, a high frequency in southern Europe, the countries bordering the Mediterranean and parts of Central and South America, and in some parts of Africa, Asia and the Pacific region as many as 20% or more of the apparently healthy population may be carriers. There is an urgent need to define the mechanisms which lead to the high carrier rate in endemic areas and to introduce methods of interruption of transmission. The management of the carrier state is a complex and vexed issue with considerable personal, social and economic implications. Guidance on the management and general recommendationss are to be found in several official reports.

The immune response

The suggestion that hepatitis B virus exerts its damaging effect on liver cells by direct cytopathic changes is inconsistent with the persistence of large quantities of the surface and core antigens in the hepatocytes of many asymptomatic and apparently healthy carriers of the surface antigen in their blood. There is, however, evidence to suggest that the pathogenesis of liver damage in the course of hepatitis B infection is related to the immune response by the host to the various structural components of the virus.

Immune complexes of surface antigen and antibody may be found in the sera of some patients during the incubation period and acute phase of hepatitis B. Immune complexes have been found in the sera of patients with fulminant hepatitis B, but only infrequently in non-fulminant infection. Immune complexes are also important in the pathogenesis of syndromes characterized by damage of blood vessels in polyarteritis nodosa, in the renal glomeruli in some forms of chronic glomerulonephritis in children and in infantile papular acrodermatitis. Surface antigen, surface antibody, core antibody and surface antigen–antibody immune complexes have been found in variable proportions of patients with virtually all the recognized chronic sequelae of acute hepatitis B. Deposits of such immune complexes have also been demonstrated in the cytoplasm and plasma membrane of hepatocytes and on or in the nuclei.

Cellular immune responses are important in determining the clinical features and course of viral infection. Cell-mediated immunity to hepatitis B antigens has been demonstrated in most patients during the acute phase of hepatitis B, and in a significant proportion of patients with surface antigen-positive chronic active hepatitis, but not in symptomless hepatitis B carriers. These observations suggest that cell-mediated immune responses may be important in terminating the infection and, under certain circumstances, in promoting liver damage and in the genesis of autoimmunity.

Evidence accumulated more recently indicates that at the time of replication of hepatitis B virus in the liver cells, the surface antigen and core antigen are expressed on the plasma membrane of infected liver cells and both cellular and immune responses are initiated. The release of large amounts of surface antigen into the circulation which follows may induce high tolerance and rapid disappearance of the immune response to this antigen. Virus particles carrying polyalbumin receptors also stimulate the formation of polymerized human serum albumin antibodies, which may prevent attachment and penetration of the virus into uninfected liver cells by reacting with the receptor on the surface of liver cells. Elimination of the virus thus depends on a combined cellular and humoral response with both receptor neutralizing polymerized human serum albumin antibodies or a similar mechanism and effective cytotoxic T-cells. Failure of either of these mechanisms would lead to chronic liver damage and viral persistence. The extent of liver damage then depends on a number of factors which include autoimmune reactions directed at native hepatocyte membrane antigens and modulation of lysis by T-cells of infected hepatocytes expressing core antigen on the surface of the cells. This would result eventually in termination of active viral replication with seroconversion to e antibody, with clinical and histological remission. On the other hand, cells with integrated viral genome do not have core antigen expressed on their surface and are protected from T-cell lysis. The destruction of hepatocytes containing integrated hepatitis B virus DNA may be dependent on an immune response to hepatitis B surface antigen, and failure of this process of elimination results in persistence of clones of cells with the potential for transformation.

Hepatocellular carcinoma

Although primary liver cancer is rare in Europe and North America, it is very common in many areas of the world including Africa and South-East Asia, and it is, therefore, among the ten most common human cancers. Review of many studies shows a highly significant excess of markers of hepatitis B infection in patients with hepatocellular carcinoma. Hepatitis B is ubiquitous in areas of the world where macronodular cirrhosis and primary liver cancer are common and where the development of the carrier state occurs most frequently. It is possible that patients with hepatocellular carcinoma are unduly susceptible to hepatitis B infection and to the development of the persistent carrier state. The question has been asked whether the infectious agent is the driver or the passenger? It has been suggested that an important factor in the aetiological association between hepatitis B infection and liver cancer may well be due to infection at an early age. Indeed, in geographical regions where the prevalence of macronodular cirrhosis and primary liver cancer is high, infection with hepatitis B virus and the carrier state occur most frequently in early life, before the defence immune mechanisms have fully developed, and asf many as 20% or more of the apparently healthy population may be carriers. It seems likely, therefore, that persistent hepatitis B infection occurs before the onset of chronic liver damage. Another possibility is that persistent infection with hepatitis B virus leads to cirrhosis and that carcinoma then arises from regenerative nodules by mechanisms in which the virus itself is not involved. However, this sequence does not explain liver cancer associated with persistent hepatitis B infection in about 20–30% of patients in the absence of cirrhosis. More recent laboratory studies have demonstrated the integration of hepatitis B viral DNA into the host chromosomal DNA molecules. In addition, several cell lines which produce hepatitis B antigen in culture have been derived from primary liver cell tumours, and at least one cell line is heterotransplantable with the production of tumours. There are several animal viruses which are phylogenetically related to human hepatitis B (the hepadnaviruses). At least two of these viruses, the woodchuck hepatitis B virus and the duck hepatitis B virus, cause primary liver cancer in their respective hosts and there are reports of hepatocellular carcinoma in infected ground squirrels. In man it is possible that liver cancer is the cumulative result of several co-factors, including genetic and hormonal factors, mycotoxins, chemical carcinogens and other environmental factors, and that hepatitis B virus acts either as a carcinogen or a co-carcinogen in persistently infected hepatocytes.

Immunization

Passive immunization

The availability of laboratory tests for hepatitis B surface antibody permitted the selection of plasma for the preparation of high titre hepatitis B immunoglobulin. Hepatitis B immunoglobulin may confer temporary passive immunity under certain defined conditions. The major indication for the administration of hepatitis B immunoglobulin is a single acute exposure to hepatitis B virus, such as occurs when blood containing surface antigen is inoculated, ingested or splashed on to mucous membranes and the conjunctiva. The optimal does has not been established, but doses in the range of 250–500 i.u. have been used effectively. It should be administered as early as possible after exposure and preferably within 48 hours, usually 3 ml (containing 200 i.u. of anti-HBs per ml) in adults. It should not be administered 7 days following exposure. It is generally recommended that two doses of hepatitis B immunoglobulin should be given 30 days apart.

Data on the use of hepatitis B immunoglobulin for prophylaxis in babies at risk of infection with hepatitis B virus are encouraging if the immunoglobulin is given as soon as possible after birth or within 12 hours of birth, and the chance of the baby developing the persistent carrier state is reduced by about 70%. More recent studies using combined passive and active immunization indicate an efficacy approaching 90%. The dose of hepatitis B immunoglobulin recommended in the newborn is 1–2 ml (200 i.u. of anti-HBs per ml).

Active immunization

Immunization against hepatitis B is required for groups which are at an increased risk of acquiring this infection. These groups include individuals requiring repeated transfusions of blood or blood products, prolonged in-patient treatment, patients who require frequent tissue penetration or need repeated access to the circulation, patients with natural or acquired immune deficiency and patients with malignant diseases. Viral hepatitis is an occupational hazard among health care personnel and the staff of institutions for the mentally-retarded and in some semi-closed institutions. High rates of infection with hepatitis B occur in narcotic drug addicts and drug abusers, homosexuals and prostitutes. Individuals working in high endemic areas are also at an increased risk of infection. Women in areas of the world where the carrier state in that group is high are another segment of the population requiring immunization in view of the increased risk of transmission of the infection to their offspring. Young infants, children and susceptible persons living in certain tropical and sub-tropical areas where present socio-economic conditions are poor and the prevalence of hepatitis B is high should also be immunized.

The repeated inability to grow hepatitis B virus in tissue culture has directed attention to the use of other preparations for active immunization. The foundation for such hepatitis B immunogens was laid by the demonstration of the relative efficacy of diluted serum containing hepatitis B virus and its antigens heated to 98°C for one minute in preventing or modifying the infection in susceptible persons.

Since hepatitis B surface antigen leads to the production of protective surface antibody, purified 22 mm spherical surface antigen particles have been developed as vaccines. These vaccines have been prepared from the plasma of symptomless carriers. Trials on protective efficacy in high-risk groups have demonstrated the value of the vaccines and their safety. There is no risk of transmission of the acquired immune deficiency syndrome (AIDS) or any other infection by vaccines derived from plasma which meet the WHO Requirements of 1981, 1983 and 1987. Local reactions reported after immunization have been minor, occurring in less than 20% of immunized individuals, and consisted of slight swelling and reddening at the site of inoculation. Temperature elevations of up to 38°C were observed in only a few individuals.

Indications for immunization against hepatitis B

The current indications for the use of hepatitis B vaccines in low prevalence areas are summarized below. The recommendations for immunization against this infection in intermediate and high prevalence regions also include the universal immunization of infants as indicated in Table 3.1.

Table 3.1 Prevalence of hepatitis B

	Northern Europe, Western Europe, Central Europe, North America	Eastern Europe, Mediterranean, USSR Central America, South America	Parts of China, South-east Asia, Tropical Africa
HBsAg	0.2–0.5%	2–7%	8–20%
Anti-HBs	4–6%	20–55%	70–95%
Neonatal infection	rare	frequent	very frequent
Childhood	infrequent	frequent	very frequent

(1) *Health care personnel in frequent contact with blood or needles*
    (a) Personnel, including teaching and training staff, directly involved over a period of time in patient care in those residential institutions for the mentally handicapped where there is a known high risk of hepatitis.
    (b) Personnel directly involved in patient care over a period of time, working in units giving treatment to patients of known high risk of hepatitis B infection.
    (c) Personnel directly involved in patient care working in haemodialysis, haemophilia and other centres regularly per-

forming maintenance treatment of patients with blood or blood products.

(d) Laboratory workers regularly exposed to increased risk from infected material.

(e) Health care personnel on secondment to work in areas of the world where there is a high prevalence of hepatitis B infection, if they are to be directly involved in patient care.

(f) Dentists and ancillary dental personnel with direct patient contact.

(2) *Patients*

(a) Patients on first entry into those residential institutions for the mentally handicapped where there is a known high incidence of hepatitis B.

(b) Patients treated by maintenance haemodialysis.

(c) Patients before major surgery who are likely to require a large number of blood transfusions and/or treatment with blood products.

(3) *Contacts of patients with hepatitis B*

(a) The spouses and other sexual contacts of patients with acute hepatitis B or carriers of hepatitis B virus, and other family members in close contact.

(4) *Other indications for immunization*

(a) Infants born to mothers who are persistent carriers of hepatitis B surface antigen (HBsAg) or who are HBsAg positive as a result of recent infection, particularly if hepatitis B *e* antigen is detectable, or HBV-positive mothers without antibody to *e* antigen (anti-*e*). The optimum timing for immunoglobulin to be given at a contralateral site is immediately at birth or within 12 hours.

(b) Health care workers who are accidentally pricked with needles used for patients with hepatitis B. The vaccine may be used alone or in combination with hepatitis B immunoglobulin as an alternative to passive immunization with hepatitis B immuno-globulin only. Studies on the efficacy of these different schedules of immunization are nearing completion.

(5) *Immediate protection*

(a) Whenever immediate protection is required, as, for example, for infants born to HBsAg-positive mothers (see 4a) or following transfer of an individual into a 'high risk' setting or after accidental inoculation, active immunization with the vaccine should be combined with the simultaneous administration of hepatitis B immunoglobulin at a different site. It has been shown that passive immunization with up to 3 ml (200 i.u. of anti-HBs per ml) of hepatitis B immunoglobulin does not interfere with an active immune response. A single dose of hepatitis B immuno-globulin (usually 3 ml for adults; 1–2 ml for the newborn) is sufficient for healthy individuals. If infection has already occurred at the time of the first immunization, virus multiplication is unlikely to be inhibited completely, but severe illness and, most importantly, the development of the carrier state of HBV may be prevented in many individuals, particularly in infants born to carrier mothers.

(6) *Immunocompromised and elderly patients*

The immune response to the current hepatitis B vaccines is poorer in immunocompromised patients and in the elderly. For example, only about 60% of patients undergoing treatment by maintenance haemodialysis develop anti-HBs. It is suggested, therefore, that patients with chronic renal damage be immunized as soon as it appears likely that they will ultimately require treatment by maintenance haemodialysis or receive renal transplant. Consideration should be given to the use of blood from healthy immunized donors with high titres of anti-HBs for the routine haemodialysis of such patients who respond poorly to immunization against hepatitis B.

(7) *Other groups at risk of hepatitis B include the following:*
   (a) Individuals who frequently change sexual partners, particularly promiscuous male homosexuals and prostitutes.
   (b) Narcotic and intravenous drug abusers.
   (c) Staff at reception centres for refugees, and immigrants from areas of the world where hepatitis B is very common, such as south-east Asia.
   (d) Although they are at 'lower risk', consideration should also be given to longterm prisoners and staff of custodial institutions, ambulance and rescue services and selected police personnel.
   (e) Military personnel are included in some countries.

Vaccines

Polypeptide vaccines

Hepatitis B polypeptide vaccines containing specific hepatitis B antigenic determinants of the major non-glycosylated peptide I of the surface antigen with a molecular weight of 22–24000 and its glycosylated form, a polypeptide with a molecular weight in the range of 22–24000 have been prepared. The individual polypeptides of the surface antigen are immunogenic, and the purified 25000 (designated as p25) and 30000 (p30) molecular weight polypeptides are effective antigens. The subunit polypeptide vaccines have been tested for safety, immunogenicity and protective efficacy in susceptible chimpanzees.

Polypeptides in monomeric solution in detergent are not a suitable form of vaccine. Consequently, a method of detergent removal which allows membrane polypeptides to reassociate into water-soluble protein micelles has been developed. Protein micelles are aggregates of polypeptides arranged so that hydrophobic regions are sequestered in the interior of the particles with the hydrophilic residues on the surface so that the resulting particulate forms are water soluble. Comparison of the immunogenicity of hepatitis B micelles with the 22 nm particle vaccine in a mouse potency assay showed that the micelles elicited a more vigorous protective surface antibody response than the intact 22 nm spherical antigen particles at all dose levels tested. Clinical trials of the polypeptide micelle vaccine are in progress.

Production of hepatitis B vaccines by r-DNA techniques

Recombinant DNA techniques have been used for expressing hepatitis B surface antigen and core antigen in prokaryotic cells (*Escherichia coli* and *Bacillus subtilis*) and in eukaryotic cells, such as mutant mouse LM cells, HeLa cells, COS cells, CHO cells and yeast cells (*Saccharomyces cerevisiae*).

Recombinant yeast hepatitis B vaccines have undergone extensive evaluation by clinical trials. The results to date indicate that this vaccine is safe, antigenic and free from side-effects (apart from minor local reactions in a proportion of recipients). The immunogenicity, using a dose of 10 μg/ml as compared with 20 μg/ml of the plasma-derived vaccine, is similar to that of the plasma vaccine. The recombinant yeast hepatitis B vaccine has now been licenced for use in many countries.

Hybrid virus vaccines

Potential live vaccines using recombinant vaccinia viruses have been constructed for hepatitis B, and also for herpes simplex, rabies and other viruses. Foreign viral DNA is introduced into the vaccinia DNA by construction of chimaeric genes. This is accomplished by homologous recombination in cells since the large size of the genome of vaccinia virus (185 000 base pairs) precludes *in vitro* gene insertion. A chimaeric gene consisting of vaccinia virus promoter sequences ligated to the coding sequence for the desired foreign protein is flanked by vaccinia virus DNA in a plasmid vector. The hepatitis B surface antigen made by vaccinia virus recombinants was similar or identical in its polypeptide composition, buoyant density, sedimentation rate and antigenicity to material obtained from the plasma of hepatitis B carriers.

The recloned vaccinia virus containing hepatitis B surface antigen coding sequences was used to vaccinate rabbits with the production of typical vaccinia lesions in the skin and high titres of hepatitis B surface antibody in the circulation. Preliminary studies in chimpanzees indicated the feasibility of using a recombinant vaccinia virus. The vaccinated chimpanzees had a secondary antibody reponse when challenged intravenously with live hepatitis B virus of a heterologous subtype, with a mild inapparent infection characterized by seroconversion to surface antibody and hepatitis B anti-core. Although the chimpanzees had little or no circulating surface antibody after vaccination when the recombinant vaccinia was growing in the skin they were immunologically 'primed'. As a result the chimpanzees had a brisk and sustained antibody response, presumably due to newly synthesized surface

67

antigen after challenge with live hepatitis B virus. IgG surface antibody and the anti-*a* responses were detected early, which is consistent with the anamnestic nature of the response.

At present, however, there is no accepted laboratory marker of attenuation or of virulence of vaccinia virus for man, either in the host directly inoculated with the virus or after several passages in the same species. Alterations in the genome of vaccinia virus which are concomitant with the selection of recombinants may alter the virulence of the virus. It has been noted, however, that interruption of the thymidine kinase gene of the virus by insertion of foreign DNA reduced its virulence for mice. Nevertheless, changes in host range or tissue tropism of vaccinia viruses may occur as a result of their genetic modification and these could be caused by changes in the virus envelope as a result of the incorporation of gene products of the foreign viral genes inserted into the vaccinia virus. The advantages of vaccinia virus recombinant as a vaccine include low cost, ease of administration by multiple pressure or by the scratch technique, vaccine stability, long shelf-life, and the possible use of polyvalent antigens. The known adverse reactions with vaccinia virus vaccines are well documented, and their incidence and severity must be carefully weighed against the adverse reactions associated with existing vaccines which a new recombinant vaccine might replace. There are also reports of a spread of current strains of vaccinia virus to contacts, and this may present difficulties. Other recombinant viruses as vectors are being explored, and in particular the oral adenovirus vaccines which have been in use for some 20 years.

Chemically synthesized hepatitis B vaccines

The development of chemically synthesized polypeptide vaccines offers many advantages in attaining the ultimate goal of producing chemically uniform, safe and cheap viral immunogens to replace many current vaccines which often contain large quantities of irrelevant microbial antigenic determinants, proteins and other material additional to the essential immunogen required for the induction of a protective antibody. The preparation of antibodies against viral proteins using fragments of chemically synthesized peptides mimicking viral amino acid sequences is now a possible and attractive alternative approach in immunoprophylaxis.

Successful mimicking of determinants of HBsAg using chemically synthesized peptides in linear and cyclical forms has been reported by several groups of investigators. Peptides have been synthesized which retain biological function and appropriate secondary structure, even though they have a limited sequence homology with the natural peptide or are much smaller. Various other studies also confirm that selected peptides corresponding to relevant epitopes of hepatitis B surface antigen may be useful as synthetic vaccines in the foreseeable future.

HEPATITIS D VIRUS (THE DELTA AGENT)

Delta antigen was initially detected as nuclear immunofluorescence in liver cells of patients with chronic hepatitis B. It is now known to be a defective, transmissible virus which requires multiplication of hepatitis B virus for its own replication. The agent is unique among human viruses, and consists of a particle measuring 35-37 nm in diameter, with the internal component containing the delta antigen surrounded by an outer protein coat of hepatitis B surface antigen. The genome of this virus is very small, consisting of a single stranded circular RNA with a molecular weight of about 500000.

Serological studies indicate a worldwide distribution of hepatitis D in association with hepatitis B virus. The infection is epidemiologically important in Italy, the Middle East (the Gulf States and Saudi Arabia), parts of Africa and South America. Epidemics with high mortality have been described in South America in association with hepatitis B. Delta infection is associated with acute and chronic hepatitis, always in the presence of hepatitis B, and superinfection in a carrier of hepatitis B virus often leads to exacerbation of severe hepatitis.

The mode of transmission of hepatitis D is similar to the parenteral spread of hepatitis B, so that serological evidence of infection is found most frequently in western Europe and North America in multiply-transfused individuals such as patients with haemophilia and in drug addicts. Non-percutaneous spread probably also occurs.

NON-A, NON-B HEPATITIS

The specific laboratory diagnosis of hepatitis A and hepatitis B has revealed a previously unrecognized form of viral hepatitis which is clearly unrelated to either type and which is referred to as non-A, non-B hepatitis. It is now the most common form of hepatitis occurring after blood transfusion and the infusion of certain plasma derivatives, particularly clotting factors, in some areas of the world. The infection has also been transmitted experimentally to chimpanzees. Although specific laboratory tests for identifying this new type of hepatitis are not yet available and the diagnosis can only be made by exclusion, there is considerable information on the epidemiology and some of the clinical features of this infection.

Non-A, non-B hepatitis has been found in every country in which it has been sought, and it shares a number of features with hepatitis B. This form of hepatitis has been most commonly recognized as a complication of blood transfusion, and in countries where all blood donations are screened for hepatitis B surface antigen by very sensitive techniques non-A, non-B hepatitis may account for as many as 90% of all cases of post-transfusion hepatitis. Outbreaks of non-A, non-B hepatitis have also been reported after the administration of blood-clotting factors VIII and IX. Non-A, non-B hepatitis has occurred in haemodialysis and other specialized units, among drug addicts and after accidental inoculation with contaminated needles and other sharp objects. In several countries a significant number of cases are not associated with transfusion, and such sporadic cases of non-A, non-B hepatitis account for 10-25% of all adult patients with recognized viral hepatitis. The route of infection or the source of infection cannot be identified in many of these patients. Males predominate as is the case with hepatitis B. Differences from the epidemiology of hepatitis B include a lack of evidence of transmission of non-A, non-B hepatitis in the family setting, and no evidence of transmission by sexual contact either heterosexual or homosexual, has been found.

Although in general the illness is mild and often subclinical or anicteric, severe hepatitis with jaundice does occur, and the infection is a significant cause of fulminant hepatitis. There is considerable evidence that the infection may be followed in many patients, and in experimentally infected chimpanzees, by prolonged viraemia and the development of a persistent carrier state. Studies of the histopathological sequelae of acute non-A, non-B hepatitis infection revealed that chronic liver damage, which may be severe, may occur in as many as 40–50% of the patients.

Clinical, epidemiological and experimental studies in several laboratories indicate that non-A, non-B hepatitis may be caused by two and possibly more than two infectious agents. Clinical evidence is based on the observation of multiple attacks of hepatitis in individual patients. Epidemiologically, short-incubation and long-incubation forms of non-A, non-B hepatitis have been described. The incubation period, however, does not appear to be a reliable index for differentiating between the two non-A, non-B types of hepatitis, and it is likely that differences in the incubation period represent differences in the infective dose. Experimental evidence for the existence of at least two distinct non-A, non-B hepatitis viruses has been obtained from recent cross-challenge experimental transmission studies in chimpanzees, but final confirmation must await the development of specific laboratory tests for non-A, non-B hepatitis and the identification and characterization of the virus(es).

EPIDEMIC NON-A HEPATITIS

Epidemic hepatitis which resembles hepatitis A, but which is serologically distinct from hepatitis A, has been reported from the sub-continent of India, central and south-east Asia, the Middle East and North Africa, Mexico and in returning travellers from these regions. The infection is acute, self-limiting and occurs predominantly in young adults. The incubation period is 30–40 days. It is more severe in pregnant women in whom it is associated with high mortality, especially during the last trimester of pregnancy. The infection is spread by the ingestion of contaminated water and probably by food, but secondary cases appear to be uncommon.

There is evidence that the virus resembles morphologically (but not serologically) hepatitis A virus, measuring approximately 27 nm in diameter. It is not transmissible to chimpanzees, unlike hepatitis A, but the infection can be transmitted experimentally to macaques. The virus is currently being characterized by its physicochemical properties. Serological tests are not yet available.

Bibliography

World-wide there have been in excess of 20000 papers published on viral hepatitis during the last decade. For example, in 1980–81 over 5000 papers were published in the English language alone. A few general references are, therefore, given below which will introduce the reader to this vast field.

World Health Organization Technical Report Series on Viral Hepatitis. (1977). No 512 (1973), No 570 (1975), No 602. (Geneva: WHO)

Zuckerman, A. J. (ed.). (1986). *Viral Hepatitis. Clinics in Tropical Medicine and Communicable Diseases.* pp. 1–461. (London: W. B. Saunders and Co)

Zuckerman, A. J. (1980). *A Decade of Viral Hepatitis. Abstracts 1969–1979.* pp. 1–501. (Amsterdam: Elsevier/North Holland)

Zuckerman, A. J. (ed.). (1988). *Viral Hepatitis and Liver Disease.* (NY: Alan R. Liss, Inc.) pp. 1–1136.

4
The Immunopathogenesis of AIDS

J. M. PARKIN AND A. J. PINCHING

INTRODUCTION

In 1981, a handful of cases of an apparently new acquired immune deficiency syndrome were reported to the Centers for Disease Control in Atlanta[1,2]. At that time it was assumed that the profound immune suppression was somehow related to aspects of the life-style of the affected individuals, as all the cases were in homosexual or bisexual men. Many theories were expounded on the immunodepressant effects of drugs, rectal exposure to allogeneic cells in semen, or sexually transmitted infections. However, as time went by, it became apparent that the disease was not confined to the group of individuals in whom it was first recognized, but was also occurring in haemophiliacs, recipients of blood transfusions, intravenous drug abusers and the sexual partners and children born to these groups. Intriguingly, inhabitants of Haiti and some central African countries also appeared to be at risk. The epidemiological pattern of infection was highly suggestive of a blood borne and sexually transmitted pathogen, and in 1983 the aetiological agent of AIDS – a novel human retrovirus Human Immunodeficiency Virus type 1 (HIV-1) was isolated[3,4]. As a direct result of intensive scientific and clinical research in conjunction with detailed epidemiological studies, our knowledge of the Acquired Immune Deficiency Syndrome (AIDS) and its causative virus, has advanced at a rate only rarely observed in other diseases which have affected man for a much greater length of time. This reflects the urgency felt as epidemiological studies revealed the rapid rate of transmission through the homosexual and drug abusing populations, and more recently the realization of the extent of disease and potential social and economic catastrophe of HIV infection in Central and East Africa. It has been said that we are fortunate that AIDS did not emerge earlier, as it is only the advances made in the last 15–20 years in techniques of viral culture and molecular biology, that have enabled us to identify, sequence and begin to genetically engineer prototype vaccines for HIV. Advances in the understanding of the immune system, particularly the cell-mediated response, have also been essential to determine not only the immunological defects of likely importance in HIV infection and, therefore, to approach immunological stimulation or reconstitution in a logical fashion, but also to study the ways in which the host's immune system controls HIV infection – information which is vital to the development of appropriate vaccination regimes.

AN OVERVIEW OF THE IMMUNOLOGICAL MANIFESTATIONS OF HIV INFECTION

The effects of HIV infection vary from asymptomatic carriage or relatively benign disorders such as persistent generalized lymphadenopathy[5], to the severe immune deficiency state of AIDS. Progressive neurological deterioration – the AIDS–dementia complex is thought to be a direct effect of HIV on cells of the nervous system[6,7], and although seen predominantly in patients with full-blown AIDS it may also occur in individuals with only minimal signs of immune deficiency. It is not yet clear what proportion of those infected will ultimately develop disease associated with HIV. Cohort studies in the USA and Europe show that the progression rate to AIDS, in asymptomatic seropositive groups is broadly 15–30% at 3 years[8-10]. However, as yet it appears that the rate of development of AIDS in these cohorts is not declining with time and that the eventual toll of disease will inevitably be higher than that reported to date. The effect of co-factors may partly explain the varying progression rates observed in different groups. Sexually transmitted disease, genital ulceration and pregnancy[11,12] have been shown to increase susceptibility to infection with HIV and/or disease progression. Genetic factors may also influence the clinical manifestations of HIV infection. Our own group has recently demonstrated a link between group-specific component phenotype and susceptibility to disease[13], although, as yet, this has not been confirmed by other investigators. Histocompatability antigen type also appears to be relevant, and early studies demonstrated an association between the possession of HLA-DR5 and the development of Kaposi's sarcoma. The association appeared to be limited to people of Mediterranean or Jewish origin[14]. More recently a link has been documented between the possession of HLA-B35 and progression to AIDS in patients with PGL.[15]

Laboratory tests have highlighted numerous defects of immune function in patients with AIDS (Table 4.1) but ultimately the relevance of these abnormalities can only be assessed in the context of the patient, in particular the response to potential pathogens both endogenous and environmental.

The clinical pattern of opportunist infections and tumours observed in patients with AIDS in the UK (Table 4.2) reflects the profound defect in cell-mediated immunity, and is reminiscent of that previously reported in patients with iatrogenic or tumour-related cellular immunosuppression, such as organ transplant recipients, those on immunosuppressant therapy for autoimmune disease, or patients with Hodgkin's lymphoma. Infections are predominantly caused by organisms that persist within cells, and which require an intact T-cell/macrophage response for eradication or maintenance of latency.

Table 4.1 Immunologic abnormalities in AIDS

I *Abnormalities that characterize the syndrome:*
    (a) Lymphopenia
    (b) Selective deficiency in CD4+ T-lymphocytes
    (c) Decreased or absent delayed cutaneous hypersensitivity to recall and new
        antigens
    (d) Elevated serum immunoglobulins, predominantly IgG and IgA in adults and
        IgM in children
    (e) Increased spontaneous immunoglobulin secretion by individual B lymphocytes

II *Consistently observed abnormalities:*
    (a) Decreased *in vitro* lymphocyte proliferative responses
        – mitogens
        – antigens
        – alloantigens; autoantigens
    (b) Decreased cytotoxic responses
        – natural killer cells
        – cell-mediated cytotoxicity (T-cell)
    (c) Decreased ability to mount a *de novo* antibody response to a new antigen
    (d) Altered monocyte/macrophage function
    (e) Elevated serum levels of immune complexes

III *Other reported abnormalities:*
    (a) Increased levels of acid-labile α-interferon
    (b) Anti-lymphocyte antibodies
    (c) Suppressor factors
    (d) Increased levels of β-$_2$ microglobulin and α-$_1$ thymosin; decreased serum thymulin
        levels

From Seligman M, Chess L, Fahey J L *et al.*[100]

Table 4.2 Opportunist infections and tumours of AIDS in the UK

Viral	**Protozoal**
Herpes simplex	*Pneumocystis carinii*
Cytomegalovirus	*Toxoplasma gondii*
Varicella zoster	*Cryptosporidium* spp.
Polyoma virus (JC/BK)	*Isospora* spp.
Bacterial:	**Neoplastic**
Salmonella typhimurium	Kaposi's sarcoma
Mycobacterium tuberculosis	Non-Hodgkin's lymphoma
M. avium-intracellulare complex	
Fungal	
Candida albicans	
Cryptococcus neoformis	
Tinea spp.	
Histoplasma capsulatum	

From Weber, J and Pinching, A[133]

In the following sections, the immunological abnormalities in AIDS and HIV infection, which are the background to the clinical manifestations, will be discussed, and the postulated mechanisms of these defects elucidated. Some of the investigations mentioned, for example phenotypic T-cell subsets and lymphocyte mitogen proliferation, are available in centres caring for AIDS patients. However, it has to be emphasized that in many cases clinical examination will detect signs of immune deficiency before there is any change in laboratory tests, and that many of the investigations described detect non-specific abnormalities which may be found in many other unrelated infections or disease states. Individuals at risk of HIV infection, such as homo/bisexual men and haemophiliacs, often have alterations in immune function without evidence of HIV infection[16,17]. The reasons for this are not known but may be related to the intercurrent infections, effects of drugs[18], and/or allogeneic stimulation by blood products in haemophiliacs or by semen during rectal exposure. Such immunological 'noise' has, therefore, to be taken into account in the interpretation of laboratory results. Indeed the investigation of patients with AIDS highlighted the limitations of the existing immunological techniques and necessitated the development of more sensitive methods to dissect the immune deficiency, monitor its natural history and follow the effects of potential therapeutic agents.

PATHOGENESIS OF HIV-INDUCED IMMUNE DEFICIENCY

To date, two strains of HIV have been isolated and sequenced. The first, HIV-1, is present in the majority of cases of AIDS in the United States, Europe and Central Africa. A second virus, HIV-2, has recently been isolated from asymptomatic individuals and patients with AIDS in West Africa, notably Guinea Bissau, Cape Verde and Senegal[19,20], and from a few documented cases in Europe[21]. This virus has approximately 43% gene homology with HIV-1 with most of the variation being in parts of the envelope region[22], antibodies to HIV-2 are, therefore, not reliably detected in the original commercially available ELISA tests. However, advances in antibody detection by ELISA using recombinant core and envelope proteins of HIV-1 and HIV-2 and 'site-directed' serology, has led to the development of assays to detect both viruses. Infection with one type of HIV does not necessarily give protection from the other, and dual infection with HIV-1 and HIV-2 is documented[23]. At present most of the work on viral pathogenicity has been performed using HIV-1, and although epidemiological data suggest that HIV-2 may have lower pathogenicity this has not yet been demonstrated by *in vitro* systems.

MECHANISMS OF CELLULAR INFECTION BY HUMAN IMMUNODEFICIENCY VIRUSES

HIV has been shown to infect only cells bearing the CD4 antigen to which it binds through its gp120 envelope protein[24]. There is substantial evidence that the CD4 molecule acts as the major cellular receptor for HIV[25,26].

Monoclonal antibodies to specific epitopes of CD4 have been shown to completely inhibit HIV infection and insertion of the CD4 gene into cells which do not constitutively express the molecule and are normally uninfectable by HIV, leads to them becoming permissive to infection[27]. However, transfection of CD4 only confers infectability in human cell lines. In a mouse model transfection and expression of the human CD4 molecule on the cell surface, induces the ability to bind virus but infection does not occur. This suggests that another molecule is required for the internalization process. Candidates are HLA-DR and Leu 8, as monoclonal antibodies to both of these antigens partially inhibit viral infection *in vitro*. However, this effect could also be a result of steric hindrance by the antibodies on viral binding to CD4, as Leu 8 and HLA-DR antigens may be closely associated with this molecule. Internalization of the virus is thought to take place by a pH independent fusion of the cell membrane and viral envelope[28]. In contrast to the binding which is dependent on the gp120 protein, fusion appears to be mediated by the transmembrane protein gp41, as HIV mutants lacking only this protein are able to bind to CD4+ cells but cannot be internalized[29]. On entering the cell the virus uncoats and releases a preformed DNA polymerase. This enzyme is named reverse transcriptase as it induces the formation of a DNA copy of the RNA genetic material of HIV (usually, transcription involving a RNA copy of DNA). The DNA provirus is then integrated into the host chromosome, initiates synthesis of virally encoded proteins and eventually new virions which then bud through the cell membrane[30]. The reverse transcriptase is, therefore, essential for viral replication, and inhibitors, for example azidothymidine (Zidovudine) or dideoxycytidine, can be used therapeutically as anti-viral agents[31,32].

Cells bearing the CD4 molecule and, therefore, susceptible to infection with HIV include 'helper' lymphocytes, monocytes, macrophages, EBV transformed B-cells and glial cells. All these cells types can be infected *in vitro*. Virus infection has been demonstrated *in vivo* in CD4+ lymphocytes, blood monocytes, tissue macrophages and dendritic cells[33-38]. It is of interest that viruses cultured from different cell types tend to have varying cell tropisms and cytopathic effects. For instance HIV isolated from lymphocytes infects and replicates well within lymphocyte lines but poorly in those derived from monocytes and *vice versa*[39,40]. It is not known whether this represents mutations of a single virus within the infected host or re-infection of the individual patient with several different HIV strains with varying tropisms. However, it is possible that the development of AIDS is caused by the emergence of a more pathogenic variant within the infected individual.

Cellular infection with HIV is associated with both quantitative and qualitative defects. One of the characteristic findings in patients with AIDS is the depletion of CD4+ T-lymphocytes which generally becomes more pronounced as the disease progresses. Several mechanisms have been suggested for this selective loss. *In vitro* infection of peripheral blood lymphocytes or cell lines with HIV, leads to the formation of multinucleated giant cells due to cell fusion and eventually to cell lysis[41,42]. Both these processes depend on the expression of the CD4 molecule[43,44]. In the case of cell fusion, it is possible that the viral envelope proteins, expressed on the cell surface and bearing the CD4 receptor site, bind the infected cell to other CD4+ cells even if uninfected[45]. The extent to which this mechanism operates *in vivo* is uncertain. Experimentally, syncytia formation in lymphocyte lines is a transient phenomenon which is not necessary for lysis[46], and lymphocyte-derived giant cells are rarely demonstrated *in vivo*. Conversely, multi-nucleated HIV infected cells, probably of macrophage origin, have been found in the brains of infected patients[47]. Other potential mechanisms of HIV-induced lysis have been proposed. Intracellular envelope proteins bind CD4 within the cytoplasm of the infected cell or at the cell membrane, and as the virus replicates this complexing may eventually become so great as to cause defects in membrane stability or fluidity. This may explain why cells expressing low levels of CD4, such as monocytes, are relatively resistant to lysis, despite productive infection. Indeed these cells may be important reservoirs of HIV, becoming infected early in the course of disease and continually releasing virus which can then infect other cells[38,48]. It is also possible that the host's immune response to HIV contributes to the development of immune deficiency as CD4 lymphopenia could be a consequence of destruction of infected helper lymphocytes by HIV specific cytotoxic T-cells. Such cells have been demonstrated *in vivo*, and could lyse HIV infected CD4+ targets which are expressing viral proteins on their surface. Alternatively, even uninfected CD4+ cells could be killed, as viral envelope proteins may adhere (without true infection) to the surface CD4 protein, including cytotoxic T-cell mediated lysis as a 'bystander' effect[49]. Whether the humoral response plays any role in the destruction of HIV-infected cells is not known, but HIV-specific antibodies to the core and particularly to the envelope may mediate antibody dependent cytotoxicity by binding to Fc receptors on antibody dependent cytotoxic cells. An antibody has also been described to an 18 kD protein which is present only on activated and HIV infected CD4+ cells. The antibody lyses these cells in the presence of complement[50]. This antibody has, to date, been found only in patients with AIDS and AIDS-related complex and not in asymptomatic patients or those with lymphadenopathy alone. Its relevance is unclear.

Infection of lymphocytes by HIV and their subsequent lysis is not only dependent on the presence of the CD4 receptor, but also on the lymphocytes being in an activated state[43]. *In vitro* this is accomplished by mitogen or antigen stimulation, techniques which have been used for virus isolation. This is likely to be important *in vivo* as lymphocyte activation in response to antigenic or allogeneic stimuli, such as during infections, pregnancy or exposure to blood products, could lead to enhanced viral replication and disease progression. This may account for the acute deterioration observed in previously asymptomatic women who become pregnant, or the increased susceptibility to HIV infection and disease progression associated with sexually transmitted disease[11]. Infectious agents may also activate HIV by other mechanisms, for example exposure to Herpes simplex virus in culture, directly upregulates the transcription of the HIV genome[51].

In addition to the depletion described above, functional defects induced by HIV infection are also likely to contribute to the immune deficiency of AIDS. Abnormalities may be caused by insertion of the viral genome at an important site in the host chromosome or the preferential transcription of viral over host DNA, with switching of the hosts' cells to produce viral proteins. The viral proteins, in turn, may interfere with cell function. Infection with HIV leads to decreased expression of the CD4 molecule due to intracellular complexing with the viral envelope[52]. As the CD4 molecule is essential for the interaction of helper lymphocytes with other cells, its loss would inevitably lead to abnormal function. Extracellular viral particles or viral products may also be intrinsically immunosuppressive, as has been shown in animal retroviral disease. In the case of HIV, incubation of the virus with normal B-lymphocytes leads to polyclonal activation and immuno-globulin production without cellular infection, which may explain the characteristic hypergammaglobulinaemia of AIDS[53].

Therefore, the primary immunological defects are likely to be a combination of the direct effects of HIV on infectable cells leading to their destruction or functional impairment and the effect of immunosuppressive viral products on uninfected cells. The close inter-relationship of the various cells within the system mean that abnormalities in one cell type will affect other cells, resulting in the loss of regulator/stimulator cell function.

IMMUNOLOGICAL ASPECTS OF CLINICAL MANIFESTATIONS OF AIDS

In adults with AIDS, the opportunist infections and tumours observed reflect the predominantly cell-mediated immune deficiency. As mentioned earlier in the chapter, the infecting organisms are those which persist intracellularly and are controlled in the immunocompetent host by the T-cell/macrophage response. From the preceeding section, it will be seen that HIV infection may abrogate this response and allow the development of a variety of infections. The common infecting organisms are the herpes viruses; HSV, VZV and CMV, yeasts such as candida and cryptococcus and protozoa, e.g. *Toxoplasma gondii, Pneumocystis carinii*, Isospora and cryptosporidia. Bacterial infections are much less common as these organisms are predominantly extracellular and controlled by the humoral response, which is generally better maintained. Exceptions are intracellular or facultative intracellular bacteria such as the *Mycobacteria* and *Salmonella* species.

In infants with AIDS the clinical picture differs as the B-cell system is immature and requires a functioning T-cell system for the development of antibody responses. Infection in early life with HIV, prevents the B-cell response from occurring. Therefore, children commonly suffer life-threatening bacterial infections particularly with encapsulated organisms such as staphylococci, pneumococci and *Haemophilus* species. Replacement therapy with intravenous immunoglobulin markedly decreases mortality from bacterial infections in this group, but has no apparent effect on the development of cellular immune defects[54].

The type of infection observed tends to change with disease progression. Early signs of immune deficiency are characterized by atypically severe infections with agents that may cause disease in immunocompetent individuals. Examples would be chronic, ulcerative herpes simplex infection requiring anti-viral therapy for control, relapsing when treatment is discontinued, the development of multi-dermatomal varicella zoster, oral candidiasis or the provocation of extensive oral or oesophageal candida infection by even short courses of antibiotics. Such findings are not diagnostic, but are poor prognostic signs in patients with HIV infection and may herald the eventual development of full-blown AIDS with a more severe opportunist infection. Tuberculosis may also behave in an 'opportunistic' fashion in individuals with HIV infection[55], causing rapidly disseminated disease often in previously fit well-nourished individuals. It has been observed that if tuberculosis is going to develop it tends to occur at an early stage of immune deficiency. This suggests that disease is due to the reactivation of an old infection. *Mycobacterium tuberculosis* is a relatively high grade pathogen and would, therefore, be expected to cause relapse when there is only a minor immune deficiency. If the tuberculosis was a new infection, as appears to be the case with disease caused by the atypical mycobacteria, it is likely that tuberculosis would appear at all stages of AIDS. Another indicator of immune deficiency is the endothelial cell neoplasm, Kaposi's sarcoma, which in the context of iatrogenic immunosuppression has been shown to correlate directly with the level of immunodeficiency, i.e. cessation of treatment can lead to regression of lesions. Patients with Kaposi's sarcoma alone without any opportunistic infections, have a relatively good prognosis, with approximately 80% surviving 2 years. In contrast, of those presenting with opportunist infections, such as *Pneumocystis carinii* pneumonia, less than 20% will survive that time. The likely explanation is that Kaposi's sarcoma commonly manifests at an early stage of immune deficiency. As the disease and immune deficiency progress, the pattern of infections changes, with usually non-pathogenic organisms such as *Pneumocystis carinii* causing overwhelming infection. Disseminated atypical mycobacterial infection and cryptosporidiosis commonly develop during the late stages of AIDS, when little immune function remains. Multiple infections are also common at all sites, although treatment of one may lead to regression of the other, perhaps by the eradication of the immunosuppressant effect of the opportunist infection concerned (personal observations). As the majority of infections are either with organisms endogenous to the host or ubiquitous in the environment, it is impossible to remove the risk of infection. However, early diagnosis and the judicious use of prophylactic agents can prolong the interval between infective episodes. The lack of appropriate immune and inflammatory responses means that the normal clinical symptoms and signs of disease may be altered or even absent in this group of patients. *Pneumocystis carinii* pneumonia may present with severe impairment of respiratory function which is in stark contrast to the minimal physical and radiological findings. Similarly, cryptococcal meningitis is commonly found in the absence of meningism or photophobia and with a lack of a cellular response in the cerebrospinal fluid. Interpretation of histological findings may also be difficult, a granulomatous response can be absent or poorly formed despite the presence of numerous mycobacteria[56]. Serological diagnosis cannot be used to detect acute infections such as CMV or toxoplasmosis.

Polyclonal B-cell activation and the inability to respond to neoantigens means that there may be a high level of specific antibody to antigens encountered a long time ago, with no IgM response or rise in antibody titre to new infecting organisms. Antibody levels, therefore, can only be used to determine past exposure to a particular organism. This may be clinically helpful in some infections such as cerebral toxoplasmosis where disease is caused by reactivation rather than re-infection, occurring almost exclusively in previously seropositive individuals. Generally, it is unwise to rely on the immune response for diagnosing infection in severely immunosuppressed patients. In most cases a tissue diagnosis by aspiration, lavage or biopsy is by far the most appropriate investigation. As many of the infections are reactivations of infections acquired in the past it is, therefore, important to take particular note of previous illnesses, and travel. The illnesses the patient develops when immunosuppressed may reflect the microbiological environment of a previous country of residence, for example the relatively common occurrence of histoplasmosis in patients from the USA.

At first sight some of the abnormalities observed in individuals with HIV infection appear incongruous. In addition to the severe immunosuppression, there are features of immune hyperactivity, manifested by the common occurrence of allergic reactions, hypergammaglobulinaemia and the presence of autoantibodies. Diseases, such as psoriasis and Reiter's syndrome which are considered to be immunologically mediated, surprisingly become more severe with HIV-related disease[57,58]. This combination of altered immune response could follow the loss of a central regulating cell, such as the CD4+ helper – lymphocyte. This would not only lead to an inability to mount and amplify an immune response, but also to impaired suppression of immune responses that are usually controlled by T-helper induced 'suppressor' T-cells. Alternatively, the hyperactivity may result from the action of HIV itself or opportunist organisms on the cells involved.

It has been noted that immunological and often neurological status may decline during episodes of opportunist infection. This may be secondary to increased HIV replication associated with lymphocyte activation in response to infection, or to direct immunosuppressive effects of the opportunist infections such as cytomegalovirus, Epstein–Barr virus and *M. tuberculosis*. These may depress the limited control that the host's immune system has over HIV and encourage further viral multiplication to occur. Similarly, when patients with HIV infection and minor immune deficiency are placed on prolonged or high dose corticosteroids there may be rapid development of opportunistic infection and failure to recover the previous immune status, even after successful treatment of the infection and cessation of steroid therapy. The relationship between HIV and the immune system is complex. In the initial stages of HIV infection the immune system appears dominant in mounting both a cellular and humoral response to the infecting agent, and is apparently able to control the replication and potential damage caused by the virus for variable lengths of time, perhaps in some cases indefinitely. However, in time, and perhaps because of the continual activation of infected lymphocytes by antigenic insults, the balance changes and a vicious cycle develops with the HIV-induced immune suppression reducing the control of the immune system over the virus and allowing further replication resulting in greater immune suppression.

THE ROLE OF THE IMMUNE SYSTEM IN THE CONTROL OF HIV INFECTION

One of the earliest serological signs in acute HIV infection is HIV antigenaemia, which usually appears within 2–4 weeks of exposure[59]. Development of an antibody response to both the core (p24) and envelope (p41) proteins usually results in loss of detectable HIV antigen[38,59]. Whether this is due to suppression of viral replication or just redistribution of antigen in immune complexes is unknown[60]. However, the former appears more likely, as at this stage it is often difficult to culture HIV either from blood or semen. With time, some patients show a progressive loss of p24 antibody associated with the re-emergence of HIV antigenaemia[61,62]. In patients with AIDS-related complex this has been shown to be a bad prognostic sign for the development of AIDS[63]. In nine patients with persistent generalized lymphadenopathy who were p24 antibody negative and HIV antigen positive at the beginning of study, six developed AIDS at 13–23 months, compared to two out of twelve in the p24 antibody positive, antigen negative group. Similarly, in a 4-year prospective study of initially asymptomatic HIV seropositive homosexual men, those with circulating p24 antibody were significantly less likely to develop AIDS[64]. It is not possible at present to know whether the loss of anti-p24 is a primary event or secondary to increased HIV replication. Neutralizing antibodies, probably to the viral envelope[65-68] have been identified in some asymptomatic individuals, usually at low titre. Their presence appears to be associated with a better prognosis[64].

During acute infection and the early stages of HIV infection there are rarely any major immunological abnormalities. However, there may be a lymphocytosis in the peripheral blood due primarily to an elevation of the CD8+ phenotype (cytotoxic/suppressor) T-lymphocytes, which is a common finding in many viral infections and is not specific to HIV. These cells are likely to have a central role in the control of the infection, as CD8+ cells from asymptomatic HIV positive individuals effectively suppress viral replication *in vitro*[69]. MHC restricted, HIV specific, cytotoxic T-cells recognizing particularly the envelope proteins of HIV have also recently been described[70-72]. These cells are found predominantly in asymptomatic carriers of the virus and are notably absent in patients with AIDS, again suggesting that they may be directly involved in viral control. Although, studies of cohorts of individuals at risk of HIV infection have shown a relative decrease in CD4 lymphocytes within the first 6 months of infection, absolute counts remain within the normal range[73]. As disease progresses the CD8+ lymphocytosis tends to be lost and a CD4+ lymphopenia develops. Therefore, the commonly quoted CD4/CD8 ratio is of little value, as it may either reflect increased CD8+ cells early in infection or decreased CD4 cells later in the disease. Absolute numbers of cells are of more direct relevance.

A proportion of patients with HIV infection, 48% at 3 years in our own study[74], will develop a syndrome of persistent generalized lymphadenopathy which primarily affects peripheral lymph nodes. Histology reveals reactive hyperplasia with markedly enlarged germinal centres, a non-specific finding in many conditions. Immunohistology of the affected lymph nodes has shown that part of the germinal centre hyperplasia is due to the infiltration of CD8+ lymphocytes. These lymphocytes are usually present in low numbers in normal lymph nodes[75]. More recently HIV has been demonstrated in the germinal centres, not in lymphocytes, but in the follicular dendritic cells[76-78]. It remains debatable whether these cells are truly infected or whether they have phagocytosed virus and have re-expressed it on their surface as part of the normal antigen-presenting function. It has been suggested that these cells could act as sources of virus, infecting circulating lymphocytes as they pass through the lymph nodes[79]. It is possible that the invasion by CD8+ lymphocytes is a response to the presence of the virus, and that these cells are locally controlling viral replication in the same way as peripheral blood CD8 cells *in vitro*. A corollary is the observation that loss of lymphadenopathy, with a pattern of follicular involution and destruction of follicular dendritic cells on histology, is commonly associated with the development of full-blown AIDS. The relative numbers of CD4+ cells in the lymph nodes is low and mirrors the counts in the blood.

EFFECTS OF HIV ON T-LYMPHOCYTES

CD4 lymphocytes

As mentioned previously not only is there a progressive depletion of CD4+ lymphocytes, but those that remain have impaired function. Investigation of their proliferative responses to mitogens such as phytohaemagglutinin (PHA), Concanavalin A (Con A) or Pokeweed mitogen (PWM) using unfractionated cells have shown deficient blast transformation in patients with HIV-related disease. These abnormal responses are not merely due to decreased numbers of a particular subset of T-cells as the response persists even when cell ratios are corrected[80]. This was initially explained on the basis of defective CD4 cell function. However, later experiments showed that the defects appeared to be due to impairment of cellular interaction rather than defects in one cell type, as similar experiments using purified populations of either CD4 or CD8 cells have shown no abnormalities in mitogen responses[81]. In contrast, there is a specific and severe deficiency of proliferative response to soluble antigens demonstrable in both unfractionated and purified CD4+ fractions[81,82]. The mechanism of these defects has not yet been fully elucidated but they may be caused by a post-signal induction effect, which would explain why mitogens are less affected than antigens, since mitogens can directly activate diacyglycerol and phosphokinase C, bypassing the specific antigen activation pathway. Studies of cell membrane function in T-cell lines have shown that infection by HIV causes depolarization of the plasma membrane, and that the cells then became refractory to stimulation by the mitogen PHA. Likewise, intracellular calcium levels were raised in infected compared to uninfected cells and did not show the normal rise following activation[83]. Some functional abnormalities, in particular the loss of proliferative response to ppd, may occur early in the course of HIV infection, before abnormalities in T-cell numbers are detected[84], Deficiency of lymphocyte function may also have prognostic significance. One study demonstrated that in initially asymptomatic individuals a low relative response to PWM was associated with a 50-fold risk factor for the development of severe disease at 10 months compared to similar patients with high proliferative responses[85]. Similarly, in a group of patients with lymphadenopathy the loss of the ability to respond to mitogenic or antigenic stimulation as measured by the production of γ-interferon, has been shown to predict the disease progression to AIDS[86].

The mixed lymphocyte response which involves helper T-cells as the major responders is also severely impaired in patients with AIDS and AIDS-related complex. The impaired response is due to a functional defect in the CD4 responder cells and not to a quantitative deficiency[87]. The addition of interleukin-2 can correct the *in vitro* defect in the majority of patients with AIDS-related complex, but only in a subset of those with AIDS[88]. Other markers of T-cell and especially CD4 cell function, for example the production of lymphokines such as γ-interferon and interleukin-2, has generally been found to be impaired[89,90]. It is likely that the γ-interferon production defects are secondary to the impaired response to proliferative signals, as the mRNA for γ-interferon is normal[91], and in some assays the addition of exogenous interleukin-2 to lymphocyte cultures reverses the defect of γ-interferon production[92]. Initial studies suggested that one of the defects in T-cell function may reside in the decreased numbers of interleukin-2 receptors on activated lymphocytes, making them unable to respond to any interleukin-2 produced[93,94]. Other studies, however, could not detect an abnormal interleukin-2 response[95]. The differences in results may have been related to the varying cell systems used. It now appears that there is no effect on mRNA of interleukin-2 receptor in HIV infected cells, but that there is down regulation of transcription of the interleukin-2 gene leading to abnormal production[91]. Whatever the mechanism, depressed proliferative responses to specific antigen and the failure of production of regulating lymphokines has profound effects on the ability to amplify antigen specific lymphocyte clones, activation of macrophages and natural killer (NK) cells by γ-interferon and the provision of help for B-cell responses to T-cell dependent antigens.

CD8 lymphocytes

The other main phenotypic subset of T-cells are the CD8+ lymphocytes which contain cells having class 1 restricted cytotoxic function and also those with suppressor activity. Suppressor function appears to be maintained, but the cytotoxic T-cell activity is abnormal. Infection of these cells has not been documented *in vivo*, therefore, the defects are likely to be secondary in nature. Cytotoxic cells help control intracellular viral infection, recognizing foreign viral proteins in the context of MHC class 1 antigens on infected cells and destroying the cells by the local production of perforins. The perforins are thought to act in a similar way to the membrane attack complex of complement, by the assembly of proteins in the membrane of the target cell to form a channel which leads to cell lysis. Individuals with HIV infection have been shown to have defective antigen-specific cytotoxic T-lymphocytes to virus infected targets[96]. In cytomegalovirus (CMV) infection, this defect was shown to become more pronounced with disease progression[97]. It is possible that the defects are partially due to the impaired production of lymphokines by helper T-cells, as the addition of recombinant interleukin-2 to the *in vitro* system leads to an improvement in function. However, the use of interleukin-2 *in vivo* has not led to such clearcut effects in combating viral infection, suggesting that the defect is more complex. Other cytotoxic cell functions such as that of NK cells [95,98] and antibody dependent cytotoxic cells are also impaired[99], but the relevance of these defects to the clinical findings is not yet clear. It is likely that the lack of T-helper derived lymphokines is an important factor in the defective NK cell cytotoxicity of tumour cell targets such as K562, and the addition of γ-interferon has been shown to partially correct the defect.

B-lymphocytes

A characteristic finding in patients with AIDS is a polyclonal hypergamma-globulinaemia involving particularly IgG and IgA and to a lesser extent IgM. The immunoglobulin levels tend to increase during asymptomatic HIV infection, and reach its height at the clinical stages of persistent generalized lymphadenopathy and AIDS-related complex, declining when AIDS develops[100]. Perversely, IgA may sometimes continue to rise. Levels of IgD are also raised and follow the same pattern of elevation as the other immunoglobulin classes but reaching relatively greater levels, with approximately an 8.8-fold rise in patients with ARC, compared to 2.5 and 1.8 for IgG and IgA, respectively[101]. The elevated IgD levels may reflect an unusual mechanism of B-cell activation, as in most diseases with polyclonal B-cell activation, IgD levels are normal or only mildly elevated. A significant amount of the immunoglobulin produced is directed against HIV, with 3% of peripheral blood B-cells in patients with AIDS-related complex and 1% in patients with AIDS secreting HIV-specific antibody. The remainder of antibody is to previously encountered pathogens or autoantibody[102]. *In vitro* peripheral blood B-cells spontaneously produce large amounts of polyspecific immunoglobulin, but become refractory to further stimulation[103].

These defects, in addition to the deficiencies in T-helper cell function, explain the inability of patients to produce an antibody response to neo-antigens, whether in the form of a controlled immunization to a novel antigen such as keyhole limpet haemocyanin, or to a pathogen or vaccine[104]. They are, therefore, functionally hypogammaglobulinaemic. Patients with AIDS may also have an absolute hypogammaglobulinaemia with respect to the IgG subclasses IgG2 and IgG4[105], and a deficiency of the IgG2 subclass is associated with a susceptibility to infection with encapsulated bacteria (personal observations). The polyclonal B-cell activation maintains high levels of antibodies to previously encountered antigens, and, therefore, may protect adults with AIDS from the severe problems that occur in infants, whose B-cell repertoire has not developed due to the lack of appropriate T-cell help. As previously mentioned in this chapter, this B-cell activation may be mediated directly by HIV. Less likely, is that the B-cell activation is due to the uncontrolled action of the Epstein-Barr virus (EBV) in the immunosuppressed host[106]. However, this cannot be the only factor as EBV negative infants with HIV infection still show hyper-gammaglobulinaemia. The high levels of circulating immune complexes[107] and auto-antibodies[108] may also be related to this phenomenon. The hyper-activity of B-cells may also contribute to the heightened allergic drug reactions which have been noted, particularly with the use of sulphonamides. The reaction is dose-related, and, therefore, unlikely to be mediated simply by a type 1 hypersensitivity reaction, type 3 mechanism possibly being involved. Despite generally low levels of total IgE[109] it has also been noted that patients with AIDS may have a recrudescence of previously quiescent atopic disease[110]. This shows a temporal association with the development of immunosuppression occurring either around the time of diagnosis of AIDS or in a prodromal phase when the patients are already showing early signs of immune deficiency, i.e. oral candidiasis, chronic ulcerative herpes simplex or varicella zoster infection. It has not commonly occurred in patients without a prior history of atopic disease, suggesting that it is not just a feature of AIDS but of immunosuppression in those already sensitized. In adults hay fever, asthma and urticaria have been common allergic phenomena, whereas in children atopic eczema is more often described[111,112].

Monocytes, macrophages and antigen presenting cells

Macrophages and antigen presenting cells have a particularly close relationship with T-helper cells, the interaction being essential for adequate function of the cellular immune response. Macrophages are poor at killing intracellular pathogens unless stimulated by the appropriate T-cell derived macrophage activating factors. Gamma-interferon may be one of the required factors, although it does not possess all the macrophage activating activity of mitogen stimulated T-cell supernatants[113]. The production of γ-interferon in response to mitogen and specific angiten is known to be abnormal in patients with AIDS. This may explain the impaired killing by macrophages of toxoplasma and mycobacteria and the failure to present antigen even to functionally normal T-cells[114]. Antigen presenting cells present antigen to specific CD4+ T-cells by the surface expression of the antigen in association with class 2 tissue antigen HLA-DR. It is only then that class 2 restricted T-helper cells can recognize and respond to the antigen. Class 2 expression is generally subnormal in patients with AIDS[115]. In the blood, the population of dendritic cells with high intensity DR expression (which are thought to be the predominant antigen presenting cells) are missing from patients with AIDS, and the cells that remain are poor antigen presenters as documented by the lack of induction of mixed lymphocyte response[116]. Likewise, the epidermal Langerhans cell also shows lack of class 2 expression[117]. It is not known whether these defects are primary or secondary to defective lymphokine production. Early clinical studies of patients with γ-interferon have suggested that it does increase DR expression on monocytes in patients with AIDS. Our own studies have revealed that even low doses of recombinant γ-interferon can restore impaired monocyte phagocytic activity[118]. However, a primary T-cell defect may be only part of the problem. Monocytes can be infected by HIV and although this does not lead to depletion, it may affect function. The level of CD4 expression by circulating monocytes is markedly decreased in individuals with HIV infection[119], and although the function of this protein in monocytes is as yet unknown the possibility remains that its loss affects function. Infection of monocytes with HIV *in vitro* has been shown to lead to alterations in the development of maturation markers and the enhanced production of interleukin-2, which are features of activation[120]. Monokine production is generally affected with impaired production of interleukin-1 and tumour necrosis factor alpha[121]. Tumour necrosis factor alpha, also termed cachectin, has potent antiproliferative and anti-infective properties, and a deficiency may play a role in the susceptibility to infection and tumour in these patients.

The high levels of circulating immune complexes may also contribute to defective function by blocking Fc receptor sites, leading to the Fc dependent abnormalities in monocytic function[122]. The mechanism of the monocyte chemotactic defect observed in drug abusers at risk of HIV infection is unknown[123].

Neutrophils

Neutroperia is a common finding in patients with HIV-related disease. This may be a consequence of bone marrow suppression related to drugs, or HIV itself, or a result of peripheral destruction in response to anti-neutrophil antibody[124]. Neutrophil function has generally been found to be normal, although some investigators have demonstrated a defect in chemotaxis[125].

OTHER IMMUNE ABNORMALITIES IN PATIENTS WITH HIV INFECTION

Many other abnormalities in various aspects of the immune system have been documented. Abnormalities in thymic hormone levels and atrophy of the thymus itself, have encouraged the use of thymic implants or hormone replacement, but have met with little successs[126,127]. However, the observation that the culture of HIV infected T-cells with thymic epithelial cells can lead to a re-expression of CD4 may be of potential therapeutic value[128]. Raised levels of an unusual acid labile α-interferon have also been described in AIDS. Whether this is due to the production by persistently virus infected cells or to antigenically stimulated cells is not known. Raised levels of α-interferon are found transiently during acute infection with HIV, and rise again later in the course of infection, correlating with the stage of disease[129]. It is possible that endogenous interferon is responsible or exacerbates some of the non-specific 'flu-like' symptoms of HIV infection. Other non-specific markers of cellular activation are also raised, such as β_2-microglobulin and neopterin.

VACCINE DEVELOPMENT

The need for an effective vaccine against HIV is clear, and much research is based on its possible future development. At present the majority of prototype vaccines employ envelope components of HIV, as antibodies to envelope have been shown to neutralize HIV *in vitro*, and would be expected to prevent viral binding to the cellular receptor. However, the envelope region is highly variable between isolates due to frequent mutation of the coding genes. It has, therefore, proved difficult to engineer a vaccine which induces antibodies that cross-react with envelope proteins from different virus isolates. An exception to this is the epitope on gp120 that binds to the CD4 molecule and which is highly conserved between clinical isolates[130], this may be a candidate for vaccine production. Despite the advances that have been made in engineering vaccines, clinical efficacy has not yet been demonstrated. Vaccination of chimpanzees (one of the few animal species infectable by HIV) induces the development of an antibody response, however, the animals are not protected from further challenge with HIV. Some investigators question the validity of any animal model, maintaining that vaccines should be used in carefully controlled trials in man. Small phase 1 trials are underway in parts of Africa and the USA to evaluate the toxicity of the available vaccines, but there is unlikely to be any information on efficacy for some years[131]. Future vaccines may be developed for alternative structural proteins such as the transmembrane or core proteins, or to the functional gene products or reverse transcriptase.

OTHER FORMS OF THERAPY

Attempts to reconstitute the immune system in those who already have immune deficiency have had variable success. Trials of immunomodulators such as interleukin-2 and γ-interferon, as well as lymphocyte transfusion and bone-marrow transplantation to replace depleted cells have only shown minor or transient benefit. The reason may be the continuing damage to the immune system by HIV, and the development of anti-viral agents active against HIV means that combination regimes are likely to yield better results.

At the present time several anti-HIV agents are under development, and some have shown encouraging results in clinical trials. Of particular interest has been the demonstration of the efficacy of the reverse transcriptase inhibitor azidothymidine (Zidovudine) in decreasing the incidence of opportunist infections and reducing mortality in patients with AIDS-related complex and AIDS[132]. Unfortunately, the high incidence of side-effects may limit its usefulness. Although such treatment does not eradicate HIV from the individual it has been shown to markedly decrease its replication. If less toxic agents are developed, they could play an important role in the prevention of disease in carriers of the virus.

CONCLUSION

AIDS has taught us much about the function of the immune system and its role not only in infection and tumour control but also in the fields of allergy and auto-immune disease. It has led us to question many previously held convictions on the immunopathogenesis of disease and to realize the limitations of laboratory assessment of immune function. This demonstrates that research into HIV has already had wide implications outside as well as within the domain of AIDS, and that unexpected benefits have arisen from this devastating but challenging disease.

References

1. Gottlieb, M. S., Schroff, R., Schanker, H. M. *et al.* (1981). *Pneumocystis carinii* pneumonia and mucosal candidiasis in previously healthy homosexual men: evidence of a new acquired cellular immunodeficiency. *N. Engl. J. Med.*, **305**, 1425–31
2. Friedman-Kein, A. E., Laubenstein, L. J., Rubinstein, P. *et al.* (1982). Disseminated Kaposi's sarcoma in homosexual men. *Ann. Intern. Med.*, **96**, 693–700
3. Barre-Sinoussi, F., Chermann, J. C., Rey, F. *et al.* (1983). Isolation of a T-lymphotropic retrovirus from a patient at risk for acquired immune deficiency syndrome (AIDS). *Science*, **220**, 868–70
4. Gallo, R. C., Salahuddin, S. Z., Popovic, M. *et al.* (1984). Frequent detection and isolation of cytopathic retroviruses (HTLV-III) from patients with AIDS and at risk of AIDS. *Science*, **224**, 500–3
5. Mildvan, D., Mathur, V. and Enlow, R., (1982). Persistent generalised lymphadenopathy among homosexual males. *Morbid Mortal Weekly Rep.*, **31**, 249
6. Ho, D. D., Rota, T. R., Schooley, R. T. *et al.* (1985). Isolation of HTLV-III from cerebrospinal fluid and neural tissues of patients with neurological syndromes related to the acquired immunodeficiency syndrome. *N. Engl. J. Med.*, **313**, 1493–7
7. Shaw, G. M., Harper, M. E., Hahn, B. H. *et al.* (1985). HTLV-III infection in brains of children and adults with AIDS encephalopathy. *Science*, **227**, 177–82
8. Weber, J. N., Wadsworth, J., Rogers, L. A. *et al.* (1986). Three-year prospective study of HTLV-III/LAV infection in homosexual men. *Lancet*, **1**, 1179–82
9. Goedert, J. J., Biggar, R. J., Weiss, S. H. *et al.* (1986). Three-year incidence of AIDS in five cohorts of HTLV-III-infected risk group members. *Science*, **231**, 992–5
10. Ragni, M. V., Tegtmeier, G. E., Levy, J. A. *et al.*, (1986). AIDS retrovirus antibodies in haemophiliacs treated with factor VIII or factor IX concentrates, cryoprecipitate, or frozen plasma: Prevalence, seroconversion rate, and clinical correlations. *Blood*, **67**, 592–5
11. Weber, J. N., McCreaner, A., Berrie, E. *et al.* (1986). Factors affecting seropositivity to human T cell lymphotropic virus type III (HTLV-III) or Lymphadenopathy Associated Virus (LAV) and progression of clinical disease in sexual partners of patients with AIDS. *Genitourin. Med.*, **62**, 177–80
12. Katzenstein, D. A., Latif, A. and Bassett, M. F., (1987). Risks for heterosexual transmission of HIV in Zimbabwe. *Third International Conference on AIDS*, June 1–5, Washington
13. Eales, L. J., Nye, K. E., Parkin, J. M. *et al.* (1987). Association of different allelic forms of group specific component with susceptibility to and clinical manifestations of human immunodeficiency virus infection. *Lancet*, **1**, 999–1002
14. Prince, M. E., Caroff, R. W., Ayoub, G. *et al.* (1984). HLA studies in acquired immune deficiency syndrome patients with Kaposi's sarcoma. *J. Clin. Immunol.*, **4**, 212–13
15. Smeraldi, R. S., Fabio, G., Luttario, A. *et al.* (1986). HLA-associated susceptibility to acquired immune deficiency syndrome in Italian patients with HIV infection. *Lancet*, **2**, 1187–9
16. Madhok, R., Gracie, A., Lowe, G. D. O. *et al.* (1986). Impaired cell mediated immunity in haemophilia in the absence of infection with human immunodeficiency virus. *Br. Med. J.*, **293**, 978–80
17. Pinching, A. J., McManus, T. J., Jeffries, D. J. *et al.* (1983). Studies of cellular immunity in male homosexuals in London. *Lancet*, **2**, 126–130
18. Goedert, J. J., Neuland, C. Y., Wallen, W. C. *et al.* (1982). Amyl nitrite may alter T lymphocytes in homosexual men. *Lancet*, **1**, 412–14

19. Clavel, F., Guetard, D., Brun-Vezinet, F. *et al.* (1986). Isolation of a new human retrovirus from West African patients with AIDS. *Science*, **233**, 343–6
20. Guenno, B. L., Jean, P., Peghini, M. *et al.*, (1987). Increasing HIV-2 associated AIDS in Senegal. *Lancet*, **2**, 972–3
21. Brucker, G., Brun-Vezinet, F., Rosenheim, M. *et al.*, (1987). HIV-2 infection in homosexual men in France. *lancet*, **1**, 223
22. Norby, E., Biberfeld, G., Albert, J. *et al.* (1987). Significance of variation between human immunodeficiency virus (HIV) isolates for serology and vaccine development. *Third International Conference on AIDS*, June 1–5, Washington
23. Rey, M. A., Girard, P. M., Harzic, M. *et al.* (1987). HIV-1 and HIV-2 double infection in French homosexual male with AIDS-related complex. *Lancet*, **1**, 388–9
24. McDougal, J. S., Kennedy, M. S., Sligh, J. H. *et al.* (1986). Binding of HTLV-III/Lav to T4+ T cells by a complex of the 110 k viral protein and the T4 molecule. *Science*, **231**, 382–5
25. Dalgleish, A. G., Beverley, P. C. L., Clapham, P. R. *et al.* (1984). The CD4 (T4) antigen is an essential component of the receptor for the AIDS retrovirus. *Nature*, **312**, 763–7
26. Klatzmann, D., Champagne, E., Chamaret, S. *et al.* (1984). T-lymphocyte T4 molecule behaves as the receptor for human retrovirus LAV. *Nature*, **312**, 767–8
27. Maddon, P. J., Dalgleish, A. G., McDougal, J. S. *et al.* (1986). The T4 gene encodes the AIDS virus receptor and is expressed in the immune system and the brain. *Cell*, **47**, 333–48
28. Stein, B. S., Gowda, S. D., Lifson, J. D. *et al.* (1987). pH-independent HIV entry into CD4-positive T cells via virus envelope fusion to the plasma membrane. *Cell*, **49**, 659–68
29. Fisher, A. G., Ratner, L., Mitsuya, M. *et al.* (1986). Infectious mutants of HTLV-III with changes in the 3′ region and markedly reduced cytopathic effects. *Science*, **233**, 655–9
30. McClure, M. O. and Weiss, R. A. (1987). Human immunodeficiency virus and related viruses. In Gottlieb *et al.*, (eds.) *Current Topics in AIDS*, pp. 95–117. (John Wiley and Sons)
31. Editorial. (1987). Zidovudine (AZT). *Lancet*, **1**, 957–8
32. Yarchoan, R., Perno, C. F., Thomas, R. V. *et al.* (1988). Phase 1 studies of 2′, 3′-dideoxycytidine in severe human immunodeficiency virus infection as a single agent and alternating with zidovudine (AZT). *Lancet*, **1**, 76–81
33. Salahuddin, S. Z., Markham, P. D., Popovic, M. *et al.* (1985). Isolation of infectious human T-cell leukaemia/lymphotropic virus type III (HTLV III) from patients with acquired immune deficiency syndrome (AIDS) or AIDS-related complex (ARC) and from healthy carriers: a study of risk groups and tissue sources. *Proc. Natl. Sci. USA*, **82**, 5530–4
34. Ho, D. D., Rota, T. R. and Hirsh, M. S., (1986). Infection of monocytes/macrophages by human T-lymphotropic virus type III. *J. Clin. Invest.*, **77**, 1712–15
35. Montagnier, L., Gruest, J., Chamaret, S. *et al.* (1984). Adaptation of lymphadenopathy-associated virus (LAV) to replication in EBV-transformed B lymphoblastoid lines. *Science*, **225**, 63–6
36. Salahuddin, S. Z., Rose, R. M., Groopman, J. E. *et al.* (1986). Human T-lymphotropic virus type III infection of human alveolar macrophages. *Blood*, **67**, 281–4
37. Tschachler, E., Groh, V., Popovic, M. *et al.* (1987). Epidermal Langerhans cells: a target for HTLV-III/LAV infection. *J. Invest. Dermatol.*, **88**, 233–7
38. Ranki, A., Valle, S. L., Krohn, M. *et al.* (1987). Long latency precedes overt seroconversion in sexually transmitted HIV infection. *Lancet*, **2**, 589–93
39. Gartner, S., Markovitz, P., Markovitz, D. M. *et al.* (1986). The role of mononuclear phagocytes in HTLV-III/LAV infection. *Science*, **233**, 215–19
40. Anand, R., Siegal, F., Reed, C. *et al.* (1987). Non-cytocidal natural variants of human immunodeficiency virus isolated from AIDS patients with neurological disorders. *Lancet*, **2**, 234–8
41. Zagury D., Bernard, I., Leonard, R. *et al.* (1986). Long-term cultures of HTLV-III infected T-cells: a model of cytopathology of T-cell depletion in AIDS. *Science*, **231**, 850–3
42. Sodroski, J., Goh, W. C., Rosen, C. *et al.*, (1986). Role of the HTLV-III/LAV envelope in syncytium formation and cytopathicity. *Nature*, **322**, 470–4
43. McDougal, J. S., Mawle, A., Cort, S. P. *et al.* (1985). Cellular tropism of the human retrovirus HTLV-III/LAV. Role of T-cell activation and expression of the T4 antigen. *J. Immunol.*, **135**, 3151–62
44. Lifson, J. D., Feinberg, M. B., Reyes, G. R. *et al.* (1986). Induction of CD4-dependent cell

fusion by the HTLV-III/LAV envelope glycoprotein. *Nature*, **323**, 725-8
45. Lifson, J. D., Reyes, G. R., McGrath, M. S. *et al.* (1986). AIDS retrovirus induced cytopathology: giant cell formation and involvement of CD4 antigen. *Science*, **232**, 1123-7
46. Somasundaran, M. and Robinson, H. L. (1987). A major mechanism of human immunodeficiency virus induced killing does not involve cell fusion. *J. Virol.*, **62**, 3114-19
47. Koenig, S., Gendelman, H. E., Orenstein, J. M. *et al.* (1986). Detection of AIDS virus in macrophages in brain tissue from AIDS patients with encephalopathy. *Science*, **233**, 1089-93
48. Popovic, M., Gartner, S. and Gallo, R. C. (1987). Mononuclear phagocytes and accessory cells in the pathogenesis of AIDS. *Third International Conference on AIDS*, June 1-5, Washington
49. Mosca, J. D., Bednarik, D. P., Raj, N. B. K. *et al.* (1987). Herpes simplex virus type-1 can reactivate transcription of latent human immunodeficiency virus. *Nature*, **325**, 67-70
50. Hoxie, J. A., Alpers, J. D., Rackowski, J. L. *et al.* (1986). Alterations in T4 (CD4) protein and mRNA synthesis in cells infected with HIV. *Science*, **234**, 1127-9
51. Schnittman, S. M., Clifford-Lane, H., Higgins, S. E. *et al.* (1986). Direct polyclonal activation of human B-cells by the acquired immune deficiency syndrome virus. *Science*, **233**, 1084-6
52. Klatzmann, D. and Gluckman, J. C. (1986). HIV infection: facts and hypotheses. *Immunol. Today.*, **7**, 291-6
53. Levy, J. (1987). Pathogenesis of HIV infection – virus: host interactions. *Third International Conference on AIDS*, June 1-5, Washington
54. Calvelli, T. A. and Rubinstein, A. (1986). Intravenous gammaglobulin in infant acquired immunodeficiency syndrome. *Pediatr. Infect. Dis.*, **5**, S207-S210
55. Pinching, A. J. (1987). The acquired immune deficiency syndrome: with special reference to tuberculosis. *Tubercle*, **68**, 65-9
56. Greene, J. B., Sidhu, G. S., Lewin, S. *et al.* (1982). *Mycobacterium avium-intracellulare:* a cause of disseminated life-threatening infection in homosexuals and drug abusers. *Ann. Int. Med.*, **97**, 539
57. Johnson, T. M., Duvic, M., Rapini, R. *et al.* (1985). AIDS exacerbates psoriasis. *N. Engl. J. Med.*, **313**, 1415
58. Duvic, M., Rios, A. and Brewton, G. W. (1987). Remission of AIDS-associated psoriasis with zidovudine. *Lancet*, **2**, 627
59. Allain, J. P., Laurian, Y., Paul, D. A. *et al.* (1986). Serological markers in early stages of human immunodeficiency virus infection in haemophilliacs. *Lancet*, **2**, 1233-6
60. Lange, J. M. A., Paul, D. A., deWolf, F. *et al.* (1987). Viral gene expression, antibody production and immune complex formation in Human Immunodeficiency Virus infection. *AIDS*, **1**, 15-20
61. Biggar, R. J., Melbye, M., Ebbesen, P. *et al.* (1985). Variation in human T lymphotropic virus III (HTLV-III) antibodies in homosexual men: decline before onset of illness related to acquired immune deficiency syndrome (AIDS). *Br. Med. J.*, **291**, 997-8
62. Lange, J. M. A., Paul, D. A., Huisman, H. G. *et al.* (1986). Persistent HIV antigenaemia and decline of HIV core antibodies associated with transition to AIDS. *Br. Med. J.*, **293**, 1459-62
63. Kenny, C., Parkin, J. M., Underhill, G. *et al.* (1987). HIV antigen testing. *Lancet*, **1**, 565-6
64. Pedersen, C., Neilsen, C. M., Vestergaard, B. F. *et al.* (1987). Temporal relation of antigenaemia and loss of antibodies to core antigens to development of clinical disease in HIV infection. *Br. Med. J.*, **295**, 567-72
65. Weber, J. N., Clapham, P. R., Weiss, R. A. *et al.* (1987). Human immunodeficiency virus infection in two cohorts of homosexual men: neutralising sera and association of anti-gag antibody with prognosis. *Lancet*, **1**, 119-22
66. Robert-Goroff, M., Brown, M. and Gallo, R. C. (1985). HTLV-III-neutralising antibodies in patients with AIDS and AIDs-related complex. *Nature*, **316**, 72-4
67. Weiss, R. A., Clapham, P. R., Weber, J. N. *et al.* (1986). Variable and conserved neutralization antigens of human immunodeficiency virus. *Nature*, **324**, 572-5
68. Lasky, L. A., Croopman, J. E., Fennie, C. W. *et al.* (1986). Neutralisation of the AIDS retrovirus by antibodies to a recombinant envelope glycoprotein. *Science*, **233**, 209-12
69. Walker, C. M., Moody, D. J., Stites, D. P. *et al.* (1986). CD8+ lymphocytes can control

HIV infection *in vitro* by suppressing virus replication. *Science*, **234**, 1563–6
70. Walker, B., Chakrabarti, S., Moss, B., *et al.* (1987). HIV env and gag specific cytotoxic T lymphocytes (CTLs) in seropositive subjects. *Third International Conference on AIDS*, June 1–5, Washington
71. Koenig, S., Earl, P., Powell, D., *et al.* (1987). Cytotoxic T cells directed against target cells expressing HIV-1 proteins. *Third International Conference on AIDS*, June 1–5, Washington
72. Weinhold, K. J., Lyerly, H. K., Matthews, T. J. *et al.* (1987). Gp 120 specific cell-mediated cytotoxicity in patients exposed to HIV. *Third International Conference on AIDS*, June 1–5, Washington 1987
73. Fahey, J. L., Giorgi, J., Martinez-Maza, O. *et al.* (1986). Immune pathogenesis of AIDS and related syndromes. In Gluckman and Vilmer (eds.). *Acquired Immunodeficiency Syndrome. International Conference on AIDS*, pp. 107–114. (Elsevier)
74. Weber, J. N., Wadsworth, J., Rogers, L. A. *et al.* (1986). Three-year prospective study of HYLV-III/LAV infection in homosexual men. *Lancet*, **1**, 1179–82
75. Janossy, G., Pinching, A. J., Bofill, M. *et al.* (1985). An immunohistological approach to persistent lymphadenopathy and its relevance to AIDS. *Clin. Exp. Immunol.*, **59**, 257–66
76. Armstrong, J. A. and Horne, R. (1984). Follicular dendritic cells and virus-like particles in AIDS-related lymphadenopathy. *Lancet*, **2**, 370–2
77. Biberfeld, P., Chayt, K. J., Marselle, L. M. *et al.* (1986). HTLV-III expression in infected lymph nodes and relevance to pathogenesis of lymphadenopathy. *Am. J. Pathol.*, **125**, 436–42
78. Tenner-Racz, K., Racz, P., Dietrick, M. *et al.* (1985). Altered follicular dendritic cells and virus-like particles in AIDS and AIDS-related lymphadenopathy. *Lancet*, **2**, 105–6
79. Tenner-Racz, K., Bofill, M., Schulz-Meyer, A. *et al.* (1986). HTLV-III/LAV viral antigens in lymph nodes of homosexual men with persistent generalised lymphadenopathy and AIDS. *Am. J. Pathol.* **123**, 9–15
80. Gluckman, J. C., Klatzmann, D., Cavaille-Coll, M. *et al.* (1985). Is there a correllation of T cell proliferative functions and surface marker phenotypes in patients with acquired immune deficiency syndrome or lymphadenopathy syndrome? *Clin. Exp. Immunol.*, **60**, 8–16
81. Lane, H. C., Depper, J. M., Greene, W. C. *et al.* (1985). Qualitative analysis of immune function in patients with the acquired immune deficiency syndrome. Evidence for a selective defect in soluble antigen recognition. *N. Engl. J. Med.*, **313**, 79–84
82. Hofmann, B., Odum, N., Platz, P. *et al.* (1985). Immunological studies in acquired immune deficiency syndrome. Functional studies of lymphocyte subpopulations. *Scand. J. Immunol.*, **21**, 235–43
83. Gupta, S. and Vayuvegula, B. (1987). Human Immunodeficiency Virus-associated changes in signal transduction. *J. Clin. Immunol.*, **7**, 486–9
84. Krohn, K., Annamari, R., Antonen, J. *et al.* (1985). Immune functions in homosexual men with antibodies to HTLV-III in Finland. *Clin. Exp. Immunol.*, **60**, 17–24
85. Hofmann, B., Lindhardt, B. O., Gerstoft, J. *et al.* (1987). Lymphocyte transformation response to pokeweed mitogen as a predictive marker for development of AIDS and AIDS-related symptoms in homosexual men with HIV antibodies. *Br. Med. J.*, **295**, 293–6
86. Murray, H. W., Hillman, J. K., Rubin, B. Y. *et al.* (1985). Patients at risk for AIDS-related opportunistic infections. Clinical manifestations and impaired gamma interferon production. *N. Engl. J. Med.*, **313**, 1504–10
87. Gupta, S. and Safai, B. (1983). Deficient autologous mixed lymphocyte reaction in Kaposi's sarcoma associated with deficiency of Leu 3+ responder T cells. *J. Clin. Invest.*, **71**, 296–300
88. Gupta, S., Gillis, M., Thornton, M. and Goldberg, M. (1984). Autologous mixed lymphocyte reaction in man. XIV. Deficiency of the autologous mixed lymphocyte reaction in acquired immune deficiency syndrome (AIDS) and AIDS-related complex (ARC). *In vitro* effect of purified interleukin-1 and interleukin-2. *Clin. Exp. Immunol.*, **58**, 395–401
89. Antonen, J., Krohn, K. (1986). Interleukin 2 production in HTLV III/LAV infection: evidence of defective antigen induced, but normal mitogen induced IL 2 production. *Clin. Exp. Immunol.*, **65**, 489–96
90. Murray, H. W., Rubin, B. Y., Masur, H. and Roberts, R. B. (1984). Impaired production of lymphokines and immune (gamma) interferon in the acquired immunodeficiency syndrome. *N. Engl. J. Med.*, **310**, 883–9

91. Fauci, A. S. (1987). Immunopathogenic mechanisms and immune response to HIV infection. *Third International Conference on AIDS*, June 1-5, Washington

92. Moore, J. L., Poiesz, B. J., Tomar, R. H. *et al.* (1985). Gamma interferon and AIDS. *N. Engl. J. Med.*, **312**, 412-13

93. Hauser, G. J., Bino, T., Rosenberg, H. *et al.* (1984). Interleukin-2 production and response to exogenous interleukin-2 in a patient with the acquired immune deficiency syndrome (AIDS). *Clin. Exp. Immunol.*, **56**, 14-17

94. Murray, J. L., Hersh, E. M., Reuben, J. M. *et al.* (1985). Abnormal lymphocyte response to exogenous interleukin-2 in homosexuals with acquired immune deficiency syndrome (AIDS) and AIDS-related complex (ARC). *Clin. Exp. Immunol.*, **60**, 25-30

95. Alcocer-Varela, J., Alarcon-Segovia, D. and Abud-Mendoza, C. (1985). Immunoregulatory circuits in the acquired immune deficiency syndrome and related complex. Production of and response to interleukins 1 and 2, NK function and its enhancement by interleukin-2 and kinetics of the autologous mixed lymphocyte reaction. *Clin. Exp. Immunol.*, **60**, 31-8

96. Sharma, B. and Gupta, S. (1985). Antigen-specific primary cytotoxic T lymphocyte (CTL) responses in acquired immune deficiency syndrome (AIDS) and AIDS-related complexes (ARC). *Clin. Exp. Immunol.*, **62**, 296-303

97. Rook, A. H., Manischewitz, J. F., Frederick, W. R. *et al.* (1985). Deficient HLA-restricted cytomegalovirus specific cytotoxic T cells and natural killer cells in patients with the acquired immunodeficiency syndrome. *J. Inf. Dis.*, **152**, 627-30

98. Hersh, E. M., Gutterman, J. U., Spector, S. *et al.* (1985). Impaired *in vitro* interferon, blastogenic and natural killer cell responses to viral stimulation in acquired immune deficiency syndrome. *Cancer Res.*, **45**, 406

99. Bender, B. S., Auger, F. A., Quinn, T. C. *et al.* (1986). Impaired antibody dependent cell-mediated cytotoxic activity in patients with the acquired immune deficiency syndrome. *Clin. Exp. Immunol.*, **64**, 166-72

100. Seligmann, M., Chess, L., Fahey, J. L. *et al.* (1985). AIDS – an immunologic reevaluation. *N. Engl. J. Med.*, **311**, 1286-92

101. Mizuma, H., Zolla-Pazner, S., Litwin, S. *et al.* (1987). Serum IgD elevation is an early marker of B cell activation during infection with the human immunodeficiency viruses. *Clin. Exp. Immunol.*, **68**, 5-14

102. Yarchoan, R., Redfield, R. R. and Broder, S., (1986). Mechanisms of B cell activation in patients with acquired immunodeficiency syndrome and related disorders. *J. Clin. Invest.*, **78**, 439-47

103. Lane, H. C., Masur, H., Edgar, L. C. *et al.* (1983). Abnormalities of B cell activation in patients with the acquired immunodeficiency syndrome. *N. Engl. J. Med.*, **309**, 453-8

104. Ammann, A. J., Schiffman, G., Abrams, D. *et al.*, (1984). B-cell immunodeficiency in acquired immune deficiency syndrome. *J. Am. Med. Assoc.*, **251**, 1447-9

105. Aucoutrier, P., Couderc, L. J., Gouet, D. *et al.* (1986). Serum immunoglobulin G subclass dysbalances in the lymphadenopathy syndrome and acquired immune deficiency syndrome. *Clin. Exp. Immunol.*, **63**, 234-40

106. Birx, D. L., Redfield, R. R. and Tosato, G. (1986). Defective regulation of Epstein–Barr virus infection in patients with the acquired immune deficiency syndrome (AIDS) or AIDS-related disorders. *N. Engl. J. Med.*, **314**, 874-9

107. Euler, H. H., Kern, P., Loeffler, H. *et al.* (1985). Precipitable immune complexes in healthy homosexual men, acquired immune deficiency syndrome and related lymphadenopathy syndrome. *Clin. Exp. Immunol.*, **59**, 267-75

108. Procaccia, S., Lazzarin, A., Colucci, A. *et al.* (1987). IgM, IgG and IgA rheumatoid factors and circulating immune complexes in patients with AIDS and AIDS-related complex with serological abnormalities. *Clin. Exp. Immunol.*, **67**, 236-44

109. Ring, J., Froschl, M., Brunner, R. and Braun-Falco, O. (1986). LAV/HTLV-III infection and atopy: serum IgE and specific IgE antibodies to environmental allergens. *Acta Dermatol Venerol (Stockh).*, **66**, 530-2

110. Parkin, J. M., Eales, L. J., Galazka, R. A. *et al.* (1987). Atopic manifestations in the acquired immune deficiency syndrome. *B. Med. J.*, **294**, 1185-6

111. Ball, L. M. and Harper, J. I. (1987). Atopic eczema in HIV-seropositive haemophiliacs. *Lancet*, **2**, 627-8

112. Scott, G. B., Buck, B. E., Leterman, J. G. *et al.* (1984). AIDS in infants. *N. Engl. J. Med.*, **310**, 76-81

113. Eales, L. J., Moshtael, O. and Pinching, A. J. (1987). Microbicidal activity of monocyte derived macrophages in AIDS and related disorders. *Clin. Exp. Immunol.*, **67**, 227–35
114. Kirkpatrick, C. H., Davis, K. C. and Horsburgh, C. R. (1984). Reduced Ia positive Langerhans' cells in AIDS (letter) *N. Engl. J. Med.*, **311**, 857–8
115. Heagy, W., Kelley, V. E., Strom, T. B. *et al.* (1984). Decreased expression of human class II antigens on monocytes from patients with acquired immune deficiency syndrome: increased expression with interferon gamma. *J. Clin. Invest.*, **74**, 2089–96
116. Eales, L. J., Farrant, J. and Pinching, A. J. (1987). Loss of peripheral blood dendritic cells in persons with AIDS and AIDS-related complex
117. Belsito, D. V., Sanchez, M. R., Baer, R. L. *et al.* (1984). Reduced Langerhans' cell Ia antigen and ATPase activity in patients with the acquired immunodeficiency syndrome. *N. Engl. J. Med.*, **310**, 1279–82
118. Parkin, J. M., Moshtael, O., Galazka, R. A. *et al.* (1986). Results of a trial of recombinant gamma interferon in patients with the acquired immune deficiency syndrome. *Second International Conference on AIDS, June, Paris*
119. Rieber, P. and Riethmuller. (1986). Loss of circulating T4+ monocytes in patients infected with HTLV-III. *Lancet*, **1**, 270
120. McCartney-Francis, N., Mizel, D., Allen, J. *et al.* (1987). Interleukin-2 (IL-2) receptor gene expression in human monocytes infected with Human Immunodeficiency Virus (HIV). *Third International Conference on AIDS*, June 1–5, Washington
121. Ammann, A. J., Palladino, M. A., Volberding, P. *et al.* (1987). Tumour necrosis factors alpha and beta in acquired immunodeficiency syndrome (AIDS) and AIDS-related complex. *J. Clin. Immunol.*, **7**, 481–5
122. Pinching, A. J. (1986). The immunology of AIDS and HIV infection. In *Clinics in Immunology and Allergy*, **6**
123. Poli, G., Bottazzi, B., Acero, R. *et al.* (1985). Monocyte function in intravenous drug abusers with lymphadenopathy syndrome and in patients with acquired immunodeficiency syndrome: selective impairment of chemotaxis. *Clin. Exp. Immunol.*, **62**, 136–42
124. Weller, I. (1987). Neutropenia and HIV infection: mechanism and value as a prognostic sign. *Vox Sang.*, **52**, 6–7
125. Nielson, H., Kharazmi, A. and Faber, V. (1986). Blood monocyte and neutrophil functions in the acquired immune deficiency syndrome. *Scand. J. Immunol.*, **24**, 291–6
126. Dardenne, M., Bach, J. F., Safai, B. *et al.* (1983). Low thymic hormone levels in patients with acquired immune deficiency syndrome. *N. Engl. J. Med.*, **309**, 48–9
127. Muscart-Lemon, F., Huygen, K., Clumeck, N. *et al.* (1983). Stimulation of cellular function by thymopentin (TP-5) in three AIDS patients. *Lancet*, **2**, 735–6
128. Schuurman, H-J., Hendriks, R. W., Lange, J. M. A. *et al.* (1986). Cultured human thymus epithelial monolayer cells induce CD4 expression on mononuclear cells of AIDS patients *in vitro*. *Clin. Exp. Immunol.*, **64**, 348–55
129. Abb, J. (1987). Interferon-alpha in sera of HIV-infected patients. *Lancet*, **2**, 1052–3
130. Sattentau, Q. J., Dalgleish, A. G., Weiss, R. A. and Beverley, P. C. L., (1986). Epitopes of the CD4 antigen and HIV infection. *Science*, **234**, 1120–3
131. Homsy, J., Steimer, K. and Kaslow, R. (1987). Towards an AIDS vaccine: challenges and prospects. *Immunol. Today*, **8**, 193–7
132. Fischl, M. A., Richman, D. D., Grieco, M. H. *et al.* (1987). The efficacy of azidothymidine (AZT) in the treatment of patients with AIDS and AIDS-related complex. A double-blind placebo-controlled trial. *N. Engl. J. Med.*, **317**, 185–91
133. Weber, J. and Pinching, A. (1986). The clinical management of AIDS and HTLV-III infection. In Miller, Weber and Green, (eds.). *The Management of AIDS Patients*. (pp. 1–33. Macmillan Press).

5
Immunology of Gonorrhoea

C. A. ISON

INTRODUCTION

Neisseria gonorrhoeae colonizes and infects the mucosal surfaces of man and is particularly well adapted to survival in the genitourinary tract. The problem with gonorrhoea is that there is no apparent natural immunity and little evidence of acquired immunity. The host response to infection is often characterized by the appearance of polymorphonuclear neutrophils (PMN). Intracellular Gram-negative cocci, first described by Neisser, are still regarded as pathognomonic for gonococcal urethritis in males. However, it is not known whether PMNs play a major role in resolving the infection.

Gonococcal infection also results in the production of gonococcal antibodies, predominately IgG and IgA, in the serum and in mucosal secretions. Gonococcal antibody is known to block adherence to epithelial cells, activate the classical complement pathway, form immune complexes and to be opsonic, but its role in modifying the course of the infection is unclear.

INCIDENCE

The annual number of reported cases of gonorrhoea in the USA is almost one million and in the United Kingdom approximately 50000. In most industrialized countries there has been a slow decline in the incidence of gonorrhoea during the last decade, which can probably be attributed to adequate therapy and increased public health measures. In recent years this decline has also been influenced by attempts to control the spread of the acquired immunodeficiency syndrome (AIDS). A decrease in the incidence of gonorrhoea in homosexual men, the main reservoir of AIDS, has been reported in Denver (32%)[1] and in New York (59%)[2]. At St Mary's Hospital, London, where a large number of homosexual and AIDS patients are seen, the total number of cases of gonorrhoea fell by 50% between 1983 and 1986, from approximately 3000 cases to 1600 per year. This decline is greatest in homosexual men, but is also evident in heterosexual men and to a lesser extent in the female population[3]. The reasons for the effect of AIDS on the incidence of gonorrhoea and other sexually transmitted infections such as syphilis[4] are complex. Increased education, particularly in the use of condoms, recommendations to modify sexual practices and reduce the number of sexual partners are probably the main causes. However, it is difficult to assess how far the fear of AIDS has affected sexual practices, promiscuity and hence the incidence of gonorrhoea in both the homosexual and heterosexual communities. It is disturbing that there is an apparent reversal of this trend in the USA where the number of cases rose in 1985 for the first time in 10 years[5].

In the developing countries such as Asia and Africa, the actual incidence is not known. However, in Africa the incidence has been estimated to be considerably higher than developed countries. Gonococcal infection in these countries is a major cause of infertility in women. In Uganda the incidence was estimated to be 10 000 cases per 100 000 population[6] which compares with 435 cases per 100 000 population in the USA in 1981[7].

ANTIBIOTIC RESISTANCE

The resurgence of interest in the immunology of gonorrhoea in part relates to the ability of the gonococcus to develop resistance to standard remedies which helps ensure the continuing prevalence of gonorrhoea. Penicillin has been the main therapy in most parts of the world for more than 40 years. Chromosomal resistance, however, was first recognized in 1963 when Reyn reported more than 50% of the strains isolated were less sensitive than in 1944[8]. The levels of resistance encountered then and in the following two decades could, nevertheless, be overcome by increasing the dosage of penicillin. The first chromosomally-mediated penicillin resistant *N. gonorrhoeae* (CMRNG) isolated from therapeutic failures were seen in an outbreak in North Carolina in 1983[9]. The gonococci were resistant to one or more milligrams of penicillin per litre, and have subsequently been isolated throughout the USA[10] and England[11]. Clinical resistance results from chromosomal mutations at a number of loci[12] and from changes in the penicillin binding proteins found in the cell envelope[13,14].

High levels of resistance due to plasmid-mediated production of the enzyme β-lactamase was first described in gonococci in 1976[15-17], and overshadowed problems with chromosomal resistance. The enzyme is a TEM-1 type β-lactamase which is encoded on plasmids of 2.9, 3.2 and 4.4 megadaltons (MD) with these plasmids being mutually exclusive[18]. The two smaller plasmids are probably deletion derivatives of the larger plasmid. The spread of these plasmids between strains is dependent on conjugal transfer mediated by a fourth plasmid of 24.5 MD known as the conjugal plasmid. The 3.2 MD and 4.4 MD plasmid originated simultaneously in Africa and the Phillipines, respectively, whereas the 2.9 MD plasmid has only recently been described[19]. Between 1976 and 1980 most infections in both the USA and United Kingdom were direct imports of the original strains. However, since 1980 the prevalence of penicillinase producing *N. gonorrhoeae* (PPNG) in the

UK has risen dramatically with apparent indigenous spread[20]. This rise reached a peak in 1983 and was followed by a slow decline in 1984 and 1985. In the USA the number of cases has continued to rise, and in 1986 PPNG were isolated from almost every state, the total number of cases being 16 648[21] with evidence of endemic foci[22]. In parts of the world where antibiotic usage is not controlled the prevalence of PPNG infections is considerably higher[23]. It has been suggested that in areas with a prevalence of greater than 5%, spectinomycin or a cephalosporin should be used as first line therapy[20].

Resistance to spectinomycin has been reported from England[24], the Phillipines[25] and from Korea[26,27]. It is thought to be chromosomally mediated, and to result from a mutation affecting the ribosome leading to resistance at concentrations of 256 mg/l or more. These have occurred in small isolated outbreaks and have not influenced the efficacy of spectinomycin therapy. It is of more concern that continued use will result in an increase in low level resistance (64–128 mg/l) and may become widespread.

In 1985, strains of N. gonorrhoeae exhibiting high levels of resistance to tetracycline, 16–64 mg/l, were first detected[28]. The resistance was subsequently found to be caused by the insertion of the tet M determinant, into the gonococcal conjugal plasmid resulting in a new plasmid of 25.2 MD[29]. This determinant has previously been found in the genus Streptococcus, Ureaplasma urealyticum, Mycoplasma hominis and Gardnerella vaginalis. Tetracycline, although not the usual treatment for gonorrhoea, is the preferred choice for chlamydial infection. The continuing ability of gonococci to evade antimicrobial therapy is alarming. Cephalosporins, such as cefuroxime, cefotaxime and ceftriaxone, still offer a suitable alternative. However, the increasing levels of chromosomal resistance and the possible link between resistance to penicillin and other β-lactam antibiotics means that approaches to therapy may need to be reassessed. The newer quinolones or combinations of antibiotics may be the way forward.

COURSE OF INFECTION

Gonorrhoea is primarily an infection of mucosal surfaces which is termed uncomplicated gonococcal infection (UGI). The majority of infections occur in the genital tract, the urethra in men and the endocervix in women. Urethritis in men can present as a mild dysuria, scanty to purulent discharge or may be asymptomatic. The prevalence of asymptomatic infection in men is unclear because they do not seek treatment and are detected only by contact tracing or routine screening, but it has been reported to be approximately 3%[30]. However, a prevalence of 40–60% has been found amongst male contacts of women with salpingitis or disseminated infection[31,32]. It is more common to find asymptomatic disease among women, although the true incidence is unknown because again it is detected through contact tracing. The spectrum of symptomatic infection in women can present with an unusual or increased vaginal discharge, dysuria and lower abdominal or pelvic pain. Although the endocervix is the primary site of infection, gonococci are also isolated from the urethra and rectum. In many instances this is caused by leakage of the endocervical secretion from the vagina and only occasionally are the urethra and rectum the primary site. Gonococci can also infect the Bartholin's and Skene's glands, cause perihepatitis and have been implicated as a cause of urethral syndrome.

Rectal infection occurs mainly in homosexual men following rectal intercourse, and can range from asymptomatic to severe symptoms including a profuse purulent discharge. Gonococci can occasionally cause prostatitis and epididymitis in men. Pharyngeal infection can occur in both men and women although the prevalence is usually low. Conjunctivitis, nowadays, is invariably an infection found in the newborn.

Complicated gonococcal infection in women occurs when gonococci spread to the upper genital tract and infect the fallopian tubes (salpingitis) and the pelvic cavity (pelvic inflammatory disease) Ectopic pregnancy and infertility are the two major sequelae. Patients who have suffered one attack have an increased risk of further episodes. Infertility can result in 10–20% of cases after one episode, rising to 60% or more after three or more episodes[33]. Invasion by the gonococci through to the bloodstream results in disseminated gonococcal infection (DGI) which can present with skin purpura or arthritis, although only some patients have a high fever. Many isolates from DGI have shared characteristics. They have a growth requirement for arginine, hypoxanthine and uracil[34], are hypersensitive to penicillin[35], resistant to killing by normal human serum[36], and have a tendency to form transparent colonies. DGI is more common in women and appears to occur either at or close to the menstrual period or during pregnancy. *N. gonorrhoeae* which form transparent colonies are isolated more frequently from the cervix, particularly at menstruation, suggesting hormones are a factor in exerting a selective pressure. Patients with a deficiency in one of the terminal components of complement, C5, C6, C7 or C8 are prone to systemic infection with Neisseria species whether *N. gonorrhoeae* or *N. meningitidis*[37,38].

The risk of transmission of infection from women to men is not clear, but has been reported to be 5% and 22% and to be greater with an increased numbers of partners or sexual exposure[39,40]. There is no reliable information on the inoculum required to cause infection, but in volunteer studies the percentage of men infected increased with inoculum size[41]. The risk of infection from men to women has been reported to vary from 50–90%[42], but no volunteer studies are possible because of the problems with sequelae. The number of gonococci present in the vagina of infected women was studied by Lowe and Kraus[43] using saline washouts and found to vary between 4.0×10^2 and 1.8×10^7. The infective dose required and the numbers of gonococci colonizing the genital tract remains largely conjectural.

Gonococcal infection occurs in two stages, attachment to the mucosa to prevent removal by the mucus stream and invasion of the epithelial cell through to the lamina propia. The initial step in attachment is to bring both the bacterial and host cell into close proximity as they are both negatively charged. Non-specific factors such as surface charge, hydrophobic interactions and pH may be important in achieving this initial association[44] which is followed by adherence to the epithelial cells by specific surface structures, primarily pili and the outer membrane protein (OMP), PII. It has been demonstrated in human fallopian tube tissue cultures that the gonococci adhere to the non-ciliated epithelial cells although it is the ciliated cells that become damaged and slough off[45]. This effect may be caused by the toxic effects of the gonococcal lipopolysaccharide[46]. In this system, the gonococci then become endocytosed by the cell where they multiply and are eventually excreted into the lamina propia, setting up a submucosal infection. There is increasing evidence that the OMP, PI, facilitates entry into the host cell[47].

IMMUNE RESPONSE

The use of sensitive detection systems has demonstrated gonococcal antibody in patients as a response to mucosal infection. There has, however, been little or no evidence of antibody preventing infection. This may be just a reflection of the ability of the gonococcus to present different antigens when it encounters protective antibody produced during a previous infection.

If the presence of antibody is to play a role in modifying the course of infection it must primarily interfere with attachment and colonization at the mucosal surface. In urethral exudates from men, IgA, IgG and to a lesser extent IgM have been detected[48-50]. Of these antibodies IgA is the first to decline after therapy, whereas IgG can still be detected 28 days later[50]. This is probably because IgG has a halflife of 42 days compared with only a few days for IgA. IgM is believed to be a rapid, short-lived response to infection. The collection of suitable mucosal samples from men, particularly convalescent, is extremely difficult, and, therefore, such results should be interpreted with caution.

In women, gonorrhoea is mainly an infection of the cervical epithelium, but saline vaginal washings collected through a speculum which contain some cervical secretion are generally used for antibody studies. The total of IgG and IgA have been shown to be present in a ratio of 2:1 in both cervical secretions[51] and vaginal washings[52], the IgA being preferentially secreted by plasma cells found mainly in the lamina propia of the endocervix[53]. Gonococcal IgG and IgA have both been found in various studies, but IgM only occasionally[52,54,55]. The antigens which stimulate an antibody response have been shown by Western blotting to be pili, lipopolysaccharide (LPS)[52,56] and the outer membrane proteins, PI and PII[56], all of which are major surface antigens. The specificity of the mucosal antibody response has been shown to vary over a 2-week-period after therapy[52]. It is not known whether this is caused by differences in the concentration of antibody between samples, or to new antigens being released by degrading bacteria stimulating a different response. In several studies the mucosal antibody response has been found to be of a lower intensity than the systemic response[52,56]. This may reflect a lower concentration of antibody or antibody being withdrawn into immune complexes and so being unavailable for detection. There is very little information on immune complexes in gonorrhoea.

Despite these findings little is known of the function of mucosal antibody. Tramont et al.[57] studied a single patient in whom vaginal secretions were adsorbed with purified pili, outer membrane complexes (OMC) and LPS. Only adsorption with pili and OMCs, but not LPS, altered the ability of the antibody to inhibit attachment of gonococci to epithelial cells in vitro.

Indirect evidence has been demonstrated by the ability of mucosal antibody, produced after vaccination of male volunteers with purified pili, to inhibit attachment[58]. In addition, the number of gonococci required to produce infection is increased in these volunteers, which suggests that the pili antibody has modified colonization[59].

The systemic response has been studied in considerably greater detail both because of the ease of obtaining sera and because the greater intensity of the response allows for easier detection. However, much of this work was initially directed towards increasing the specificity and sensitivity of antibody tests for screening populations. There is overwhelming evidence that infected patients have increased levels of serum IgG, IgM and IgA, and that the IgA is secretory[60] which implies absorption from the mucosa. Sera from patients with both disseminated and uncomplicated gonorrhoea contain antibodies directed against pili[61] and LPS[62,63], but antibody to PI appears to be more prevalent in disseminated infection[62,63]. Experiments designed to detect different subclasses of IgG in sera from women with uncomplicated gonorrhoea or pelvic inflammatory disease have shown IgG_1 antibodies were directed mainly to pili and IgG_3 antibodies to pili and LPS. Very little IgG_2 was detected against gonococcal antigens (Crabtree, L. and Ison, C. A., unpublished observations). The studies of the specificity of the immune response have used a variety of techniques, most of which give relative differences in the amounts of antibody but do not give true quantitative differences. The source of antigen in these studies may also influence the results. Laboratory adapted strains have been used, but because of the antigenic heterogeneity shown by the gonococcus it may be better to use the patient's infecting strain. The results obtained by these two antigens may, therefore, not be identical.

Men with gonorrhoea appear to have less serum antibody than women. The majority of men are symptomatic and treated within 3–7 days of infection, whereas female infections are commonly of a longer duration, and this could affect both the intensity and nature of the antibody response.

In mucosal infections the gonococcal antibody found in the serum is assumed to be absorbed from the mucosa, and is without a primary function in modifying the host's defence against gonorrhoea. However, natural (see below) and immune antibodies may protect against the systemic spread of gonococci by activating the complement pathway, resulting in cell death. The classical pathway of C1, 4, 2 and 3, appears to be more important than the alternative pathway in which C3 is activated by properdin[64]. It is the late acting component C9 which attacks the membrane causing holes and subsequent lysis, hence the susceptibility to neisserial infection of patients who lack C9 or the precursors in the cascade C5a, 6, 7 and 8. In order for gonococci to spread systemically they need to avoid this bactericidal activity of serum. Gonococci isolated from disseminated infection are, not surprisingly, resistant to serum killing[65,66]. Of the major surface antigens, lipopolysaccharide is the dominant cell component involved in serum resistance[67,68]. This has recently been supported by evidence that a genetic locus involved in LPS structure[69] appears identical with one of the loci which influence serum susceptibility, sac-3[70]. Resistance to killing is also believed to be associated with a surface component which binds non-immune human IgG. The bound IgG then blocks the antigen(s) involved in the activation of the classical complement pathway. The main antigens involved appear to be PI[71] and PIII[72].

Gonococcal antibody is known to be opsonic and enhance the uptake of gonococci by polymorphonuclear cells (PMN) presumably leading to intracellular killing. IgG or IgM antibodies can attach to gonococci and then activate the complement pathway. This results in the presence of C3b fragments on the gonococcal membrane which are recognized by receptors on the PMNs thereby initiating the phagocytic process. The evidence for this has been obtained using immune or non-immune sera and PMN from non-infected individuals[73]. It must be remembered that phagocytic killing is not as important as the bactericidal activity of serum in protection against systemic infection and, therefore, care should be taken in comparing the *in vitro* results with the situation in the mucosal infection. Pili and the OMP, PII, are believed to have antiphagocytic functions, but, as yet, the mechanisms are not fully understood[73].

Gonococci are known to be killed by natural cytotoxity and antibody-dependent cell-mediated cytotoxic mechanisms[74]. These results were obtained using non-immune human peripheral mononuclear cells and immune sera. Gonococci are mucosal pathogens and, therefore, these results will need to be repeated using mucosal antibody and mononuclear cells.

VACCINES

Production of antibody in response to a vaccine has been considered as an alternative or supplement to chemotherapy because of the persistance of gonococcal infection despite adequate therapy and control measures. It is not feasible to use such a vaccine to protect the whole population, but it could be targeted at high risk groups, such as homosexual men with a large number of partners, military personnel, patients with repeated infection and prostitutes. However, it has been recommended that the first priority of a vaccine should be the prevention of pelvic inflammatory disease, because of both the sequelae and economic consequences[75]. Prevention of asymptomatic infection in males would be the second aim.

With these priorities in mind, the question arises whether an animal model is necessary or suitable for testing potential vaccines or, if human volunteers are essential, which group should be used. Animal models for experimental infection with gonorrhoea have been studied using a range of animals including chick embryos, mice and chimpanzees[76-80]. The insertion of plastic chambers in guinea pigs has provided much useful information on potential virulence determinants[81,82]. However, it is still not possible to reproduce a model of genital infection of gonorrhoea in any animal including the chimpanzee. Man is the only natural host and reservoir for *N. gonorrhoeae*, and even the chimpanzee has some increased resistance. A suitable alternative to animal models would be the use of human fallopian tube organ culture[83,84], which has been used so successfully in studies of pathogenesis[85]. However, establishing this technique is technically demanding and has only been achieved in a few centres. The use of endocervical organ cultures may be more relevant but needs further characterization.

Potential vaccines will, therefore, need to be tested in human volunteers, preferably adolescent women. This will probably only be feasible in countries where prostitution is legal and organized in order to produce a high prevalence population that can be effectively monitored. In the absence of this population, candidate vaccines have and could be tested in male volunteers. The aim would be to demonstrate an increase in the infective dose required for urethral infection to occur. A potential vaccine should show protection in this manner against both the homologous strain used for production of the vaccine and heterologous strains.

Gonorrhoea is primarily an infection of mucosal surfaces, and consequently the aim of any vaccine should be to prevent colonization by interrupting the mechanisms by which gonococci adhere, invade and cause inflammation. The antibody produced by a vaccine that will achieve this function will need to be produced at the mucosal surface. Antibody has been demonstrated in volunteer experiments with potential vaccines but this has often been systemic rather than mucosal. The relationship between the types and functions of the two antibodies is still unclear, and more emphasis needs to be given both to the study of mucosal immunity and the monitoring of its presence during vaccine trials. It is not known whether the production of protective immunity to more than one strain is possible or which class or isotype of antibody is required. Indirect evidence of protection was obtained by Buchanan et al.[86] who demonstrated that women with salpingitis did not become re-infected with gonococci of the same serotype.

Candidates which have been considered for a vaccine are mainly situated on the outer surface of the gonococcus as this is in contact with the host's immune response. Most attention has centred on the use of pili because they are the primary mediators of attachment. Kellogg showed in 1963[87] that piliated, but not non-piliated, gonococci could infect male volunteers and this was the first indication that pili were a major virulence factor. Pili are proteinaceous surface appendages, 6 nm in diameter and 1–4 μm in length and consist of up to 10000 identical subunits, termed pilin. Pili are invariably found on fresh clinical isolates but are lost on repeated subcultures[88]. This phase variation from piliated to non-piliated occurs at high frequency, but the reverse occurs less frequently[89]. A number of antigenically different pili have been described in vitro[90,91] which are thought to help evade the host's immune response in vivo[92] and possibly confer specificity for different mucosal surfaces[93].

Purified pili from a single strain have been used both in volunteer[41] and clinical trials[94]. Homologous antibody was demonstrated but the vaccine did not protect a large number of men when given parenterally. Pili have been shown to have conserved and variable sequences which in the intact molecule are immunorecessive and immunodominant, respectively[95]. The use of whole purified pili will produce antibody to the immunodominant portion of the molecule which is responsible for antigenic variation and, therefore, it is not surprising that protection to heterologous strains was not produced. Recent work has shown that synthetic peptides spanning common, normally immunorecessive regions of the pilus will produce polyclonal antibody that can inhibit attachment of both homologous and heterologous gonococci to epithelial cells *in vitro*[96]. A vaccine to a common pilin peptide may be a real possibility.

The outer membrane protein, PI, has been the second candidate studied for a vaccine. It is a major constituent of the outer membrane, approximately 60% of the total weight and has been shown to act as a porin, probably when complexed with PIII[97]. More recently it has been demonstrated that PI has the ability to transfer from the gonococcal membrane into erythrocyte ghosts and lipid bilayers[47]. It is possible that this insertion into eukaryotic membranes is important in the internalization of gonococci by epithelial cells, and, therefore, antibody to PI could be important in mucosal infection by preventing this process. Purified PI is weakly immunogenic, and the amount of antibody produced relates directly to the amount of antigen given[86]. However, PI remains a potential candidate for a vaccine because it is the predominant protein in the cell envelope and only a limited number of serotypes exist. Conserved epitopes have been demonstrated on both PrIA and PrIB molecules, and monoclonal antibodies raised to these epitopes were protective in bactericidal and opsonic assays *in vitro*[98,99]. It should, therefore, be possible to use these portions of the molecule as vaccines and theoretically induce protection in the host against a large number of strains.

The OMP, PII, is another surface exposed protein whose presence enhances the attachment of gonococci to epithelial cells and which is known to be immunogenic in the natural infection[56]. PII is a family of heat modifiable proteins of molecular weight 24–32000 with 0–6 different PIIs expressed in a single strain[97]. Gonococci have the ability to switch the expression of PII on or off (phase variation) or change the species of PII (antigenic variation) both occurring at high frequency[89]. The antigenic diversity of this group of proteins may help the gonococcus evade the host's immune response or confer tissue tropism. However, it is this variability that has limited its potential as a vaccine candidate. PIIs are thought to have conserved common peptides, but these are probably buried in the membrane, and it is the unique peptides, responsible for antigenic variation, that are surface exposed[100]. If the conserved region of PII produces antibody in the host which could be shown to interfere with colonization, it may then become a more serious vaccine candidate.

Since an effective vaccine has not been produced, the search continues for an antigen that is conserved within and between strains and to which antibody is produced during an infection. In recent years a number of proteins have emerged that fulfil these criteria, including the OMP, PIII; antigen H8: the 37 kD iron-regulated protein and anaerobically expressed proteins. PIII has been the best studied of these proteins. It is characterized by its ability to change molecular weight in the presence of a reducing agent, and has been found in all strains tested[97]. The antigen H8 was first identified by its reactivity with a monoclonal antibody, its presence having not previously been evident on SDS-polyacrylamide gels[101]. It is a heat modifiable protein, of MW 20–21000, which has been demonstrated in all strains of *N. gonorrhoeae* and *N. meningitidis* and in some strains of *N.*

lactamica tested but whose function is unknown.

There is much interest in the iron-regulated[102] and anaerobic proteins[103] which are expressed under conditions thought to be closer to the environment *in vivo*. Antibodies have been demonstrated to these proteins in patients although their function is as yet unknown[104,105]. IgA_1 protease, which is an enzyme produced by the pathogenic, but not commensal neisseriae, splits antibodies of the IgA_1 subclass[106] and has also been considered. IgA antibodies have been detected in vaginal secretions of infected patients, and hence production of this protease has led to the belief that it is a virulence determinant. Its role in the pathogenesis of gonorrhoea is still unproven but it remains a potential antigen probably within a multivalent vaccine.

DETECTION OF ANTIBODY

There has been a continual search for a serological test for gonorrhoea to detect antibody in patient's serum. Such a test has the potential of overcoming the problems of culture, of avoiding the necessity for pelvic examination in women and of screening large populations. Culture still provides the definitive diagnosis of gonorrhoea, although the sensitivity is influenced by the quality and transport of the specimen and by the prevalence of strains of *N. gonorrhoeae* sensitive to vancomycin, an antibiotic used in selective culture media. The sensitivity of culture is believed to be between 80 and 90%[107,108] but can fall as low as 40%[109]. Culture requires the collection of specimens by trained personnel and in women, a pelvic examination. A serological test would need a blood sample which could be obtained by less qualified staff and repeat samples could be collected more easily. It would be particularly useful in people who would not normally be cultured for *N. gonorrhoeae*, such as in ante-natal or family planning clinics. Asymptomatic reservoirs, which are believed to be important in the spread of gonorrhoea, may be identified by such a screening method.

However, the ideal serological test for gonorrhoea remains elusive. A successful test is dependent on three main factors, sensitivity, (a positive result in patients with gonorrhoea), specificity, (a negative result in patients without gonorrhoea) and the prevalence of gonococcal infection in the population, which directly effects the predictive values*[110]. If a test is to be useful in

---

Sensitivity, specificity and predictive value

$$\text{Sensitivity} = \frac{\text{Number of 'infected' patients with positive test}}{\text{Total number of 'infected' patients tested}} \times 100$$

$$\text{Specificity} = \frac{\text{Number of 'non-infected' patients with negative test}}{\text{Total number of 'non-infected' patients tested}} \times 100$$

Predictive value of a positive test:
$$\frac{\text{Number of 'infected' patients with positive test}}{\text{Total number of patients with a positive test}} \times 100$$

Predictive value of a negative test:
$$\frac{\text{Number of 'non-infected' patients with a negative test}}{\text{Total number of patients with a negative test}} \times 100$$

screening populations where the prevalence is low, the sensitivity and specificity must be greater than 90%. For example, if the prevalence is 1% and the sensitivity and specificity are 95% the predictive value of a positive test would be 16%, but in a population with a prevalence of 5% the predictive value would be 50%. A large number of gonococcal infections would be missed in both these instances, but of greater concern is the number of false positives that would be found. with a specificity of 95% for every 1000 people screened who do not have gonorrhoea, 50 would give a false positive result. This is unacceptable for the diagnosis of a sexually transmitted infection. It is possible that a serological test could be used to reduce the number of patients who need to be screened by culture, but the emotive aspects associated with recalling and examining low-risk patients also make this approach difficult. It has been suggested that the lack of specificity might be overcome by the use of two unrelated antigens used in parallel[111]. A true positive serum would react with both antigens, whereas a false positive with only one.

Two problems are associated with designing a serological test, the choice of a suitable antigen which will detect antibody directed only to the infecting organism but that is shared by all strains and a convenient and sensitive detection system.

The choice of antigen is particularly difficult in gonorrhoea because the gonococcus has diverse antigens and yet has common antigens with other species of Neisseria especially *N. meningitidis*. Consequently, a number of antigens have been used including whole bacteria, lipopolysaccharide, pili and outer membrane extracts. Complement fixation tests were the first to be used as systems of detection, but these have now been superseded by the more sensitive techniques of immunofluorescence, enzyme-linked and radio-immunoassay.

Complement fixation tests used whole bacteria either from a number of strains[112,113] or a single strain[114], and had the advantage of providing all the surface antigens simultaneously. The sensitivity of these tests was low in uncomplicated infection, ranging from 10 to 50% even in high-risk populations. However, in complicated infections, the sensitivity was relatively high, approximately 60%, and in the absence of an alternative, the test was used in this context for many years. The specificity was high, 91–100%, when the control sera were obtained from patients attending sexually transmitted disease clinics. Whole cells of *N. gonorrhoeae* strain 9 have been used in indirect immunofluorescence (IIF) tests[115,116]. This particular strain was used because it is reported to have antigens common to most strains of gonococci but none which cross-react with other species of Neisseria[117]. This test gave very promising results particularly for the detection of IgG antibodies, with sensitivities of 98–100% and specificities of 92–94% in different populations. However, it was not recommended for the diagnosis of patients with a past history of gonorrhoea.

An enzyme-linked immunosorbent assay (ELISA) using whole gonococci attached to microtitre trays with poly-L-lysine was developed to detect IgG antibodies[118]. Although the sensitivity of this assay is much lower than the IIF it does not detect antibodies from previous infections, and might, therefore, have greater diagnostic potential.The ELISA may be improved by careful choice of a single strain or the use of a number of different strains.

The use of a purified antigen was tried in order to attempt to overcome the detection of cross-reactive antibodies to other commensal neisseriae and Gram-negative organisms. Of the potentially useful antigens, pili have been used most often and the antibodies have been detected using ELISA[119,120], radio-immunoassay (RIA)[121,122] and indirect haemagglutination[123]. The results show that pili from a single strain are unlikely to detect antibody in more than 80% of infected patients and that pili isolated from a selection of strains are more successful. This latter approach was used by Reimann et al.[124] and had a sensitivity of 82% in women and 59% in men with a specificity of 77% in the control group. Lipopolysaccharide[125-127] and outer membrane extracts[60,128] have been used as semi-purified antigens, but as with pili provide no real advantage over whole bacteria.

Many of the antibody tests for gonorrhoea have presented similar problems. Host factors influence the level of the response, including sex, race and history of previous infection. In quantitative assays a marked overlap is always seen between infected and non-infected patients which creates difficulty in defining the end-point for a positive test. If the level is set too high, too many infected patients will be missed, and if it is set too low, too many false-positives will be obtained.

The search for a serological test for gonorrhoea is now in abeyance. The low sensitivities, specificities and predictive values have shown them to be unacceptable in low prevalence populations and of limited use in complicated infections. The only current need for a serological test is to monitor the antibody produced in response to a potential vaccine.

USE OF ANTIBODY

Despite the lack of success in using patient's antibody for the diagnosis of gonorrhoea, polyclonal and monoclonal antibodies have been raised to gonococcal antigens with the aim of improving the detection, identification and serological classification of *N. gonorrhoeae*.

Gonococcal infections are diagnosed by the Gram stain, showing the presence of intracellular Gram-negative cocci, and culture of *N. gonorrhoeae*. The Gram stain is used to give a rapid presumptive diagnosis and to ensure appropriate therapy, whereas culture is used for confirmation and is regarded as the definitive diagnosis. The sensitivity of Gram stain compared to culture in men with a urethral discharge is high, greater than 98%, but in women and asymptomatic men falls to 40–50%[129-131]. Culture on media such as New York City medium requires up to 48 hours incubation, and the subsequent identification and antibiotic susceptibility testing a further 24 hours.

Polyclonal and monoclonal antibodies have been used to develop tests to detect gonococcal antigens in clinical samples to provide an alternative to the standard methods. An ELISA using a polyvalent antiserum to *N. gonorrhoeae* (Gonozyme: Abbott Labs) has been evaluated by many workers. Urethral and cervical samples are immersed in a storage fluid which is then added to beads onto which the gonococci and gonococcal antigens are adsorbed. Rabbit anti-gonococcal antibody is added, and any antigen/

antibody complexes formed are detected by goat antibody to rabbit immunoglobulin conjugated to horseradish peroxidase. A peroxidase substrate is added and colour development read photometrically. The intensity of the colour is directly related to the amount of gonococcal antigen in the original sample.

In comparison with culture, this test has a sensitivity between 87–100% and a specificity of 99.4–100% in symptomatic men[131–141]. Although the sensitivity is high it is difficult to imagine a role for this test in the routine diagnosis of gonorrhoea in men because the Gram stain is relatively inexpensive, will give a result while the patient waits and gives comparable results to the ELISA in experienced hands.

In women, the sensitivity and specificity are lower than in men, and there are greater discrepancies between results from different groups[133–137,140,141]. Gonococci detected by culture, but not ELISA, could be caused by inadequate specimen collection or to low numbers of organisms. However, the number of specimens giving a false-positive result in the ELISA is perhaps of more concern. The culture may be negative because of poor specimen collection or to the failure of the organism to grow on selective culture media[142]. The ELISA will detect non-viable gonococci persisting in the genital tract after therapy which would account for some false-positives, and thus makes it unsuitable as a test of cure[135]. However, it seems probable that many of the false-positives are due to cross-reacting antigens on the resident microbial flora[132]. As discussed before if the specificity is not very high the number of false-positives in a low prevalence population would be alarmingly high. Monoclonal antibodies raised to the major outer membrane protein, PI, have been used in a direct immunofluorescence (IF) test for gonococcal antigen[143]. In men, this test again offered no advantage over the Gram stain. In women, the specificity was high and the sensitivity was 72% and 88% after testing single and duplicate cervical smears, respectively. This reagent offered a considerable improvement on the use of the Gram stain for rapid diagnosis, but the sensitivity was not high enough to replace culture, and it is not yet commercially available.

Both the ELISA and IF systems aimed to replace culture as the definitive diagnosis for male and female gonorrhoea. However, their greatest potential is to replace the Gram stain for the rapid, presumptive diagnosis of gonorrhoea in women where infection is often asymptomatic and the Gram stain has a low sensitivity.

Antibody has been used more successfully in the identification of *N-gonorrhoeae* in the laboratory. Both polyclonal and monoclonal antibodies have been used in co-agglutination reagents[144]. Staphylococci rich in protein A bind IgG subclasses 1, 2 and 4 non-specifically by the Fc portion. If staphylococci coated with gonococcal antibodies are then mixed with a boiled suspension of gonococci, visible agglutination results. This test was originally developed using polyclonal antibodies raised in rabbits, but gave problems of specificity reacting with some strains from other species of Neisseria. The newer monoclonal reagent, however, has a high sensitivity (97%) and specificity (97%). A number of commercial reagents are available (Phadebact, Pharmacia: Gonogen, New Horizons) and have replaced carbohydrate utilization tests in some laboratories because of their ease of use and reliability.

A similar approach has used a fluorescent label attached to the gonococcal antibody, but commercially available reagents using polyclonal antibodies were never fully specific and consequently were seldom used. Monoclonal antibodies have only recently been included into this type of reagent (GC Microtrak: Syva, USA) but it has resulted in a greater specificity and sensitivity[145].

Monoclonal antibodies have the potential to overcome the major problems of false-positives encountered with polyclonal antibodies so that more of these rapid immunologically based tests are likely to become available.

Antibodies have been used in attempts to produce a serological typing scheme for *N. gonorrhoeae*. It has proved very difficult to produce good reproducible typing schemes that have sufficient discrimination to enable epidemiological studies to be carried out. Auxotyping has been used extensively[146], but of the 35 types described only four are common. Serological typing schemes have centred on antibodies raised to the outer membrane protein, PI. In a micro-immunofluorescence system using polyclonal antibodies Wang et al.[147] divided gonococci into three groups A, B and C. A co-agglutination system divided gonococci into three analogous groups designated WI, WII and WIII, and thus provided a rapid and inexpensive technique of serotyping[148]. An ELISA serotyping system which was more complex and time consuming to use, recognized nine serotypes, serotypes 1, 2 and 3 corresponding to WI, serotypes 4, 5, 6 and 7 to WII, and serotype 9 to WIII[149]. Serotype 8 strains belonged predominately to serogroup WII, but a few strains belong to WIII. Peptide mapping of protein I showed two biochemical types existed, IA and IB, corresponding to serogroups WI and WII/WIII, respectively[150]. Monoclonal antibodies raised to epitopes on PrIA and PrIB have been used to create a standard panel of 12 antibodies to produce a serotyping scheme that is reproducible and has good discrimination[151]. Bygdeman et al.[152,153] have used a similar approach with a greater number of antibodies. Discrimination can be enhanced by combining auxotyping and serotyping, two genetically distinct characteristics, to give auxotype/serovar (A/S) classes. These systems are currently being used to distinguish between treatment failures and re-infection, to identify mixed infection, to monitor antibiotic resistance and to help choose relevant strains for the production of a vaccine. The reagents are available internationally, and consequently it is now possible to monitor movement of strains on a global basis.

CONCLUSION

There has been a considerable interest in the pathogenesis and immunology of gonococcal infections during the last decade, mainly directed at producing an effective vaccine. However, the gonococcus has proved to be more difficult and interesting than expected. It continues to evolve and adapt itself to evade both the host's immune response and our efforts to provide adequate control measures. The suitable vaccine remains elusive, but will be needed in the future if the gonococcus continues developing antibiotic resistance. The only way forward to such a vaccine is a full understanding of the immune response and its role in modifying colonisation.

ACKNOWLEDGEMENTS

I would like to thank N. Woodford for his help and encouragement in the preparation of this chapter and G. Hadfield for her contributions.

References

1. Judson, F. N. (1983). Fear of AIDS and gonorrhoea rates in homosexual men. *Lancet*, **2**, 159

2. Schultz, S., Firedman, S., Kristal, A., and Sencer, D. J. (1984). Declining rates of rectal and pharyngeal gonorrhoea - New York City. *MMWR*, **33**, 295

3. Gellan, M. C. A. and Ison, C. A. (1986). Declining incidence of gonorrhoea in London: A response to the fear of AIDS. *Lancet*, **2**, 920

4. Krogh von, G., Hellstrom, L. and Bottinger, M. (1986). Declining incidence of syphilis among homosexual men in Stockholm. *Lancet*, **2**, 920-1

5. Zenilman, J. M., Cates, W. and Morse, S. A. (1986). *Neisseria gonorrhoeae:* An old enemy rearms. *Infectious and Medical Disease Letters for Obstetrics and Gynecology*, **VIII**, Suppl., 2-9

6. Osoba, A. O. (1981). Sexually transmitted diseases in tropical Africa: a review of the present situation. *Br. J. Vener, Dis.*, **57**, 89-94

7. Donegan, E. A. (1985). Epidemiology of gonococcal infection. In Brooks, G. F. and Donegan, E. A. (eds.). *Gonococcal Infection*, pp. 181-198. (London: Edward Arnold)

8. Reyn, A. (1963). Current problems in the diagnosis and therapy of gonorrhoea from a laboratory point of view. *Acta Dermatol. Venerol.*, **43**, 380-93

9. Faruki, H., Kohmescher, R. N., McKinney, D. and Sparling, P. F. (1985). A community based outbreak of infection with penicillin resistant *Neisseria gonorrhoeae* not producing penicillinase (chromosomally mediated resistance). *N. Engl. J. Med.*, **313**, 607-11

10. Rice, R. J., Biddle, J. W., Jean Louis, Y. A., DeWitt, W. E., Blount, J. H. and Morse, S. A. (1986). Chromosomally mediated resistance in *Neisseria gonorrhoeae* in the United States: Results of surveillance and reporting, 1983-1984. *J. Infect. Dis.*, **153**, 340-5

11. Ison, C. A., Gedney, J. and Easmon, C. S. F. (1987). Chromosomal resistance of gonococci to antibiotics. *Genitourin. Med.*, **63**, 239-43

12. Cannon, J. G. and Sparling, P. F. (1984). The genetics of the gonococcus. *Annu. Rev. Microbiol.*, **38**, 111-33

13. Dougherty, T. J., Koller, A. E. and Tomasz, A. (1980). Penicillin-binding proteins of penicillin-susceptible and intrinsically resistant *Neisseria gonorrhoeae*. *Antimicrob. Agents Chemother.*, **18**, 730-7

14. Barbour, A. G. (1981). Properties of penicillin-binding proteins in *Neisseria gonorrhoeae*. *Antimicrob. Agents Chemother.*, **19**, 316-22

15. Phillips, I. (1976). B-lactamase producing penicillin-resistant gonococcus. *Lancet*, **2**, 656-7

16. Percival, A., Corkhill, J. E., Ayra, O. P., Rowlands, J., Alergant, C. D., Rees, E. and Annels, E. H. (1976). Penicillinase producing gonococci in Liverpool. *Lancet*, **2**, 1379-82

17. Ashford, W. A., Golash, R. G. and Hemming, V. A. (1976). Penicillinase producing *Neisseria gonorrhoeae. Lancet*, **2**, 657-8

18. Brunton, J., Clare, D. and Meier, M. A. (1986). Molecular epidemiology of antibiotic resistance plasmids of *Haemophilus* species and *Neisseria gonorrhoeae*. *Rev. Infect. Dis.*, **8**, 713-24

19. Embden, J. D. A. van, Desssens-Kroon, M. and van Kilingeren, B. (1985). A new B-lactamase plasmid in *Neisseria gonorrhoeae*. *J. Antimicrobial Chemother.*, **15**, 247-50

20. McCutchan, J. A., Adler, M. W. and Berrie, J. R. H. (1982). Penicillinase-producing *Neisseria gonorrhoeae* in Great Britain 1977-81: alarming increase in incidence and recent development of endemic transmission. *Br. Med. J.*, **285**, 337-40

21. Center for Disease Control. (1987). Antibiotic-resistant strains of *Neisseria gonorrhoeae*. *MMWR*, **36** (Suppl. 55), 1–18
22. Jaffe, H. W., Biddle, J. W., Johnson, S. R. and Wiesner, P. J. (1981). Infections due to penicillinase-producing *Neisseria gonorrhoeae* in the United States. 1976–1980. *J. Infect. Dis.*, **144**, 191–7
23. Brown, S., Warninissorn, T., Biddle, J., Panikabutra, K. and Traisupa, A. (1982). Antimicrobial resistance of *Neisseria gonorrhoeae* in Bangkok: is single-drug treatment passe. *Lancet*, **2**, 1366–8
24. Ison, C. A., Littleton, K., Shannon, K. P., Easmon, C. S. F. and Phillips, I. (1983). Spectinomycin resistant gonococci. *Br. Med. J.*, **287**, 1827–9
25. Ashford, W. A., Potts, D. W., Adams, H. J. U., English, J. C., Johnson, S. R., Biddle, J. W., Thornsberry, C. and Jaffe, H. W. (1981). Spectinomycin-resistant penicillinase producing *Neisseria gonorrhoeae*. *Lancet*, **2**, 1035–7
26. Center for Disease Control. (1983). Spectinomycin-resistant-penicillinase-producing *Neisseria gonorrhoeae*. *MMWR*, **32**, 51
27. Piziak, M. V., Woodbury, C., Berliner, D., Takafuji, E., Kirkpatrick, J., Opal, S. and Tramont, E. (1984). Resistant trends of *Neisseria gonorrhoeae* in the Republic of Korea. *Antimicrob. Agents Chemother*, **25**, 7–9
28. Knapp, J. S., Zenilman, J. M., Biddle, J. W., Perkins, G. H., DeWitt, W. E., Thomas, M. L., Johnson, S. R. and Morse, S. A. (1987). Frequency and distributions in the United States of *Neisseria gonorrhoeae* with plasmid-mediated, high-level resistance to tetracycline. *J. Infect. Dis.*, **155**, 819–22
29. Morse, S. A., Johnson, S. R., Biddle, J. W. and Roberts, M. C. (1986). High-level tetracycline resistance in *Neisseria gonorrhoeae* is result of acquisition of streptococcal *tetM* determinant. *Antimicrob. Agents Chemother.*, **30**, 664–70
30. Handsfield, H. H., Lipman, T. D., Harnisch, J. P., Tronca, E. and Holmes, K. K. (1974). Asymptomatic gonorrhoea in men: diagnosis, natural course, prevalence and significance. *N. Engl. J. Med.*, **290**, 117–23
31. McCormack, W. M. (1981). Clinical spectrum of infection with *Neisseria gonorrhoeae*. *Sex. Transm. Dis.*, **8**, 305–7
32. Eschenbach, D. A. and Holmes, K. K. (1979). The etiology of acute pelvic inflammatory disease. *Sex. Transm. Dis.*, **6**, 244–7
33. Westrom, L. (1980). Incidence, prevalence, and trends of acute pelvic inflammatory disease and its consequences in industrialised countries. *Am. J. Obstet. Gynecol.*, **138**, 880–92
34. Knapp, J. S. and Holmes, K. K. (1975). Disseminated gonocóccal infections caused by *Neisseria gonorrhoeae* with unique nutritional requirements. *J. Infect. Dis.*, **132**, 204–8
35. Weisner, P. J., Handsfield, H. H. and Holmes, K. K. (1973). Low antibiotic resistance of gonococci causing disseminated infection. *N. Engl. J. Med.*, **228**, 1221–2
36. Schoolnik, G. K., Buchanan, T. M. and Holmes, K. K. (1976). Gonococci causing disseminated gonococcal infection are resistant to the bactericidal action of normal human sera. *J. Clin. Invest.*, **58**, 1163–73
37. Petersen, B. H., Lee, T. J., Snyderman, R. and Brooks, G. F. (1979). *Neisseria meningitidis* and *Neisseria gonorrhoeae* bacteremia associated with C6, C7 or C8 deficiency. *Ann. Intern. Med.*, **90**, 917–20
38. Lee, T. J., Utsinger, P. D., Snyderman, R., Yount, W. J. and Sparling, P. F. (1978). Familial deficiency of the seventh component of complement associated with recurrent bacteremic infections due to *Neisseria*. *J. Infect. Dis.*, **138**, 359–68
39. Holmes, K. K. (1973). Gonococcal infection: clinical, epidemiologic and laboratory prospectives. *Adv. Int. Med.*, **19**, 259–85
40. Holmes, K. K., Johnson, D. W. and Trostle, H. J. (1970). An estimate of the risk of men acquiring gonorrhoea by sexual contact with infected females. *Am. J. Epidemiol.*, **108**, 136–44
41. Brinton, C. C., Bryan, J., Dillon, J-A., Guerina, N., Jacobson, L. J., Labik, A., Simon, L., Levine, A., Lim, S., McMichael, J., Polen, S., Rogers, K., To, A. C-. C. and To, S. C-. M. (1978). Uses of pili in gonorrhoea control: Role of bacterial pili in disease, purification and properties of gonococcal pili and progress in the development of a gonococcal pilus vaccine for gonorrhoea. In Brooks, G. F., Gotschlich, E. C., Holmes, K. K., Sawyer, W. D. and Young, F. E. (eds.). *Immunobiology of Neisseria gonorrhoeae*, pp. 155–78 (Washington,

DC: American Society of Microbiology)
42. Wright, D. J. M. and Daunt, O. (1973). How infectious is gonorrhoea? *Lancet*, **1**, 208
43. Lowe, T. L. and Kraus, S. J. (1976). Quantitation of *Neisseria gonorrhoeae* from women with gonorrhoea. *J. Infect. Dis.*, **133**, 621-6
44. Watt, P. J. and Ward, M. E. (1980). Adherence of *Neisseria gonorrhoeae* and other *Neisseria* species to mammalian cells. In Beachey, E. H. (ed.). *Receptors and Recognition, Bacterial Adherence*, Vol. B6, pp. 251-88 (London: Chapman and Hall)
45. McGee, Z. A., Melly, M. A., Gregg, C. R., Horn, R. G., Taylor-Robinson, D., Johnson, A. P. and McCutchan, J. A. (1978). Virulence factors of gonococci: studies using human fallopian tube organ cultures. In Brooks, G. F., Gotschlich, E. C., Holmes, K. K., Sawyer, W. D. and Young, F. E. (eds.). *Immunobiology of Neisseria gonorrhoeae*, pp. 258-62 (Washington, DC: American Society of Microbiology)
46. Gregg, C. R., Johnson, A. P., Taylor-Robinson, D., Melly, A. and McGee, Z. A. (1981). Host species specific damage to oviduct mucosa by *Neisseria gonorrhoeae* lipopolysaccharide. *Infect. Immun.*, **34**, 1056-8
47. Blake, M. S. (1985). Implications of the active role of gonococcal porins in disease. In Schoolnik, G. K. (ed.). *The Pathogenic Neisseriae*, pp. 251-8 (Washington, DC: American Society of Microbiology)
48. Kearns, D. H., O'Reilly, R. J., Lee, L. and Welch, B. G. (1973). Secretory IgA antibodies in the urethral exudate of men with uncomplicated urethritis due to *Neisseria gonorrhoeae*. *J. Infect. Dis.*, **127**, 99-101
49. Kearns, D. H., Sibert, G. B., O'Reilly, R., Lee, L. and Logan, L. (1973). Paradox of the immune response to uncomplicated gonococcal urethritis. *N. Engl. J. Med.*, **289**, 1170-4
50. McMillan, A., McNeillage, G. and Young, H. (1979). Antibodies to *Neisseria gonorrhoeae*: a study of the urethral exudates of 232 men. *J. Infect. Dis.*, **140**, 89-95
51. Tjokonegoro, A. and Sirisnha, S. (1975). Quantitative analysis of immunoglobulins and albumin in the secretion of the female reproductive tract. *Fertil. Steril.*, **26**, 413-17
52. Ison, C. A., Hadfield, S. G., Bellinger, C. M., Dawson, S. G. and Glynn, A. A. (1986). The specificity of serum and local antibodies in female gonorrhoea. *Clin. Exp. Immunol.*, **65**, 198-205
53. Rebello, R., Green, F. H. Y. and Fox, H. (1975). A study of the secretory immune system of the female genital tract. *Br. J. Obstet. Gynaecol.*, **82**, 812-16
54. O'Reilly, R. J., Lee, L. and Welch, B. G. (1976). Secretory IgA antibody response to *Neisseria gonorrhoeae* in the genital secretions of infected females. *J. Infect. Dis.*, **133**, 113-25
55. McMillan, A., McNeillage, G., Young, H. and Bain, S. S. R. (1979). Secretory antibody response of the cervix to infection with *Neisseria gonorrhoeae*. *Br. J. Vener. Dis.*, **55**, 265-70
56. Lammel, C. J., Sweet, R. L., Rice, P. A., Knapp, J. S., Schoolnik, G. K., Heilbron, D. C. and Brooks, G. F. (1985). Antibody-antigen specificity in the immune response to infection with *Neisseria gonorrhoeae*. *J. Infect. Dis.*, **152**, 990-1001
57. Tramont, E. C., Ciak, J., Boslego, J., McChesney, D. C., Brinton, C. C. and Zollinger, W. (1980). Antigenic specificity of antibodies in vaginal secretion during infection with *Neisseria gonorrhoeae*. *J. Infect. Dis.*, **140**, 23-31
58. Tramont, E. C., Sadoff, J. C., Boslego, J. W., Ciak, J. and McChesney, J. (1981). Gonococcal pilus vaccine: studies of antigenicity and inhibition of attachment. *J. Clin. Invest.*, **68**, 881-8
59. Brinton, C. C., Brown, A. and Rogers, K. (1980). The development of a neisserial pilus vaccine for gonorrhoea and meningococcal meningitis. In Weinstein, L. and Fields, B. N. (eds.). *Seminars in Infectious Diseases IV: Bacterial Vaccines*. pp. 140-59 (New York: Thieme-Stratton)
60. Ison, C. A. and Glynn, A. A. (1979). Classes of antibodies in acute gonorrhoea. *Lancet*, **1**, 1165-8
61. Hadfield, S. G. and Glynn, A. A. (1982). Analysis of antibodies in local and disseminated *Neisseria gonorrhoeae* infections by means of gel-electrophoresis derived ELISA. *Immunology*, **47**, 283-8
62. Hadfield, S. G. and Glynn, A. A. (1984). Application of immunoblotting to the differentiation of specific antibodies in gonorrhoea. *Immunology*, **51**, 615-21
63. Hook, E. W., Olsen, D. A. and Buchanan, T. M. (1984). Analysis of the antigen specificity

of the human serum immunoglobulin G immune response to complicated infection. *Infect. Immun.*, **43**, 706–9

64. Ingwer, I., Petersen, B. H. and Brooks, G. (1978). Serum bactericidal action and activation of the classical and alternate complement pathways by *Neisseria gonorrhoeae*. *J. Lab. Clin. Med.*, **92**, 211–20

65. Schoolnik, G. K., Buchanan, T. M. and Holmes, K. K. (1976). Gonococci causing disseminated gonococcal infection are resistant to the bactericidal action of normal human sera. *J. Clin. Invest.*, **58**, 1163–73

66. Brooks, G. F., Israel, K. S. and Petersen, B. H. (1976). Bactericidal and opsonic activity against *Neisseria gonorrhoeae* in sera from patients with disseminated infection. *J. Infect. Dis.*, **134**, 450–62

67. Tramont, E. C., Sadoff, J. C. and Wilson, C. (1977). Variability of the lytic susceptibility of *Neisseria gonorrhoeae* to human sera. *J. Immunol.*, **118**, 1843–51

68. Ward, M. E., Lambden, P. R., Heckels, J. E. and Watt, P. J. (1978). The surface properties of *Neissereia gonorrhoeae*: determinants of susceptibility to antibody complement killing. *J. Gen. Microbiol.*, **108**, 205–12.

69. Stephens, D. S. and Shafer, W. M. (1987). Evidence that the serum resistance genetic locus *sac-3* of *Neisseria gonorrhoeae* is involved in lipopolysaccharide structure. *J. Gen. Micrbiol.*, **133**, 2671–8

70. Shafer, W. M., Guymon, L. F. and Sparling, P. F. (1982). Identification of a new genetic site (*sac-3*) in *Neisseria gonorrhoeae* that affects sensitivity to normal human serum. *Infect. Immun.*, **35**, 764–9

71. James, J. F., Zurlinden, E., Lammel, C. J. and Brooks, G. F. (1982). Relation of protein I and colony opacity to serum killing of *Neisseria gonorrhoeae*. *J. Infect. Dis.*, **145**, 37–44

72. Rice, P. A., Tam, M. R. and Blake, M. S. (1985). Immunoglobulin G antibodies in normal human serum directed against protein III block killing of serum-resistant *Neisseria gonorrhoeae* by immune human serum. In Schoolnik, G. K. (ed.). *The Pathogenic Neisseriae*, pp. 427–34 (Washington, DC: American Society of Microbiology)

73. Brooks, G. F. (1985). Pathogenesis and immunology of gonococcal infection. In Brooks, G. F. and Donegan, E. A. (eds.). *Gonococcal Infection* (London: Edward Arnold)

74. Floyd-Reising, S. A., Cooper, M. D. and Moticka, E. J. (1985). Natural and antibody-dependant cell-mediated activity against *Neisseria gonorrhoeae* by peripheral blood lymphocytes in humans. In Schoolnik, G. K. (ed.). *The Pathogenic Neisseriae*, pp. 508–514 (Washington, DC: American Society of Microbiology)

75. Schoolnik, G. K. and McGee, Z. (1985). Gonococcal vaccine development strategies: summary of the recommendations of a National Institutes of Health Vaccine Panel. In Schoolnik, G. K. (ed.). *The Pathogenic Neisseriae*, pp. 329–331 (Washington, DC.: American Society of Microbiology)

76. Bummgarner, L. R. and Finkelstein, R. A. (1973). Pathogenesis and immunology of experimental gonococcal infection: virulence of colony types of *Neisseria gonorrhoeae* for chicken embryos. *Infect. Immun.*, **8**, 919–24

77. Salit, I. E. and Gotschlich, E. C. (1978). Gonococcal color and opacity variants: virulence for chicken embryos. *Infect. Immun.*, **22**, 359–64

78. Corbeil, L. B., Wunderlich, A. C., Corbeil, R. R., McCutchan, J. A., Ito, J. I. and Braude, A. I. (1979). Disseminated gonococcal infection in mice. *Infect. Immun.*, **26**, 984–90

79. Kita, E., Matsuura, H. and Kashiba, S. (1981). A mouse for the study of genital gonococcal infection. *J. Infect. Dis.*, **143**, 67–70

80. Kraus, S. J., Brown, W. J. and Arko, R. J. (1975). Acquired and natural immunity to gonococcal infection in chimpanzees. *J. Clin. Invest.*, **55**, 1349–56

81. Veale, D. R., Smith, H., Witt, K. A. and Marshall, R. B. (1975). Differential ability of colonial types of *Neisseria gonorrhoeae* to produce infection and an inflammatory response in subcutaneous perforated plastic chambers in guinea pigs and rabbits. *J. Med. Microbiol.*, **8**, 325–35

82. Parsons, N. J., Penn, C. W., Veale, D. R. and Smith, H. (1980). The complexity of immunogenicity of *Neisseria gonorrhoeae* in the guinea pig subcutaneous chamber model. *J. Gen. Microbiol.*, **118**, 523–7

83. Ward, M. E., Watt, P. J. and Robertson, J. N. (1974). The human fallopian tube: a laboratory model for gonococcal infection. *J. Infect. Dis.*, **129**, 650–9

84. Melly, M. A., Gregg, C. R. and McGee, Z. A. (1981). Studies of toxicity of *Neisseria gonorrhoeae* for human fallopian tube mucosa. *J. Infect. Dis.*, **143**, 423-31
85. Gregg, C. R., Melly, M. A., Hellerqvist, C. G., Coniglio, J. G. and McGee, Z. A. (1981). Toxic activity of purified lipopolysaccharide of *Neisseria gonorrhoeae* for human fallopian tube mucosa. *J. Infect. Dis.*, **143**, 432-9
86. Buchanan, T. M., Eschenbach, D. A., Knapp, J. S. and Holmes, K. K. (1980). Gonococcal salpingitis is less likely to recur with *Neisseria gonorrhoeae* of the same outer membrane antigenic type. *Am. J. Obstet. Gynecol.*, **138**, 978-80
87. Kellogg, D. S., Peacock, W. L., Deacon, W. E., Brown, K. and Pirkle, C. L. (1963). *Neisseria gonorrhoeae*. I. Virulence genetically linked to colonial variation. *J. Bacteriol.*, **85**, 1274-9
88. Swanson, J., Kraus, S. J. and Gotschlich, E. C. (1971). Studies on gonococcus infection. I. Pili and zones of adhesion: their relation to gonococcal growth patterns. *J. Exp. Med.*, **134**, 886-906
89. Sparling, P. F., Cannon, J. G. and So, M. (1986). Phase and antigenic variation of pili and outer membrane Protein II of *Neisseria gonorrhoeae*. *J. Infect. Dis.*, **153**, 196-201
90. Lambden, P. R., Heckels, J. E., McBridge, H. and Watt, P. J. (1981). The isolation and identification of novel pilus types produced by variants of *Neisseria gonorrhoeae* P9 following selection *in vivo*. *FEMS Microbiol. Lett.*, **10**, 339-41
91. Hagblom, P., Segal, E., Billyard, E. and So, M. (1985). Intragenic recombination leads to pilus antigenic variation in *Neisseria gonorrhoeae*. *Nature*, **315**, 156-8
92. Zak, K., Diaz, J-L., Jackson, D. and Heckels, J. E. (1984). Antigenic variation during infection with *Neisseria gonorrhoeae*: detection of antibodies to surface proteins in sera of patients with gonorrhoea. *J. Infect. Dis.*, **149**, 166-73
93. Lambden, P. R., Robertson, J. N. and Watt, P. J. (1980). Biological properties of two distinct pilus types produced by isogenic variants of *Neisseria gonorrhoeae* P9. *J. Bacteriol.*, **141**, 393-6
94. Tramont, E. C., Boslego, J. W., Chung, R., McChesney, D., Ciak, J., Sadoff, J., Piziak, M., Brinton, C. C., Wood, S. and Bryan, J. (1985), Parental gonococcal pilus vaccine. In Schoolnik, G. K. (ed.). *The Pathogenic Neisseriae*. pp. 316-22 (Washington, DC: American Society of Microbiology)
95. Schoolnik, G. K., Tai, J. Y., Rothbard, J. and Gotschlich, E. C. (1983). A pilus peptide for the prevention of gonorrhoea. *Prog. Alleg.*, **33**, 314-31
96. Rothbard, J. R., Fernandez, R., Wang, R., Teng, N. N. H. and Schoolnik, G. K. (1985). Antibodies to peptides corresponding to a conserved sequence of gonococcal pilins block bacterial adhesion. *Proc. Natl. Acad. Sci. USA.*, **82**, 915-19
97. Blake, M. S. and Gotschlich, E. C. (1983). Gonococcal membrane proteins: speculation on their role in pathogenesis. *Prog. Alleg.*, **33**, 298-313
98. Virji, M., Zak, K. and Heckels, J. E. (1986). Monoclonal antibodies to gonococcal outer membrane protein IB: use in the investigation of the potential protective effect of antibodies directed against conserved and type-specific epitopes. *J. Gen. Microbiol.*, **132**, 1621-9
99. Virji, M., Fletcher, J. N., Zak, K. and Heckels, J. E. (1987). The potential protective effect of monoclonal antibodies to gonococcal outer membrane protein IA. *J. Gen. Microbiol.*, **133**, 2639-46
100. Judd, R. C. (1985). Structure and surface exposure of Protein IIs of *Neisseria gonorrhoeae* JS3. *Infect. Immun.*, **48**, 452-7
101. Cannon, J. G., Black, W. J., Nachamkin, I. and Stewart, P. W. (1984). Monoclonal antibody which recognises an outer membrane antigen common to the pathogenic *Neisseria* species but not to most non-pathogenic *Neisseria* species. *Infect. Immun.*, **43**, 994-9
102. Meitzner, T. A., Luginbuhl, G. N., Sandstrom, E. C., and Morse, S. A. (1984). Identification of an iron regulated 37000 dalton protein in the cell envelope of *Neisseria gonorrhoeae*. *Infect. Immun.*, **45**, 410-16
103. Clark, V. L., Campbell, L. A., Palermo, D. A., Evans, T. M. and Klimpel, K. W. (1987). Induction and repression of outer membrane proteins by anaerobic growth of *Neisseria gonorrhoeae*. *Infect. Immun.*, **55**, 1359-64
104. Morse, S. A., Mietzner, T. A., Schalla, W. O., Lammel, C. J. and Brooks, G. F. (1987). Serum and vaginal antibodies against the major iron-regulated protein in women with gonococcal pelvic inflammatory disease or uncomplicated infection. In Poolman, J. (ed.).

Gonococci and Meningococci. (In press)
105. Clark, V. L., Klimpel, K. W., Thompson, S. and Knapp, J. (1987). Anaerobically expressed outer membrane proteins of *Neisseria gonorrhoeae* are recognised by antibodies in the sera of PID patients. In Poolman, J. (ed.). *Gonococci and Meningococci.* (In press)
106. Mulks, M. H. and Plaut, A. G. (1978). IgA protease production as a characteristic distinguishing pathogenic from harmless *Neisseriaceae*. *N. Engl. J. Med.*, **299**, 973–6
107. Caldwell, J. G., Price, E. V., Pazin, G. J. and Cornelius, C. E. (1971). Sensitivity and reproducibility of Thayer–Martin culture medium in diagnosing gonorrhoea in women. *Am. J. Obstet. Gynecol.*, **109**, 463–8
108. Schmale, J. D., Martin, J. E. and Domescik, G. (1969). Observations on the culture diagnosis of gonorrhoea in women. *J. Am. Med. Assoc.*, **210**, 312–14
109. Johnson, D. W., Holmes, K. K., Kvale, P. A., Halverson, C. W. and Hirsch, W. P. (1969). An evaluation of gonorrhoea case finding in the chronically infected female. *Am. J. Epidemiol.*, **90**, 438–48
110. Vecchio, T. J. (1966). Predictive value of a single diagnostic test in unselected populations. *N. Engl. J. Med.*, **274**, 1171–3
111. Glynn, A. A. and Ison, C. A. (1981). Enzyme immunoassays in bacteriology. In Voller, A., Bartlett, A. and Bidwell, E. (eds.). *Immunoassays for the 80s.* pp. 431–40 (Lancaster: MTP)
112. Magnusson, B. and Kjellander, J. (1965). Gonococcal fixation test in complicated and uncomplicated gonorrhoea. *Br. J. Vener. Dis.*, **41**, 127–31
113. Danielsson, D., Thyresson, N., Falk, V. and Barr, J. (1972). Serologic investigation of the immune response in various types of gonococcal infection. *Acta Dermatol. Venerol.*, **52**, 467–75
114. Oranje, A. P., Iseriet, C. O. A., de Roo, A., Stolz, E. and Michel, M. F. (1983). Antibodies to gonococcal pili in women with asymptomatic gonorrhoea. *Br. J. Vener. Dis.*, **59**, 85–8
115. Welch, B. G. and O'Reilly, R. J. (1973). An indirect immunofluorescent antibody technique for the study of uncomplicated gonorrhoea. I. Methodology. *J. Infect. Dis.*, **127**, 69–76
116. McMillan, A., McNeillage, G., Young, H. and Bain, S. R. (1979). Serum immunoglobulin response in uncomplicated gonorrhoea. *Br. J. Vener. Dis.*, **55**, 5–9
117. O'Reilly, R. J., Welch, B. G. and Kellogg, D. S. (1973). An indirect fluorescent antibody technique for the study of uncomplicated gonorrhoea. II. Selection and characterisation of the strain of *N. gonorrhoeae* used as an antigen. *J. Infect. Dis.*, **127**, 77–83
118. Ison, C. A., Hadfield, S. G. and Glynn, A. A. (1981). Enzyme-linked immunosorbent assay (ELISA) to detect antibodies in gonorrhoea using whole cells. *J. Clin. Pathol.*, **34**, 1040–3
119. Young, H. and Low, A. C. (1981). Serological diagnosis of gonorrhoea: detection of antibodies to gonococcal pili by enzyme-linked immunosorbent assay. *Med. Lab. Sci.*, **38**, 41–7
120. Oranje, A. P., Reimann, K., Eijk, R. V., Schouter, H. J. A., Roo, A., Tideman, G. J., Stolz, E. and Michel, M. F. (1983). Gonococcal serology: A comparison of three different tests. *Br. J. Vener. Dis.*, **59**, 47–52
121. Buchanan, T. M., Swanson, J., Holmes, K. K., Kraus, S. J., Gotschlich, E. C. (1973). Quantitative determination of antibody to gonococcal pili. *J. Clin. Invest.*, **52**, 2896–909
122. Oates, S. A., Falker, W. A., Joseph, J. M. and Warfel, L. E. (1977). Asymptomatic females: Detection of antibody activity to gonococcal pili antigen by radio-immunoassay. *J. Clin. Microbiol.*, **5**, 26–30
123. Reimann, K., Lind, I. and Andersen, K. E. (1980). An indirect haemagglutination test for demonstration of gonococcal antibodies using pili as antigen. *Acta Path. Microbiol. Scand. Sect. C*, **88**, 155–62
124. Reimann, K., Oranje, A. P. and Michel, M. F. (1982). Demonstration of antigenic heterogeneity of *N. gonorrhoeae* pili antigens using human sera in the test system. *Acta Path. Microbiol. Scand. Sect. C.*, **90**, 47–50
125. Watt, P. J., Ward, M. E. and Glynn, A. A. (1971). A comparison of serological tests for the diagnosis of gonorrhoea. *Br. J. Vener, Dis.*, **47**, 448–51
126. Ward, M. E. and Glynn, A. A. (1972). Human antibody response to lipopolysaccharides from *N. gonorrhoeae*. *J. Clin. Pathol.*, **25**, 56–9
127. Fletcher, S., Miller, R. and Nicol, C. S. (1973). Study of the passive haemagglutination test for gonorrhoea. *Br. J. Vener. Dis.*, **49**, 508–10
128. Brodeur, B. R., Ashton, F. E. and Diena, B. B. (1982). Enzyme-linked immunosorbent

assay with polyvalent gonococcal antigen. *J. Med. Microbiol.*, **15**, 1–9

129. Handsfield, H. H., Lipman, T. O., Harnisch, J. P., Tronca, E. and Holmes, K. K. (1974). Asymptomatic gonorrhoea in men. Diagnosis, natural course, prevalence and significance. *N. Engl. J. Med.*, **290**, 117–123

130. Goodhart, M. E., Ogden, J., Zaidi, A. A., and Kraus, S. J. (1982). Factors affecting the performance of smear and culture tests for the detection of *Neisseria gonorrhoeae*. *Sex. Transm. Dis.*, **9**, 63–9

131. Burns, M., Rossi, P. H., Cox, D. W., Edwards, T., Kramer, M. and Kraus, S. J. (1983). A preliminary evaluation of the Gonozyme test. *Sex. Transm. Dis.*, **10**, 180–3

132. Manis, R. D., Harris, B. and Geiseler, P. J. (1984). Evaluation of Gonozyme, an enzyme immunoassay for the rapid diagnosis of gonorrhoea. *J. Clin. Microbiol.*, **20**, 742–6

133. Danielsson, D., Moi, H. and Forslin, L. (1983). Diagnosis of urogenital gonorrhoea by detecting gonococcal antigen with a solid-phase enzyme immunoassay (Gonozyme). *J. Clin. Pathol.*, **36**, 674–7

134. Demitriou, E., Sackett, R., Welch, D. F. and Kaplan, D. W. (1984). Evaluation of an enzyme immunoassay for the detection of *Neisseria gonorrhoeae* in an adolescent population *J. Am. Med. Assoc.*, **252**, 247–50

135. Nachamkin, I., Sondheimer, S. J., Barbagallo, S. and Barth, S. (1984). Detection of *Neisseria gonorrhoeae* in cervical swabs using the Gonozyme enzyme immunoassay. Clinical evaluation in a university family planning clinic. *Am. J. Clin. Pathol.*, **82**, 461–5

136. Papasian C. J., Bartholomew, W. R. and Amsterdam, D. (1984). Validity of an enzyme immunoassay for the detection of *Neisseria gonorrhoeae* antigens. *J. Clin. Microbiol.*, **19**, 347–50

137. Papasian, C. J., Bartholomew, W. R. and Amsterdam, D. (1984). Modified enzyme immunoassay for detecting *Neisseria gonorrhoeae* antigens. *J. Clin. Microbiol.*, **20**, 641–3

138. Rudrik, J. T., Waller, J. M. and Britt, E. M. (1984). Efficacy of an enzyme immunoassay with uncentrifuged first voided urine for detection of gonorrhoea in males. *J. Clin. Microbiol.*, **20**, 577–8

139. Schachter, J., McCormack, W. M., Smith, R. F., Parks, R. M., Bailey, R. and Ohlin, A. C., (1984). Enzyme immunoassay for diagnosis of gonorrhoea. *J. Clin. Microbiol.*, **19**, 57–79

140. Stamm, W. E., Cole, B., Fennell, C., Bonin, P., Armstrong, A. S., Herrmann, J. E. and Holmes, K. K. (1984). Antigen detection for the diagnosis of gonorrhoea. *J. Clin. Microbiol.*, **19**, 399–403

141. Granato, P. A. and Roefaro, M. (1985). Comparative evaluation of enzyme immunoassay and culture for the laboratory diagnosis of gonorrhoea. *Am. J. Clin. Pathol.*, **83**, 613–18

142. Mirrett, S., Reller, L. B. and Knapp, J. S. (1981). *Neisseria gonorrhoeae* strains inhibited by vancomycin in selective media and correlation with auxotype. *J. Clin. Microbiol.*, **14**, 94–9

143. Ison, C. A., McClean, K., Gedney, J., Munday, P. E., Coghill, D., Smith, R., Harris, J. R. W. and Easmon, C. S. F. (1985). Evaluation of a direct immunofluorescence test for the diagnosis of gonorrhoea. *J. Clin. Pathol.*, **38**, 1142–5

144. Young, H. and Reid, K. G. (1984). Immunological identification of *Neisseria gonorrhoeae* with monoclonal and polyclonal antibody coagglutination reagents. *J. Clin. Pathol.*, **37**, 1276–81

145. Ison, C. A., Tanna, A. and Easmon, C. S. F. (1988). Evaluation of a fluorescent monoclonal antibody reagent for culture confirmation of *Neisseria gonorrhoeae*. *J. Med. Microbiol.*, **26**, 121–3.

146. Catlin, B. W. (1973). Nutritional profiles of *Neisseria gonorrhoeae*, *Neisseria meningitidis* and *Neisseria lactamica* in chemically defined media and the use of growth requirements for gonococcal typing. *J. Infect. Dis.*, **128**, 178–94

147. Wang, S. P., Holmes, K. K., Knapp, J. S. and Kyzer, D. (1977). Immunologic classification of *Neisseria gonorrhoeae* with immunofluorescence. *J. Immunol.*, **119**, 795–803

148. Sandstrom, E. G. and Danielsson, D. (1980). Serology of *Neisseria gonorrhoeae* classification by coagglutination. *Acta Path. Micro. Scand. Sect. B.*, **88**, 27–38

149. Buchanan, T. M. and Hildebrandt, J. F. (1981). Antigen-specific serotyping of *Neisseria gonorrhoeae*: characterisation based upon principal outer membrane protein. *Infect. Immun.*, **32**, 1483–9

150. Sandstrom, E. G., Chen, K. C. S. and Buchanan, T. M. (1982). Serology of *Neisseria*

gonorrhoeae coagglutination serogroups WI and WII/III correspond to different outer membrane protein I molecules. *Infect. Immun.*, **38**, 462–70

151. Knapp, J. S., Tam, M. R., Nowinski, R. C., Holmes, K. K. and Sandstrom, E. G. (1984). Serological classification of *Neisseria gonorrhoeae* with use of monoclonal antibodies to gonococcal outer membrane protein 1. *J. Infect. Dis.*, **150**, 44–8

152. Bygdeman, S. M., Gillenius, E-C. and Sandstrom, E. C. (1985). Comparison of two different sets of monoclonal antibodies for the serological classification of *Neisseria gonorrhoeae*. In Schoolnik, G. K. (ed.). *The Pathogenic Neisseriae*. pp. 31–36 (Washington, DC: American Society of Microbiology)

153. Sandstrom, E. C., Lindell, P., Harfast, B., Blomberg, F., Ryden, A-C. and Bygdeman, S. (1985). Evaluation of a new set of *Neisseria gonorrhoeae* serogroup W-specific monoclonal antibodies for serovar determination. In Schoolnik, G. K. (ed.). *The Pathogenic Neisseriae*. pp. 26–30 (Washington, DC: American Society of Microbiology)

6
Chlamydial Genital Infections

M. A. MONNICKENDAM

Chlamydia trachomatis causes a wide range of diseases in the human genital tract and eye. Infection in females extends from asymptomatic cervicitis to perihepatitis and acute salpingitis with subsequent infertility. In males, infection causes asymptomatic urethritis, severe urethritis and acute epididymitis. Both males and females can develop chlamydial proctitis, and genital infection may be followed by reactive arthritis. Babies born to infected mothers may be infected but asymptomatic, they may develop neonatal chlamydial ophthalmia (NCO) or neonatal chlamydial pneumonitis (NCP). Lymphogranuloma venereum (LGV) may present as painless genital ulceration, but this can be followed by lymphadenitis and the genito-ano-rectal syndrome. Ocular infections range from mild inclusion conjunctivitis and punctate keratitis associated with chlamydial genital infections, to blinding trachoma, transmitted from eye to eye in rural populations in many developing countries.

Chlamydial genital infection is very common in both industrialized and developing countries. Estimates of the prevalence of chlamydial genital infections are likely to be underestimates because infections are frequently asymptomatic and are, therefore, undetected. In the United Kingdom, there were over 155000 reported cases of non-specific (non-gonococcal) genital infection (NSGI) in 1984, consisting of 111500 cases in men and 43500 cases in women[1]. If half of these cases of NSGI were caused by *C. trachomatis*[1], then there were approximately 77500 cases of chlamydial genital infection. In the United States of America, it has been estimated that there are two million cases of non-specific urethritis (NSU) in men each year[2]. If half are caused by *C. trachomatis*, there are approximately one million cases of chlamydial urethritis. If the ratio of male to female cases is the same in the United States as in the United Kingdom, the number of female cases is approximately 390500. This adds up to an annual total of approximately 1400000 cases of chlamydial genital infection in the United States. Acute salpingitis is becoming common, particularly in younger women. It is estimated that there are 83000 cases of salpingitis in England and Wales each year[3].

117

C. trachomatis is implicated in about two-thirds of these cases[4], so that there are 55000 cases of chlamydial salpingitis in England and Wales each year. It is estimated that each year over one million babies throughout the world develop NCO and just under half a million develop NCP[5]. Lastly, it is estimated that in the Third World, 500 million people have trachoma, two million of whom are blind[6].

The ways in which *C. trachomatis* can cause such a wide range of diseases are not well-understood. The type of disease which develops depends on factors such as the site of infection, the *C. trachomatis* biovar and host responses to infection. The aim of this article is to discuss what is known about how *C. trachomatis* affects the host and how to develop improved methods of diagnosis, management and prevention.

CLASSIFICATION, LIFE CYCLE AND ANTIGENS

Chlamydiae are divided into *C. trachomatis* and *C. psittaci*. The classification of chlamydiae and the diseases which they cause in humans are listed in Table 6.1. *C. trachomatis* is a human pathogen which does not normally infect other mammals, except for one strain which was isolated from mice (mouse pneumonitis agent). *C. trachomatis* causes three major forms of disease; trachoma, NSGI and associated diseases and LGV. *C. psittaci* includes a group of human pathogens, which presently comprise *C. IOL-207* and TWAR strains. These were first isolated from the eyes of children with trachoma, one in Iran and the other in Taiwan, and have since been identified as a cause of respiratory tract infection in adults[7]. However, most strains of *C. psittaci* are normally pathogens of birds and mammals and only occasionally infect humans.

Chlamydiae are Gram-negative bacteria which are obligate parasites of eukaryotic cells. *C.trachomatis* serovars A–K infect the mucosal epithelia of the urethra, cervix, rectum and eye, whereas serovars L_1, L_2 and L_3 infect lymphoid tissue. *C. trachomatis* is commonly grown in McCoy cells, HeLa cells and L cells, which are usually treated with cytostatic agents such as ionizing radiation, 5-iodo-2[1]-deoxyuridine, cycloheximide or mitomycin-C because members of the trachoma biovar grow better in non-dividing cells than in multiplying cells. The complex chlamydial life-cycle has been elucidated in cell culture[8]. The infectious form is known as the elementary body (EB) which is approximately 200–300 nm in diameter. The EB is taken up into the host cell, where it enlarges to form the non-infectious reticulate body (RB), which is 800–1000 nm in diameter. The RB is metabolically active and divides by binary fission, giving rise to more RBs, which later condense into EBs. The processes of division and condensation into EBs take place within a characteristic intracellular inclusion body (IB). Mature IBs can be released to the external environment by exocytosis[9]. Under the most favourable nutritional conditions of cell culture, the growth cycle takes 48–72 hours. *C. trachomatis* trachoma biovars also grow in human endometrial and ectocervical cell culture[10] and in human fallopian tube fragments in organ culture[11]. EBs, RBs and IBs are also found in cervical epithelial cells in biopsy specimens[12]. The duration of the

Table 6.1 Chlamydiae and human diseases

Species, biovars, serovars and strains	Tissue	Disease
C. trachomatis trachoma biovar, serovars A,B,Ba,C	conjunctiva	trachoma
C. trachomatis trachoma biovar, serovars D,E,F,G,H,I,J,K	conjunctiva respiratory tract genital tract other tissues	ophthalmia neonatorum, inclusion conjunctivitis, nasopharyngeal infection, pneumonia, cervicitis, salpingitis, urethritis, epididymitis, proctitis, perihepatitis, Reiter's syndrome
C. trachomatis lymphogranuloma venereum biovar, serovars L_1, L_2, L_3	lymphoid tissue	lymphogranuloma venereum
C. psittaci strains IOL–207, TWAR	conjunctiva respiratory tract	keratoconjunctivitis, acute respiratory infection
C. psittaci strain psittacosis agent	respiratory tract	pneumonia
C. psittaci strain feline keratoconjunctivitis agent	conjunctiva	keratoconjunctivitis
C. psittaci strain ovine abortion agent	placenta and fetus	abortion

chlamydial growth cycle *in vivo* is not known, but it is likely to be longer than the *in vitro* cycle, since conditions are unlikely to be optimal for chlamydial growth.

The chlamydial genome contains 600–850 kilobase pairs, sufficient to specify approximately 600 proteins[13]. *C. trachomatis* is antigenically complex, with genus or group-, species-, sub-species and serovar or type-specific antigens. Analysis has concentrated on EBs because they are stable and can be obtained in reasonable quantities. There are also antigens associated with the intracellular growth cycle, including antigens in the host cell membrane and antigens released into the external environment.

C. trachomatis EBs contain several types of antigens. The genus-specific antigen used in the complement-fixation (CF) test was the first one to be described. The CF-test was the earliest serological test for the diagnosis of chlamydial infections and was originally developed to diagnose psittacosis[14]. The genus-specific antigen is a lipopolysaccharide (LPS). The acidic component of chlamydial LPS is 2-keto-3-deoxyoctanoic acid, but it migrates more slowly than the 2-keto-3-deoxyoctanoic acid from salmonella LPS and is probably a different stereoisomer[15]. Antibodies raised against chlamydial LPS react strongly with the inner core of *Salmonella typhimurium* LPS, as do antibodies from patients with LGV, psittacosis and chlamydial salpingitis[16]. Similarly, antibodies against *S. typhimurium* LPS react with *C. trachomatis* LPS. Chlamydial LPS can agglutinate mouse and rabbit erythrocytes, but not human or guinea pig erythrocytes[17,18]. The major constituent of the outer membrane protein is a species-specific antigen termed major outer membrane protein (MOMP)[19]. Antibodies raised against MOMP prepared from L₂ EBs neutralize the infectivity of serovar L₂ EBs for cells in cultue[20]. Monoclonal antibodies raised against LPS and the species-specific antigen in MOMP are used to detect *C. trachomatis* EBs in smears of ocular and genital material. Although monoclonal antibodies are highly specific, there are cross-reactions between the monoclonal antibody against *C. trachomatis* MOMP and several other species of bacteria[21,22]. Protein A of *Staphylococcus aureus* non-specifically binds the Fc portion of monoclonal antibodies raised against *C. trachomatis* MOMP[21]. MOMP also contains sub-species and serovar-specific antigens[23]. Serovar-specific antigens include proteins of various sizes including MOMP and lipids. The nature of serovar-specific antigens has been recently reviewed[24]. Sub-species and serovar-specific antigens can be detected using the micro-immunofluorescence (micro-IF) test. These sub-species antigens have been used to divide *C. trachomatis* into the B and C complexes and 15 serovars. These are A, B, Ba, C, D, E, F, G, H, I, J, K, L_1, L_2, L_3. The B complex contains serovars B, Ba, D, E, F, G, L_1 and L_2, the C complex contains serovars A, C, H, I, J, K and L_3[25-27]. Different serovars are associated with different forms of infection. Serovars A, B, Ba and C are associated with trachoma, serovars D–K cause NSGI and associated infections and serovars L_1, L_2, and L_3 cause LGV.

When assessing serological results, it is important to know whether the antibodies detected are against group, species, sub-species or serovar-specific antigens. If, for example, a group antigen is being used to screen for NSGI, then antibodies against *C. psittaci*, including IOL-207 and TWAR strains, will be detected as well as antibodies against *C. trachomatis*. This can lead to the prevalence of NSGI being overestimated. LGV EBs or IBs are commonly used in single-antigen tests because they both cross-react with antibodies against most other serovars although the degree of cross-reactivity varies[27]. Tests using EBs of several serovars detect sub-species and serovar-specific antibodies. A comparison has been made of an indirect immunofluorescence (indirect-IF) test using L_2 IBs, with the micro-IF test using EBs of various serovars. The indirect-IF test was more sensitive, detecting antibodies in a greater number of sera and giving higher titres. However, the micro-IF test was more specific[28].

The choice of a serological test for the diagnosis of chlamydial genital infections must depend on the prevalence of chlamydial infections in the population. However, all tests will produce false-positive and false-negative results and single results must be considered together with the history, symptoms and signs before arriving at a diagnosis. The micro-IF test with EBs from a range of *C. trachomatis* and *C. psittaci* strains, will distinguish between infections caused by the two species, but the preparation of a range of antigens is long and laborious. In our laboratory, the need for compromise between a complex highly specific test and a simple test for routine diagnosis of chlamydial genital infection on the United Kingdom, has led to a modification of the micro-IF test. The *C. psittaci* strain IOL-207 and a pool of *C. trachomatis* serovar D–K EBs are used because the prevalence of trachoma and LGV is low, chlamydial NSGI is common and the prevalence of respiratory tract infections caused by IOL-207 is rising[29]. There may be false-positive results because of cross-reactions with sera from patients with other *C. trachomatis* and *C. psittaci* infections, and false-negative results in patients with low levels of antibodies specific to EBs of only one serovar in the pool. However, there are probably only a small number of misleading results.

In recent year, radio-immunoassay (RIA) and enzyme immunoassay (EIA) methods have been found to be of particular use in routine serological screening tests for chlamydial infections, as the reading of results can be automated and end-points determined objectively.

Other antigens have been detected only during the intracellular stages of the *C. trachomatis* life-cycle. A genus-specific antigen has been found on the surface of cells containing inclusions and on adjacent membranous material, the identification of the antigen and location depends on the method of fixation and staining[30]. Antigens have also been found in cell-culture medium from infected cultures. They comprise serovar-specific antigens with phosphate-specific esterase activity[31] and a heterogeneous genus-specific glycolipid with a wide molecular weight range which is distinct from the LPS present in chlamydial EBs[32].

Studies of chlamydial antigens have been handicapped for many years by the presence of contaminating host-cell antigens and the difficulties of producing chlamydial antigens in bulk. The advent of monoclonal antibodies, immunoblotting techniques and gene cloning now allows the analysis of chlamydial antigens and chlamydial antibodies in greater detail.

CELLULAR AND SUB-CELLULAR INTERACTIONS BETWEEN
C. TRACHOMATIS AND HUMANS

C. trachomatis EBs have to reach susceptible cells, attach and enter them before they can commence their intracellular growth cycle. *C. trachomatis* serovars L_1, L_2 and L_3 cause genital ulcers and later infect lymphoid tissue. Since they cause ulcers, it is probable that they can reach susceptible cells through breaks in the skin or mucosal epithelium. The identity of these susceptible cells is not known. L_2 EBs can attach to B-lymphocytes[33], which presumably carry the infection to the lymphoid tissue. *C. trachomatis* serovars D–K infect mucosal epithelial cells, causing urethritis in males and cervicitis in females. These EBs presumably possess efficient methods of attachment to the surface mucus, and for moving through it to the underlying mucosal epithelial cells in the male urethra to avoid being washed out during urination. In the female genital tract, there is not the same need for rapid attachment. However, since only cervical epithelial cells are susceptible to infection, EBs must reach the cervix, attach to the mucus and move through it to reach the cells underneath, but nothing is yet known about this mechanism.

Non-immune defence mechanisms

Once infection has occurred, there are several non-immune biochemical and cellular mechanisms which can inactivate *C. trachomatis* EBs. The biochemical mechanisms are listed in Table 6.2, which shows that there are some conflicting results. These studies have been carried out *in vitro*, using EBs of several serovars. It is not known whether differences between *in vitro* assay systems contribute towards these conflicting results, or whether EBs of different serovars have differing susceptibilities.

Biochemical mechanisms

Seminal plasma reduces the infectivity of serovar F or L_2 EBs in cell culture[34,35]. Analysis of seminal plasma components shows that spermine, cupric chloride and zinc chloride have inhibitory activity against serovar F. Seminal plasma also contains lysozyme which may affect chlamydial growth. Lysozyme obtained from human urine stimulates the growth of serovar F, while pre-incubation of serovar L_2 EBs with hen egg-white lysozyme inhibits growth[36]. In contrast, hen egg-white lysozyme appears to have no effect when incubated with EBs of various serovars before inoculation, nor does it affect the growth of serovar F in cells which are incubated in medium containing hen egg-white lysozyme[37]. It is not clear whether these conflicting results are caused by the use of lysozyme from different sources. Hormones affect growth of *C. trachomatis* in cells. Incubation of cells with cortisol before inoculation stimulates the growth of an untyped cervical isolate and inhibits the growth of serovar L_2, while incubation of cells with cortisol after inoculation stimulates the growth of serovar L_2[38,39]. When oestrogens are present during inoculation and incubation, they do not alter the binding

Table 6.2 Non-immune factors and growth of *C. trachomatis*

Factor	Serovar	Effect on growth of C. trachomatis in cells	Reference
Seminal plasma	F	inhibition	34
	L_2	inhibition	35
Seminal plasma components			
Spermine	F	inhibition	34
$CuCl_2$, $ZnCl_2$	F	inhibition	34
Lysozyme (hen egg white)	L_2	inhibition	36
	A,B,C,F,L_2	no effect (pre-inoculation treatment of EBs)	37
	F	no effect (post-inoculation treatment of cells)	37
(human urine)	F	stimulation (post-inoculation treatment of cells)	34
Hormones			
Cortisol	cervical isolate	stimulation (pre- and post-inoculation treatment of cells)	38
	L_2	inhibition (pre-inoculation treatment of cells)	39
	L_2	stimulation (post-inoculation treatment of cells)	39
Oestrogens	D, LGV isolate	stimulation	40
progesterone, testosterone and other hormones	D, LGV isolate	no effect	40
Blood	NSU isolate	inhibition (some individuals) no effect (others)	41
Interferon			
Non-immune chick	NCO isolate	inhibition (in eggs)	44
Non-immune mouse	L_2	inhibition	43
Non-immune mouse	D	inhibition	45
Non-immune mouse	L_1	inhibition	46
Mouse	L_1	inhibition	47
Human	L_2	inhibition	48

of serovar D or LGV EBs to cells, but the number of IBs is doubled[40]. Progesterone, testosterone and other hormones have no effect on the growth of *C. trachomatis*[40]. Some individuals have non-immune inhibitory factors in their blood. EBs of an isolate obtained from a patient with NSU were incubated with sera from individuals with very low or undetectable levels of chlamydial antibodies (measured with an indirect-IF test), and four out of twelve individuals had inhibitory activity[41].

Although *C. trachomatis* is a bacterium, it induces the production of the anti-viral agent interferon and is sensitive to its effects. Interferon production is induced by infection of HeLa and L-cell cultures with several serovars, and interferon is present in blood obtained from mice for about 24 hours after the intravenous injection of EBs[42,43]. Non-immune chick interferon inhibits the replication in eggs of *C. trachomatis* serovar E and a strain isolated from NCO[44], and non-immune mouse interferon inhibits the growth of several serovars in L-cells[43,45,46]. Mouse and human γ-interferon also inhibit the growth of *C. trachomatis* L_1 and L_2[47,48]. Several stages of the intracellular growth cycle are inhibited by interferon[46,48,49].

Cellular mechanisms

The infected host mounts a considerable cellular response to *C. trachomatis*. There is evidence that some cells can inactivate *C. trachomatis* EBs. *In vitro* studies have shown that polymorphonuclear (PMN) leukocytes rapidly inactivate *C. trachomatis* EBs serotypes B and L_2, which are taken up into vacuoles and degraded[50–52]. There is disagreement about the effects of sera on this reaction. The attachment of serovar E and EBs into PMN cells is not enhanced by heat-inactivated human chlamydial antisera, unlike the chemiluminescent response of PMN cells, which is markedly enhanced by serovar- but not group-specific antisera[53]. In contrast, the chemiluminescent response of PMN cells to serovar L_2 EBs is increased by human sera with or without complement or chlamydial antibodies[54]. It is possible that some of these differences may reflect differences in the non-specific inactivating ability of different sera[41]. Incubation of serovar L_2 EBs with peripheral blood monocytes also produces a decrease in infectivity, but they can replicate in monocyte-derived macrophages[55]. It is not known whether other *C. trachomatis* serovars can also replicate in macrophages.

There are also non-specific interactions between *C. trachomatis* and lymphocytes. The addition of L_2 EBs to human peripheral blood mononuclear leukocytes increases the amount of immunoglobulins secreted into the medium and the number of immunoglobulin-producing cells. There is a further increase in the number of immunoglobulin-producing cells when cultures are depleted of monocytes. Live L_2 EBs and formalin-fixed EBs are equally effective. However, these immunoglobulins lack antichlamydial activity[56]. L_2 EBs stimulate the incorporation of radio-labelled thymidine into B-lymphocytes. There is no correlation between these stimulatory effects and levels of chlamydial antibodies in donors' sera, indicating that these responses do not reflect previous exposure to *C. trachomatis*. These results show that *C. trachomatis* can stimulate non-immune polyclonal responses[56]. Detailed analysis has shown that about half of the B-lymphocytes and less than 10% of T-lymphocytes bind L_2 EBs and that B-cells do not support the growth of *C. trachomatis*[33]. It is not known whether other *C. trachomatis* serovars can elicit similar responses.

Specific immune responses

Humoral responses to *C. trachomatis* infection have been studied extensively because it is easy to collect and store blood and discharges (exudates), and because the tests are relatively simple and easy to quantify and standardize. Chlamydial antibodies have been found in blood and local exudates. The anti-chlamydial activities of chlamydial antibodies include complement-fixation[14] and neutralization of infectivity[57]. Neutralizing antibodies have been detected in blood and tears of patients with trachoma and may also be present in blood and local discharges from patients with chlamydial genital infections.

The presence of cellular immune responses was originally elicited by skin tests. Various *in vitro* tests have been developed which correlate with skin tests. The *in vitro* tests require a substantial number of lymphocytes, which are usually obtained from peripheral blood. The tests are complicated functional assays which are difficult to standardize for comparative purposes. It has been assumed that the responses of peripheral blood lymphocytes reflect responses of lymphocytes at the site of infection, but this may not apply in chlamydial infections.

There are some indications of the role of the immune responses from studies of chlamydial ocular infections in humans and animal models[58]. The cellular immune responses are important in clearing primary infection and restricting chlamydial growth in re-infection. Secretory IgA prevents re-infection, and when it disappears from the conjunctiva, re-infection can occur although it tends to be shorter than primary infection. Transfer of serum IgG containing chlamydial antibodies does not protect animals from re-infection. Repeated re-infection is characterized by chronic inflammation and conjunctival scarring.

Immune responses do not provide good protective immunity to ocular chlamydial infection, since people living in areas where trachoma is hyperendemic are susceptible to repeated re-infection. Vaccine trials have demonstrated that vaccines are largely ineffective, producing, at best, only short-lived benefit. Immune responses may contribute to the development of tissue damage in trachoma, since blinding disease is only found in areas where the rate of re-infection is very high and some vaccines have a deleterious effect on the development of trachoma[59,60].

The genital tract of a person with an infected partner or partners may be considered to be analogous to the eye of a person with trachoma, since both are subjected to multiple episodes of chlamydial infection. Immune responses evoked by genital chlamydial infection may be protective, but may also cause damage to tissues.

RESPONSES TO LYMPHOGRANULOMA VENEREUM INFECTION

LGV is endemic in developing countries in East and West Africa, India and parts of South East Asia, South America and the Caribbean, whilst it is sporadic in the rest of Asia and South America and in industrialized countries[61]. The prevalence of LGV is not known. LGV is caused by the LGV biovar comprising serovars L_1, L_2 and L_3, which infect lymphatic tissues. The primary lesion is generally a transient asymptomatic ulcer or 'haircut lesion' on the penis or vagina, which suggests that LGV infects through damaged tissues and that the susceptible cells are in the submucosa. Primary LGV can also present as urethritis or cervicitis. The secondary stage comprises fever, an acute lymphadenitis with bubo formation known as the inguinal syndrome, with or without acute haemorrhagic proctitis. In some patients, the secondary stage is followed by the development of chronic inflammation, fistulae, rectal strictures and genital elephantiasis, known as the anogenito-rectal syndrome[61]. There are a few studies of the aetiology of genital ulcerations in developing countries. In Swaziland, for example, *C. trachomatis* was isolated from the ulcer base in eight patients (5%)[62] and a diagnosis of LGV was made in 12% of patients with genital ulcers, while in Kenya it was isolated from only one out of 30 women with genital ulcers[63].

Infection with LGV agents evokes humoral and cellular immune responses. The first immunological test for the diagnosis of chlamydial infections was the Frei test, which was introduced as a diagnostic skin test for LGV[64]. The original antigen was a suspension of pus obtained from buboes of patients with LGV. This was replaced by heat-inactivated mouse brain extracts, obtained from mice which had been given an intracerebral LGV infection, and later by LGV grown in yolk sacs of embryonated hens' eggs. The yolk-sac antigen could be produced in bulk and was much more reliable, sensitive and specific than the antigens from mouse-brains[65,66]. The CF test, which was first used for the diagnosis of psittacosis[14] was later used to diagnose LGV[67]. A comparison of mouse-lung antigen and hen-egg antigen using sera from patients with a clinical history of LGV who were Frei-test positive showed that hen-egg antigen appeared to be more potent[67]. A significant rise in CF-antibody titre during the disease is unusual in LGV because most patients present with acute lymphadenitis, which is a secondary manifestation of LGV[68]. Cross-reactions between sera of patients with LGV or psittacosis and LGV and psittacosis antigens were observed. Some patients with psittacosis were Frei-test positive[69]. Another study showed that psittacosis, ornithosis, meningopneumonitis, feline and mouse pneumonitis strains could all be used in place of LGV strains for the Frei test[70]. These results indicate that the CF test and the Frei test detect responses to chlamydial group antigens.

LGV EBs attach to lymphocytes *in vitro*[33] and LGV may spread in this way from the primary lesion to lymphoid tissue. LGV EBs may also be carried by lymphocytes into the circulation where they can react with serum antibodies, followed by activation of complement, producing some of the systemic features of LGV.

The introduction of the micro-IF test has shown that LGV isolates can be grouped into three serovars, L_1, L_2 and L_3 and that most isolates are L_2[26]. Patients with LGV have much higher titres of antibodies than patients with uncomplicated genital infections caused by the trachoma biovar and these antibodies are broadly cross-reactive[71]. Immunoblotting studies of sera from patients with LGV react to a wide range of EB surface antigens, with the major proportion of antibodies reacting with MOMP[72]. Although LGV infection evokes immune responses, they are not necessarily effective at terminating infection. *C. trachomatis* has been isolated from perianal lesions in a patient 20 years after LGV was diagnosed[73]. Patients with LGV often have high levels of immunoglobulins in their blood, particularly IgA, indicating that LGV infection causes non-specific stimulation of immuno-globulin production *in vivo* as well as *in vitro*[56,74]. Non-specific stimulation may also cause chronic inflammatory reactions and the enlargement of lymph nodes which are found iN LGV.

At present, we have very little understanding of the disease process in LGV. It is not known how many patients develop complicated LGV or what factors contribute towards the development of these complications. Nothing is known about the relative prevalence of the three serovars L_1, L_2 and L_3 whether they are all equally virulent or if they are associated with different forms of LGV.

RESPONSES TO NON-SPECIFIC GENITAL INFECTIONS CAUSED BY *C. TRACHOMATIS* SEROVARS D–K

C. trachomatis serovars D–K cause about 50% of NSGI[1]. Infection in women is associated with cervicitis, urethritis and proctitis, and can spread, producing endometritis, salpingitis, perihepatitis and infertility. In men, infection produces urethritis, epididymitis, and proctitis. Some individuals develop reactive arthritis. Infection can be asymptomatic, mild, moderate or severe and can be transmitted to the eye by fingers, causing adult chlamydial ophthalmia. Infection can also be transmitted from mothers to their babies, who acquire infection through contact with infected cervical discharges during birth. Infected babies may be asymptomatic or develop NCO or NCP. The reasons why some individuals have an asymptomatic infection while others have severe disease is not known. There may be differences in virulence between different strains and serovars of *C. trachomatis* as well as differences between responses to infection individuals, which may predispose some people to severe disease. At present, it is not known to what extent such differences exist or if they are responsible for the varying severity of disease. It is important, therefore, to treat asymptomatic patients to prevent transmission to others who may be at risk of developing severe disease.

NSGI caused by *C. trachomatis* serovars D–K evokes humoral and cellular immune responses. However, the Frei test and CF test which were widely used for the diagnosis of LGV are not useful for diagnosing NSGI caused by *C. trachomatis*. In a survey of patients with chlamydial genital infection and their consorts[75], it was found that only 9% had a positive reaction to the Frei test and 6% a significant level of CF-antibodies. More recently, it was reported[76] that 26% of women from whose cervices *C. trachomatis* was isolated, and 23% of women from whom *C. trachomatis* was not isolated, had CF-antibody titres of 16 or more, indicating that the CF test is an insensitive indicator of NSGI associated with *C. trachomatis* infection. The micro-IF test is far more sensitive than the CF test and has been widely used for the serological diagnosis of NSGI caused by *C. trachomatis* serovars D–K[71]. *In vitro* tests for cellular immune responses appear to be more sensitive than the Frei test, since lymphocyte stimulation and leukocyte migration inhibition are evoked by L_2 EBs in the majority of patients with proven or probable chlamydial infection[77]. It is not clear, however, whether these results reflect specific T-lymphocyte proliferation, stimulated by L_2 EBs or non-specific proliferation of the B-lymphocyte[56].

Infection in women

Chlamydial cervicitis does not always evoke symptoms and signs. In a study in the United Kingdom[78], only 51% of women from whom *C. trachomatis* was isolated had symptoms. Cervical ectopy was found in 70% of women, and 37% had endocervical mucopus. There was a significant association between cervical ectopy, mucopus, and large quantities of *C. trachomatis*. Most women who had more than 10000 inclusion forming units (IFU) of *C. trachomatis* per monolayer had ectopy and mucopus (75% and 66%, respectively) compared with 36% and 58%, respectively, in women who had less than 10 IFU[79]. Some women who develop complicated chlamydial genital infection have chlamydial cervical infection, but failure to isolate *C. trachomatis* from the cervix does not exclude *C. trachomatis* as a cause of upper genital tract infection. In Sweden[80], *C. trachomatis* was isolated from the fallopian tubes of five women with salpingitis and from the cervices of four of them. Isolates were also obtained from the endometrium of eight women with acute salpingitis and the cervices of six of them[81]. There has recently been a report[82] of three women who had upper genital tract infection caused by *C. trachomatis*, but from whose cervices *C. trachomatis* was not isolated. One of these women had a hysterectomy because of persistent irregular vaginal bleeding which may have been caused by her undiagnosed infection. There is no correlation between the severity of tubal inflammation and the presence of *C. trachomatis* in the cervix[80]. Serological studies have shown that infertility, ectopic pregnancy and failure of *in vitro* fertilization and embryo replacement are all associated with *C. trachomatis* infection[83–85].

Biopsy specimens from patients with chlamydial cervicitis, show that there is cellular infiltration consisting of PMN cells, lymphocytes and plasma cells[86–89]. Lymphoid follicles with germinal centres are present in cervical biopsies from women with follicular cervicitis whose partners have NSU[90]. Non-specific severe inflammatory cellular atypia occurs in cervical smears from 38% women from whom *C. trachomatis* is isolated, compared with 18% of women with negative cultures and this difference is statistically significant[91]. The presence of transformed lymphocytes or histiocytes in cervical smears correlates with the presence of *C. trachomatis* in the cervix[92]. Endometrial biopsies from patients with chlamydial salpingitis show cellular infiltration with plasma cells and PMN cells[81], while the fallopian tubes are infiltrated with lymphocytes and PMN cells[93,94].

Non-immune factors are important in protecting against chlamydial genital infection and in preventing the spread of infection to the upper genital tract. The use of oral contraceptives is associated with a two to three-fold increase in cervical *C. trachomatis* infection[95]. It would be reasonable to expect a corresponding increase in chlamydial salpingitis with resultant infertility in women who take oral contraceptives. However, oral contraceptives appear to modify the manifestations of complicated infection. In a Swedish study[96], 40% of patients with chlamydial salpingitis used oral contraceptives, whereas none of the 12 patients with chlamydial perihepatitis used them. Acute chlamydial salpingitis is more likely to develop within 7 days of the onset of menses than at any other stage of the menstrual cycle. This suggests that the spread of chlamydial cervical infection is favoured by conditions at this time[97]. Childbirth and termination of pregnancy also potentiate the spread of chlamydial infection to the upper genital tract. In a study in the United Kingdom[98], 4% of women with chlamydial cervicitis developed salpingitis, whereas 67% of women whose babies developed NCO, subsequently developed salpingitis. In Norway, *C. trachomatis* was isolated from the cervices of 13% of women undergoing termination of pregnancy; 20% of these women subsequently developed salpingitis, whereas only 2% of women from whom *C. trachomatis* was not isolated developed salpingitis[99].

Chlamydial genital infections evoke humoral and cellular immune responses in women. Humoral immune responses consist of systemic and local responses, the systemic responses comprising chlamydial IgM and IgG antibodies in serum, the local responses comprising chlamydial IgA and IgG antibodies in genital secretions. Seroconversion or a four-fold rise in titre between acute and convalescent sera are not commonly seen in patients with chlamydial cervicitis because infections are often asymptomatic or are mild at onset, so that patients present late. A provisional serological diagnosis of chlamydial cervicitis can be made on single specimens using the micro-IF test, particularly in populations with a low prevalence of chlamydial genital infections. The presence of chlamydial antibodies in serum IgM, or high levels of antibodies in serum IgG ($1 > 32$), or chlamydial IgG or IgA antibodies in secretions, indicate current chlamydial genital infection. In London, these criteria included 77% of women from whose cervices *C. trachomatis* was isolated, 49% of whom had chlamydial antibodies in serum IgM, 40% had high levels of chlamydial antibodies in serum IgG, 74% had chlamydial IgG in cervical secretions and 57% had chlamydial IgA in cervical secretions[29]. The presence of chlamydial IgA antibodies in cervical secretions, detected by radio-immunoassay (RIA) using L_2 EBs, may be a very useful diagnostic test, since high levels were found in 35% of women from whose cervices *C. trachomatis* was isolated and only 6% of women from whom it was not isolated[100]. Immunoblotting studies have shown that women with chlamydial cervicitis have antibodies to *C. trachomatis* MOMP[101].

Women with complicated chlamydial genital infections have higher titres of chlamydial antibodies, presumably reflecting exposure to much larger amounts of chlamydial antigens compared with women who have uncomplicated infections. In a study in London[102], 55% of sera from women with salpingitis contained chlamydial IgG with a geometric mean titre of 99, while 7% had contained chlamydial IgM. In comparison, 29% of the sera from women with uncomplicated genital infections had chlamydial IgG with a geometric mean titre of 58, and 19% of sera from women attending a gynaecological clinic had chlamydial IgG with a geometric mean titre of 33. None of the sera from the women in these two groups contained chlamydial IgM. Chlamydial antibodies were found in cervical secretions in 26% of women with salpingitis, 10% of women with uncomplicated genital infection and 1% of women attending a gynaecological clinic. In another study[103], there was a correlation between the severity of salpingitis and high titres of antibodies against *C. trachomatis*. It was found that 73% of women with severe salpingitis had chlamydial IgG in serum at a titre of 64 or more, compared with 48% of women with moderate salpingitis, 43% of women with mild salpingitis and 11% of controls. There was also a correlation between the severity of salpingitis and mean antibody levels. The geometric mean titre of chlamydial IgG in serum was 527 in patients with severe salpingitis, 189 in patients with moderate salpingitis and 63 in patients with mild disease. High levels of chlamydial IgG and IgA antibodies were also found in fluid aspirated from the pouch of Douglas[103]. It has been reported that chlamydial antibody titres, detected using a modified micro-IF test, are significantly higher in patients with chlamydial salpingitis and perihepatitis than in patients with chlamydial salpingitis only, the geometric mean titres being 1021 and 69, respectively[96]. Chlamydial IgG and IgA antibodies, detected using an indirect-IF test with L_2 IBs as antigen, appear to persist in serum for several years after an episode of chlamydial salpingitis treated with appropriate antibiotics. Most of these women did not have recurrent salpingitis, but it is not clear whether their partners also received antichlamydial therapy[104].

Although skin tests indicate that only a few patients with chlamydial genital infection develop cellular immune responses, these results conflict with those obtained using *in vitro* tests, which indicate that the majority develop cellular immune responses. In a study of men and women with uncomplicated *C. trachomatis* genital infections, a comparison of lymphocyte transformation stimulated by serovar E or L_2 EBs showed that responses to the two serovars were highly correlated, while stimulation by L_2 RBs was 'less well correlated'. In untreated women, the lymphocyte stimulation index was significantly higher in those who had chlamydial antibodies in their sera, irrespective of whether or not *C. trachomatis* was isolated from their cervices. These women were not given antichlamydial treatment, and when retested 3–4 weeks later, showed no significant change in the lymphocyte stimulation index[105]. In a subsequent study, it was found that women with large amounts of *C. trachomatis* (more than 10^4 IFU per ml transport medium) had significantly higher lymphocyte stimulation indices than women with smaller amounts, presumably reflecting exposure to larger amounts of *C. trachomatis* antigens[106]. In women with laparoscopically-confirmed acute salpingitis and cervical *C. trachomatis* infection, significant lymphocyte transformation was stimulated by serovar I and L_2 EBs compared with controls. The response to serotype L_2 EBs was greater than the response to serotype I EBs[107].

Table 6.3 *C. trachomatis* cervical infections in women of different ages

| Group studied | Country | C. trachomatis isolation rate (%) | | | | Reference |
		< 19 years	20–24 years	25–29 years	> 30 years	
Pregnant women	Sweden	10.0	8.7	6.0	3.9	108
Puerperal women	Sweden	24.0	10.2	3.4	5.7	108
Puerperal women	Sweden	7.1	3.7	2.3	0.5	109
Puerperal women	Norway	15.6	17.9	10.6	1.9	99
Puerperal women	Norway	25.8	8.9	} 2.3		110
Women attending sexually transmitted diseases clinic	USA	> 30*	15*	10*	10*	114

*These figures are approximations which were read off a histogram

131

There are several observations that rates of *C. trachomatis* isolation from the cervix are higher in younger than in older women, and some of these are summarized in Table 6.3. In a study of pregnant and puerperal women in Sweden, *C. trachomatis* was isolated from 10% and 24%, respectively of women aged 19 years or less, from 9% and 10%, respectively, of women aged 20–24 years, from 6% and 3%, respectively of women aged 25–29 years, and from 4% and 6%, respectively, of women aged 30 years or more[108]. Other studies of puerperal women in Sweden and in Norway have produced similar results[99,109,110]. Similar observations have been made in the USA. In a study of high-risk pregnant women[111], *C. trachomatis* was isolated from 33% of those aged less than 20 years, compared with 16% of those aged more than 21 years, a difference which is statistically significant. In a prospective study of women undergoing termination of pregnancy[112], women from whom *C. trachomatis* was isolated had a mean age of 18 years. They were significantly younger than women from whom *C. trachomatis* was not isolated, who had a mean age of 22 years. In another study of women seeking abortion in the USA, 64% of women from whom *C. trachomatis* was isolated were less than 20 years of age. This percentage was significantly higher compared with women from whom *C. trachomatis* was not isolated, 38% of whom were less than 20 years old[113]. In women attending a clinic for sexually transmitted diseases, there was a correlation between age and the isolation of *C. trachomatis* which was isolated from approximately 35% in women aged 15 years or less, 30% of women aged 16–19 years, 15% of women aged 20–24 years and about 10% of women aged 25 years or more[114].

It has also been reported that large amounts of *C. trachomatis* (>1000 IFU per monolayer) were isolated from 40% of women aged less than 20 years compared with 13% of all the women studied[79]. However, another study failed to confirm the correlation between the amount of *C. trachomatis* isolated from the cervix and age[115].

Younger women are more likely to develop complicated infection than older women. In a study in Norway, 40% of women with *C. trachomatis* cervical infection aged 19 years or under developed salpingitis after termination of pregnancy, compared with 16% of women aged 20–24 years, 13% of women aged 25–29 years, and no women aged 30 years or more[99]. In another Scandinavian study, *C. trachomatis* was isolated from the cervix and fallopian tubes of 53% and 10%, respectively, of women with salpingitis aged 20 years or less, compared with 34% and 7%, respectively, of women with salpingitis aged 21 years or more[80].

It may be that the increased isolation rate and the large amount of *C. trachomatis* isolated from younger women indicate that these younger women lack protective responses, which older women may have developed presumably as a result of previous exposure to *C. trachomatis*. However, this assumes that the rate of exposure to *C. trachomatis* is the same in all age groups. This may not be so, since peak rates of sexual activity occur around 25 years of age. Younger women with *C. trachomatis* cervical infection also appear to be more likely to develop complicated infection, which indicates that lack of protective responses rather than hypersensitivity causes complicated infection. The nature of these protective responses is not known.

There are some indications as to the roles of immune responses in chlamydial genital infections in women. Comparison of the amount of *C. trachomatis* recovered from the cervix with levels of local and systemic chlamydial antibodies in women with uncomplicated infection has produced some interesting correlations. The numbers of women with chlamydial IgM in their sera increases proportionately with the amount of *C. trachomatis* recovered from the cervix. This suggests that a minimum quantity of *C. trachomatis* is required to trigger the production of chlamydial IgM in serum. It also suggests that chlamydial IgM antibodies neither control nor limit infection. There is no relation between high levels ($>1/64$) of chlamydial IgG antibodies in serum and the amount of *C. trachomatis* recovered from the cervix. However, there is a reciprocal relationship between the amounts of *C. trachomatis* and levels of chlamydial antibodies in local secretions, particularly secretory IgA. This implies that local antibodies may be important in reducing shedding of *C. trachomatis*[106]. A long-term study of women with chlamydial salpingitis has shown that chlamydial cervical IgA antibodies, detected using an indirect-IF test with L_2 IBs, tend to be less common in women who subsequently become infertile than in women who are either fertile or voluntarily infertile. While the difference between the groups was not statistically significant, this trend suggests that cervical IgA antibodies may prevent the spread of chlamydial infection[104]. An immunoblotting study of antibodies from infertile women, fertile women and women attending a gynaecological clinic revealed several differences. Sera from infertile women reacted more frequently with LPS and two other antigens than sera from the other two groups of women. All the women had similar titres of chlamydial antibodies measured by an indirect-IF test with L_2 IBs as antigen, and all their sera reacted with MOMP[116]. Titres of chlamydial antibodies were significantly lower in sera from pregnant women with chlamydial cervical infection who developed acute salpingitis following termination of pregnancy compared with women who did not develop salpingitis (geometric mean titres 14.9 and 41.6, respectively). In addition, those who developed acute salpingitis lacked chlamydial IgA antibodies in serum to high molecular weight antigens[117]. Immunoblotting analysis showed that there were qualitative and quantitative differences between sera from these two groups of women. Antibodies to three antigens (100, 31 and 29 kD) only occurred in women who did not develop salpingitis. These women often had more antibodies to other chlamydial antigens than those who developed salpingitis. However, there was no relation between levels of chlamydial neutralizing antibodies in sera and the development of salpingitis[118]. These results suggest that certain specific antibodies may limit chlamydial genital infections in women. A comparison of chlamydial antibodies from younger and older women might reveal which antibodies are related to resistance to salpingitis.

Infection in men

C. trachomatis causes urethritis, epididymitis, proctitis and pharyngeal infection in men and is associated with infertility.

The urethra is the most common site of *C. trachomatis* genital infection, which can be asymptomatic or present as urethritis. Asymptomatic infection may be common. *C. trachomatis* was isolated from 11% of sexually active asymptomatic men in the USA Army and 3–6 weeks later, none of these men had developed signs or symptoms of infection[119]. In men attending a clinic for sexually transmitted diseases from whom *C. trachomatis* was isolated, symptoms were found in 73% of the heterosexual and 35% of homosexual men, while 16% and 35% respectively, had signs but no symptoms, and the remainder were without symptoms or signs[120]. Some of these asymptomatic men were followed-up. The majority remained free of symptoms, yet *C. trachomatis* could still be isolated from them for several more weeks[121]. In a study in New Orleans[122], men who attended hospital because of minor trauma were screened for *C. trachomatis* urethral infection and 11% had asymptomatic infection. Men with asymptomatic *C. trachomatis* infection any act as a reservoir of infection whose size and importance is probably underestimated.

Chlamydial infection can spread from the urethra and produce epididymitis. In a study of men with chlamydial urethritis in the USA, 1% had concomitant acute epididymitis at their initial visit. No additional cases of epididymitis occurred when antichlamydial therapy was delayed until their second visit[120]. In two studies in the United Kingdom, *C. trachomatis* was detected in urethral smears from men with acute epididymitis in 38% in the first study[123] and 25% in the second[124].

Chlamydial genital infections in men evoke humoral and cellular immune responses. Seroconversion or a four-fold rise in titre establishes the diagnosis. In a study of men experiencing their first known episode of urethritis in Seattle[125], it was found that 55% of men from whom *C. trachomatis* was isolated and 5% of men from whom *C. trachomatis* was not isolated developed chlamydial antibodies or had a four-fold rise in titre using a micro-IF test. However, these serological criteria are often not fulfilled because many men present late or have mild disease. Analysis of a single specimen allows only a provisional diagnosis to be made. In the same study, chlamydial IgM antibodies were detected using the micro-IF test in sera from 16 out of 20 men during their first attack of urethritis from whom *C. trachomatis* was isolated, and in sera from 4% of men from whom *C. trachomatis* was not isolated. This Chlamydial IgM was present only transiently[125]. However, the absence of chlamydial antibodies does not exclude a diagnosis of chlamydial urethritis. In a study carried out in London[126], only 54% of men with urethritis from whom *C. trachomatis* was isolated, had antibodies in serum detected with the micro-IF test. Some of the antibody-negative men may have been tested before antibody production had begun, producing an overestimate of the number of men who fail to produce antibodies. The titre of chlamydial antibodies in men with urethritis is lower than in women with cervicitis. The geometric mean titre of serum antibodies was 37 in men with urethritis from whom *C. trachomatis* had been isolated, compared with 66 in women with cervicitis again from whom *C. trachomatis* had been isolated. In a further study in Seattle[127], comparing men and women from whom *C. trachomatis* had been obtained, men with urethritis had a mean serum titre of 21 compared with a mean serum titre of 101 in women with cervicitis. These findings suggest that men are exposed to lower doses of *C. trachomatis* antigens than women, or that they are less efficient at producing chlamydial antibodies. Antibodies have also been detected in urethral secretions of men with chlamydial urethritis using RIA with L_2 EBs antigen. Sixty-five per cent of men from whom *C. trachomatis* was isolated had high levels of IgA in urethral secretions, 31% had intermediate levels and 4% had low levels, while only 15% of men from whom *C. trachomatis* was not isolated had high levels of antibodies, 32% had intermediate levels and 53% had low levels. This test could be useful for screening of populations with a low prevalence of urethritis caused by *C. trachomatis*[100].

Serological studies suggest that *C. trachomatis* infection is associated with infertility in men. Chlamydial IgG antibodies were detected using an enzyme-immune assay (EIA) method using L_2 EBs as antigen, in sera from 47% of subfertile men who reported previous genito-urinary infection, compared with 28% of subfertile men and 26% of fertile men without such a history[128]. Chlamydial IgA antibodies have also been detected in semen using RIA, with L_2 IBs as antigen. This method detected antibodies in 51% of infertile men with excessive numbers of PMN cells in their semen, compared with 27% of infertile men and 23% of fertile men with normal seminal PMN cell counts. Significantly more men in the first group had antibodies[129]. Immuno-blotting analysis of sera from men with urethritis from whom *C. trachomatis* was isolated, show that IgG in acute-phase sera reacts only with MOMP, whereas IgG in convalescent-phase sera reacts with a wider range of antigens from L_2 EBs[130].

Cellular immune responses have also been detected following chlamydial urethritis. The lymphocyte stimulation index was significantly higher in men from whom *C. trachomatis* was isolated, compared with those from whom *C. trachomatis* was not isolated or those without circulating chlamydial antibodies. When treated patients returned 3–4 weeks later, the lymphocyte stimulation index had fallen significantly[105]. However, positive skin tests were found in only a minority of men with urethritis and from whom *C. trachomatis* was isolated[75].

Younger men appear to be more susceptible to *C. trachomatis* genital infection than older men. In patients from Seattle[120], *C. trachomatis* was isolated from 18% of heterosexual and homosexual men with urethritis aged 18 years or less, 14% of men aged between 19 and 25, 10% of men aged 25–29 and 4% of men aged over 29. A study was carried out in Sweden[131] of men with acute urethritis. *C. trachomatis* was isolated from 71% of patients aged 25 years or less and from 17% of men aged 26 or more. *C. trachomatis* is also associated with significantly more asymptomatic infections in younger men. Karam and colleagues[122] in New Orleans, found that the average age of asymptomatic men from whom *C. trachomatis* was isolated was 22 years, which was significantly lower than the average age of the asymptomatic men from whom *C. trachomatis* was not isolated. *C. trachomatis* epididymitis also occurs more often in younger men which was 28 years in the United Kingdom. In a survey in London[123], *C. trachomatis* was associated with 48% of cases in men aged under 35 years and 15% of cases in men aged over 35, while in a survey in Leeds[124], *C. trachomatis* was associated with 45% of cases in men under 35 years and 9% of cases in men over that age. These qualitative findings are supported by quantitative studies. Large numbers of *C. trachomatis* (4500 IFU or more per monolayer) were obtained from 32% of teenage men with urethritis and from 18% from men aged 20 or more. The quantities of *C. trachomatis* in the infective exudates were similar in both heterosexual partners, and declined with age[115]. This parallels the decline in the prevalence of *C. trachomatis* infection with increasing age. These observations suggest a degree of protective immunity in older men, presumably caused by previous exposure. The development of protective immunity is also reflected in the rates of isolation of *C. trachomatis* from men experiencing their first episode of NSU compared with those with recurrent episodes. In a London study[132], the isolation rates from men with no previous episodes of NSU, or from men with a past history of gonococcal urethritis were 56% and 58% respectively, while in men who had had two previous recorded episodes of NSU, the isolation rate fell to 12%.

Reactive Arthritis

Chlamydial genital infection is sometimes associated with the development of reactive arthritis. It is far more common in men than in women and occurs in approximately 1% of men with NSU[133]. The possession of the histocompatibility antigen HLA-B27 predisposes the development of reactive arthritis (see Chapter 2). It has been estimated that 80% of patients with reactive arthritis have the HLA-B27 antigen, using data pooled from several studies[133], but in a London study[134], 47% of men with reactive arthritis had HLA-B27 antigen compared with 6% of men with uncomplicated NSU and 7% of healthy controls. It is not certain whether *C. trachomatis* is present in the affected joints. *C. trachomatis* has occasionally been isolated from joints, more frequently from specimens inoculated into hens' eggs than from specimens inoculated into cell cultures[133]. *C. trachomatis* EBs have recently been detected in synovial fluid using a fluorescein-labelled monoclonal antibody against *C. trachomatis* MOMP[135]. This implies that *C. trachomatis* probably spreads from the genital tract to joints in patients with reactive arthritis. *C. trachomatis* has not been detected in other lesions associated with reactive arthritis, such as circinate balanitis[136].

Chlamydial antibodies and cellular immune responses to *C. trachomatis* have been detected in reactive arthritis. When men with reactive arthritis were compared to those with uncomplicated NSU, *C. trachomatis* was isolated from 36% and 37% respectively. Chlamydial IgM antibodies were present in sera from 37% and 42% respectively. However, 73% of men with reactive arthritis had significant levels of chlamydial IgG antibodies in their sera, with a geometric mean titre of 48, compared with 50% of men with NSU who had a titre of 8. In the men from whom *C. trachomatis* was associated, the geometric mean titres of chlamydial IgG, in the men with reactive arthritis compared to those with uncomplicated urethritis were 188 and 15, respectively. The high levels of chlamydial antibodies were not caused by polyclonal activation because levels of antibodies against measles, rubella and influenza viruses were not raised[134], so they probably reflect exposure to large quantities of *C. trachomatis*. In another study from the Seattle group[137], chlamydial antibody levels were compared in men from whom *C. trachomatis* was isolated. The geometric mean titre was 70 in with reactive arthritis, which was significantly higher than the mean titre of 25 in the men with urethritis but without arthritis. There was no correlation between antibody levels and the presence of the HLA-B27 antigen. Cellular immune responses have been detected using peripheral blood mononuclear cells. Lymphocyte transformation, stimulated by serovar L_2 EBs, was significantly greater in men with reactive arthritis than those with NSU[137]. Synovial mononuclear cells from patients with reactive arthritis also respond to chlamydial antigen[138].

It seems that being male, having the histocompatibility antigen HLA-B27 and acquiring chlamydial genital infection, all predispose to the development of reactive arthritis. However, reactive arthritis does occur in women and also occur in the absence of the HLA-B27 antigen.

Infection in immunosuppressed adults

C. trachomatis infection is not a major problem in immunosuppressed patients, suggesting that *C. trachomatis* is not harboured in a latent form after episodes of genital infection. There are a few reports of the isolation of *C. trachomatis* from the respiratory tract of immunosuppressed patients with pneumonia. It was isolated from transbronchial biopsies or bronchial washings of three patients with acquired immune deficiency syndrome (AIDS) who had pneumonia. They all had chlamydial IgG antibodies in their sera, and one also had chlamydial IgM. However, all three patients had concomitant respiratory infection with *Pneumocystis carinii*. *C. trachomatis* was associated with less than 1% of episodes of pneumonia in patients with AIDS, suggesting that it is not a major respiratory pathogen in these patients[139].

Chlamydial genital infection and children

Effects on fetal development

There are conflicting reports about the effects of chlamydial genital infection in pregnant women and on their babies. Some studies suggest that infection is associated with preterm rupture of membranes, preterm labour and low birth-weight[140-142]. Other studies have not found any association[110,143-145].

Neonatal chlamydial infection

Pregnant women who have chlamydial genital infection can transmit their infection to their babies, who acquire it through contact with infected cervical discharges during birth. The most common form of neonatal chlamydial infection (NCI) is NCO, but upper and lower respiratory tract, genital tract and rectal infections also occur. The prevalence of NCI reflects the prevalence of chlamydial genital infections in pregnant women, which, in turn, reflects the prevalence of chlamydial genital in infections in the population.

Surveys of ophthalmia neonatorum (ON) and NCO have given some widely differing figures. Surveys in the last 10 years include three studies in the United Kingdom. In two studies, the incidence of NCO was very low. In a suburb of outer London, the incidence of ON was 8% and no cases of NCO were found[146]. In Southampton, the incidence of ON was 12% and C. trachomatis was isolated from only one out of 54 cases[147]. In contrast, C. trachomatis was isolated from half of babies with ON in a study in inner London[148]. In a Swedish study[149], 14% of infants with ON had NCO, which usually developed within one month of birth. In an American study[150], where penicillin and tetracycline prophylaxis were given shortly after birth, the incidence of ON was less than 1%, and NCO was diagnosed in 3% of cases of ON. In two American studies of babies with ON[151,152], NCO was diagnosed in 46% of babies less than 2-months-old and 73% of those less than 1-month-old.

Prospective studies of pregnant women with untreated C. trachomatis infection in the USA, show that 8–22% of their babies develop NCP[153]. NCP is less common in Western Europe. In London, for example, two cases of NCO followed by NCP have been reported[154], and in a study in Sweden[109], there were no cases of NCP in a total of 39 babies with NCO. Other pathogens have been isolated from babies with NCP. These include such viruses as cytomegalovirus, respiratory syncytial virus and Bordetella pertussis[155]. These infections may exacerbate symptoms and signs of NCP[153]. C. trachomatis has been isolated from middle ear fluids obtained from babies with NCP and serous otitis media[156]. A prospective study[157] showed a higher rate of otitis media, gastroenteritis, conjunctivitis and pneumonitis in babies from whose mothers C. trachomatis was isolated, composed with babies whose mothers were not infected.

Prospective studies show that some babies acquire NCI from their mothers and some develop NCO or NCP, while others remain asymptomatic. Several factors may account for these differences. Some mothers may resolve their C. trachomatis genital infection after being tested but before the birth of their babies, so that their babies are not exposed to C. trachomatis during birth. Some babies may not acquire NCI from their mothers because the amount of viable C. trachomatis in their mothers' cervical secretions may be too small to infect them. It is possible that some serovars of C. trachomatis are more infectious for neonatal tissues. This hypothesis can be tested by comparing the relative frequencies of the different serovars in NCI and chlamydial genital infection. Preliminary evidence, based on analysis of chlamydial antibodies in sera from 16 pairs of parents of babies with NCO indicates that serovar K is associated with 25% of infections[126]. A comparison of sera from 35 mothers whose babies who had NCO, compared with 95 women with chlamydial cervicitis suggests that serovars G and K are more common and serotypes D and D/E were less frequent in the mothers than in the women with cervicitis[158]. There may, therefore, be differences in tissue tropism between different serovars. Babies with NCI have been born to mothers from whom C. trachomatis has not been isolated. In a prospective study of pregnant women, NCI occurred in four babies born to women from whom C. trachomatis was isolated and in three babies born to women from whom C. trachomatis was not isolated. It is possible that the mothers of these three babies acquired their chlamydial genital infection between the time when they were tested and the birth of their babies. However, this is unlikely, since all three women had antibodies in their cervical secretions when they were tested[159]. In another study[155], four cases of NCI occurred in babies born to women from whom *C. trachomatis* was not isolated and who had chlamydial IgG antibodies in their sera. These observations indicate that in order to interrupt maternal transmission of chlamydial infection to neonates, teatment should be given to all pregnant women who have antibodies to *C. trachomatis* and not only to those from whom *C. trachomatis* has been isolated. Babies who acquire NCI from their mothers but who do not develop NCO or NCP are likely to remain undiagnosed and untreated. Some of these babies become chronically infected and *C. trachomatis* can be repeatedly isolated from them for many months[160].

Mothers with chlamydial genital infections can transfer chlamydial IgG antibodies to their babies through the placenta. If chlamydial antibody titres in the sera of mothers are compared with those of their babies, aged 2–4 weeks, there is a close correlation between the levels, implying that the babies' antibodies are acquired from their mothers[159]. In another study[161], levels of chlamydial IgG antibodies in maternal sera and cord blood were virtually identical. They differed by a two-fold dilution or less in 93%, and by a four-fold dilution in only 7%. This difference lies within the range of experimental error in the system. In contrast, although chlamydial IgM antibodies were present in 25% of maternal sera, they were not present in cord blood[161]. A study of 393 cord blood specimens in London, showed that 18% had IgG antibodies against *C. trachomatis*, but none had chlamydial IgM or IgA antibodies[159]. A survey in Liverpool of 23 babies with NCO whose mothers were seropositive showed that only three babies (13%) had antibodies in the first week of life[161] which suggests that lack of maternal antibodies may make babies more prone to NCO. Chmalydial secretory IgA antibodies have been detected in colostrum and milk, using EIA with serovar L_2 EBs as antigen. While chlamydial antibody levels in colostrum and milk were closely related, there was no relation between chlamydial secretory IgA antibody levels in milk and IgA antibodies in serum, suggesting that antibodies in milk are locally produced[162]. Babies can, therefore, acquire chlamydial IgA antibodies from their mothers during breast-feeding, and these antibodies may be protective. There are no studies comparing the incidence of NCI, NCO and NCP in breast-fed and bottle-fed babies.

The presence of maternally-derived chlamydial IgG antibodies in babies means that these antibodies do not necessarily confirm a diagnosis of NCI. Chlamydial antibodies in tears may be more useful if it can be shown that they are made by the baby and are not passively acquired from the mother's colostrum or milk. In one study[163], tear antibodies were absent at birth, but developed in four out of eight babies with NCO and three out of ten babies without NCO born to mothers from whom *C. trachomatis* had been isolated. In another study[158], all babies who had NCO, NCP or nasopharyngeal infection developed chlamydial antibodies in tears and nasopharyngeal secretions, as did some babies who were clinically normal. These two studies detected mainly IgG chlamydial antibodies with the micro-IF test, using antihuman globulin as the second antibody. Chlamydial IgM antibodies can develop in babies with NCO and NCP but they are not always found. Only 11% of babies with NCO had these IgM antibodies in their sera. Chlamydial IgM was detected, using a simplified micro-IF test, in 35% of babies with pneumonia, and *C. trachomatis* was isolated from 46% of these babies. Much higher levels of chlamydial IgM antibodies have been found in babies with NCP compared with babies with NCO or asymptomatic nasopharyngeal infection[161]. Chlamydial IgM antibodies have also been detected in babies with NCP using an indirect-IF test with serovar I RBs as antigen or EIA with serovar L_2 MOMP as antigen. EIA using serovar L_2 RBs, or LPS from *Salmonella minnesota* as antigen was much less sensitive in this study[164]. Chlamydial IgM antibodies have also been detected by micro-IF or EIA, using L_2 EBs as antigen, in babies with NCP, but not in babies with NCO[165]. The presence of chlamydial IgM antibodies is, therefore, a useful diagnostic test for NCP. The higher prevalence and titres of chlamydial IgM antibodies in babies with NCP presumably reflects their exposure to much larger quantities of chlamydial antigens than babies with NCO.

Non-specific stimulation of immune responses has also been reported in babies with NCP. These babies have much higher levels of total IgM, IgG and IgA in their sera than babies with afebrile viral pneumonia[155]. Babies with NCP also have increased numbers of blood lymphocytes with IgM or IgG in their cytoplasm. Lymphocytes from these babies produce considerable amounts of IgM, IgA and IgG when cultured, but these immunoglobulins have no detectable anti-chlamydial activity. In contrast, lymphocytes from normal babies and babies with other respiratory infections or NCO do not secrete immunoglobulins *in vitro*[166]. These observations indicate that *C. trachomatis* serovars D–K can cause non-specific stimulation of B-lymphocytes *in vivo* similar to that seen in LGV[74].

Although chlamydial IgM antibodies have been detected using a modified micro-IF test in young children with lower respiratory tract infection or infectious mononucleosis, *C. trachomatis* could not be isolated from them. It was concluded that this represented non-specific stimulation of B-lymphocytes by pathogens[167]. However, production of chlamydial IgM antibodies may have been stimulated by infection with *C. 207* or TWAR strains in some of these cases.

INFECTIONS IN DEVELOPING COUNTRIES

NSGI is the most prevalent infection associated with *C. trachomatis* in Western Europe and the USA. In some developing countries, all three forms of infection caused by *C. trachomatis* occur; trachoma caused by serovars A–C, NSGI by serovars D–K and LGV. Sexually transmitted diseases are more prevalent in developing than in industrialized countries and complications are more common and severe[168]. In developing countries, confirmation of chlamydial genital infections by laboratory tests is limited mainly to major hospitals and clinics with suitably equipped laboratories. In Table 6.4, chlamydial genital infections caused by *C. trachomatis* serovars

Table 6.4 Chlamydial genital infections in developing countries

General features of sexually transmitted diseases in developing countries[168]	Non-specific genital infection*	Lymphogranuloma venereum
(1) More prevalent in developing countries	common in many African countries, e.g. Kenya[236,169], Ethiopia[237], Sudan[238], Nigeria[239], Ghana[177], Gambia[170], common in India[171], Singapore[172], common in urban populations of Iran[173,174], common in Australian aborigines[175] and American Indians[176]	endemic in some countries, e.g. East and West Africa, India[61]
(2) Different relative frequencies in developing countries	more common than gonorrhoea in some countries, e.g. Ghana[177]; less common than gonorrhoea in some countries, e.g. Gambia[170], Kenya[169]; Swaziland[186]	common cause of genital ulceration in some countries e.g. Swaziland[186]
(3) Complications more common and severe in developing countries	common cause of salpingitis or infertility in some countries, e.g. Gambia[179], Gabon[180], common cause of ophthalmia neonatorum in some countries, e.g. Gambia[170], Central African Republic[181], Kenya[182], but not in others, e.g. Zambia[183]	Severe disease more common in countries where LGV is endemic

*Chlamydial Infection confirmed by culture or serology

D–K and LGV in particular countries, are compared with the general features of sexually transmitted diseases in developing countries.

Infections caused by serovars D–K and LGV

Although data on the prevalence of these infections in developing countries is limited, there seems to be a considerable variation between different countries[169–176], see Table 6.4.

NSGI is now more common than gonococcal infection in the United Kingdom[1], Sweden and the USA[5] and probably throughout Western Europe. In developing countries, the relative frequencies are very variable. *C. trachomatis* was isolated more often than *Neisseria gonorrhoeae* from Ghanaian women attending a gynaecological clinic (5% and 3%, respectively) and from post-partum women in a maternity ward (8% and 3%, respectively). Serological tests showed that 25% of these post-partum women had antibodies to *C. trachomatis*[177]. *N. gonorrhoea* is more common than *C. trachomatis* in other developing countries. In Nairobi for example, *N. gonorrhoeae* was isolated from 26% and *C. trachomatis* from 7% of women attending a clinic for sexually transmitted diseases[169]. In a survey in Swaziland[178], 80% of men with urethritis had gonococcal urethritis, 6% had NSU and *C. trachomatis* was isolated from 3% of patients. Serological testing using a modified micro-IF test did not aid the aetiological diagnosis of urethritis in these patients because many of them had antibodies which cross-reacted with all three pools of *C. trachomatis* (A–C, D–K, L$_1$, L$_2$ and L$_3$), regardless of whether they had gonococcal, non-gonococcal or no 'objective' urethritis.

The prevalence and severity of complications resulting from genital infection with *C. trachomatis* serovars D–K in developing countries is not known. It is generally believed that both *C. trachomatis* and *N. gonorrhoeae* are major causes of salpingitis and infertility in African women. Chlamydial IgG antibodies, detected using an ELISA technique with serovar L$_1$ EBs, were found in 68% of infertile women and 35% of fertile women in Gambia[179]. However, trachoma is also common in Gambia, and this test does not distinguish between antibodies to serovars A–C which cause trachoma and serovars D–K. The prevalence of chlamydial genital infection may, therefore, have been overestimated. A study of women with salpingitis in Gabon revealed that *C. trachomatis* could be isolated from 26%, while, using a simplified micro-IF test, 86% had chlamydial antibodies, and 49% had titres greater than 256[180]. *C. trachomatis* is a major cause of ON in some African countries. It was isolated from 35% of babies with ON in Gambia[170], 29% of babies with ON in Central African Republic[181] and 17% of babies with ON in Kenya[182]. In Zambia, it was isolated from only 6% of babies with ON[183].

These findings illustrate the fragmentary state of our knowledge, and they also show that there are clearly considerable differences between developing countries. Very little is known about many other African, Latin American, Middle Eastern and Far Eastern countries.

LGV is endemic in some developing countries[61]. The prevalence of LGV and the proportion of people who subsequently develop severe disease in different countries is not known, but presumably severe disease is more common where LGV is endemic than in countries where it is sporadic.

Interactions between trachoma and chlamydial genital infections

In some developing countries, all three forms of infection caused by *C. trachomatis* occur: trachoma, NSGI and LGV. Although there are indications that in industrialized countries, men and women with NSGI may develop protective immunity, it is not known whether this also occurs in patients with trachoma or LGV, and if this immunity protects against other forms of disease. Serovars A–C and D–K can infect the eye, and they could therefore, be associated with trachoma and NCO. In Gambia, trachoma and genital infections are common. Serotyping of isolates from patients with chlamydial NSGI or NCO and serological analysis of sera from patients with trachoma all indicate that genital infections are associated with serovars D–K and L_2, and trachoma is associated with serovars A and B[184]. However, it is not clear whether genital infection and trachoma occur in the same populations or different sub-populations. In Iran, where trachoma is endemic in rural populations[185], serological studies show that chlamydial genital infection is only common in urban populations[175,176]. In both Gambia and Iran, different serovars continue to be associated with different forms of infection. It is not known, however, whether individuals are actually exposed to serovars causing different forms of disease in these two countries, let alone whether they are protected. In Southern Africa, all three forms of *C. trachomatis* infection occur. A comparison of urban white and black patients with urethritis in Johannesburg, with black patients with urethritis in Swaziland, showed that while *C. trachomatis* was isolated from 2% of white patients and 14% of black patients in Johnnesburg, chlamydiae were isolated from only 3% of black patients with urethritis in Swaziland[186]. In contrast, *C. trachomatis* (presumably serovars L_1, L_2 and L_3) is a common cause of genital ulceration in Swaziland, where it was isolated from 10% of patients[186], but from only one out of 102 black men with genital ulceration in Johannesburg and one out of 100 black women[187,188]. These observations suggest that genital infections caused by serovars D–K, L_1, L_2 and L_3 tend to be mutually exclusive and that immune responses to these infections may be broadly protective.

ANIMAL MODELS

The study of animal models bridges the gap between interactions between host and pathogen at the cellular level and chlamydial infection in humans.

The first step in developing an animal model of an infectious disease is to find a species which is susceptible to the pathogen, or alternatively, a species which has a natural pathogen which produces disease resembling the human disease. The first approach uses the same pathogen, but the animal/pathogen relationship is an unnatural one, and may be very different from the human/pathogen relationship. The second approach uses a different pathogen, but the animal/pathogen relationship is a natural one. The two approaches are complementary, and both have been used to probe chlamydial genital infections. Non-human primates, rabbits and mice have all been used to study *C. trachomatis* genital infections in unnatural hosts, while the guinea pig infected with guinea pig inclusion conjunctivitis (GPIC) agent, the cat infected with feline keratoconjunctivitis (FKC) agent and the mouse infected with mouse pneumonitis (MoPn) agent have been used to study infection in natural hosts.

C. trachomatis infections in unnatural hosts

Non-human primates

Males and females of several species of non-human primates have been used to study *C. trachomatis* genital infections. Infection of male or female chimpanzees, grivet monkeys and marmosets with isolates obtained from patients with chlamydial salpingitis or urethritis (serovars D/E, I and K) elicit a mild PMN and mononuclear cell response[189–193].

Most female marmosets develop chlamydial IgM and IgG antibodies in their sera following vaginal inoculation with a strain of *C. trachomatis* isolated from a patient with NSU, although titres are low and the antibodies are not strain-specific[194]. These animals remain susceptible to vaginal re-infection with the strain used in the initial infection or a serovar H strain, but the duration of re-infection is shorter. These animals, therefore, have partial protective immunity. Antibody titres are boosted by re-infection, and the higher the titre of antibodies in sera, the shorter the duration of re-infection. Following re-infection, inflammation persists for several weeks, despite rapid clearance of *C. trachomatis*[195].

Studies in grivet monkeys have shown that the spread of serovar K infection from the cervix to the fallopian tubes requires an intact genital tract[192]. Repeated cervical re-infection of grivet monkeys with serovar K produces a cervicitis characterized by redness, friability and mucopurulent discharge[196]. These features are common in women with chlamydial cervicitis[78] and suggest that repeated *C. trachomatis* infection may be necessary for the development of cervicitis.

Direct inoculation of *C. trachomatis* serovars E and F into fallopian tubes of pig-tailed macaques produces mild clinical signs of tubal inflammation, associated with infiltration of mononuclear cells and deciliation of epithelial cells. The inflammation is self-limiting, subsiding within 35 days after inoculation. Animals produce chlamydial IgM and IgG antibodies in their sera. *C. trachomatis* can be re-isolated from the fallopian tubes and cervix, and chlamydial secretory IgA is present in cervical secretions during cervical infection[197]. Repeated cervical infection with various serovars (D, F, J) does not produce visible salpingitis at laproscopy. However, when a single direct tubal inoculation is administered after repeated cervical infection, severe tubal disease develops with extensive adhesions and tubal obstruction[198].

Repeated clinical observation and tissue sampling of the upper genital tract presents considerable technical problems. An ingenious method of overcoming this problem is the technique of transplanting fragments of oviductal fimbriae into the skin. The tissue fragments are then walled-off, forming cysts. This model has been used to study chlamydial genital infection in cynomolgus and rhesus monkeys, and complements studies in the intact genital tract. Serovar E infection of subcutaneous pockets containing fimbrial fragments produces redness and swelling of the pockets, and *C. trachomatis* can be re-isolated from the transplanted tissue. Cellular infiltration first consists of PMN cells, followed by lymphocytes. Chlamydial IgM antibodies appear in sera but are short-lived and are followed by IgG[199].

Primary urethral infection of male chimpanzees and baboons with serovars D, D/E and an isolate from a patient with chlamydial urethritis leads to the development of chlamydial antibodies in sera[189,190,200]. Baboons develop a degree of protection against urethral re-infection, no matter whether the same or different strains are used[194].

Inoculation of *C. trachomatis* serovar K into the spermatic cords of male grivet monkeys produces acute inflammation of the spermatic cord, epididymis and testicles with urethral discharge containing PMN cells. Histological studies[201] have shown that the wall of the spermatic cord is infiltrated with PMN cells and lymphocytes, and the lumen of the cord is reduced in diameter and contains an exudate with lymphocytes and desquamated cells.

C. trachomatis serovar D/E obtained from a baby with NCP inoculated into the upper respiratory tract of infant baboons produces nasopharyngitis and pneumonitis. This may be a useful model of chlamydial infections in babies[202].

Rectal infection of male cynomolgus monkeys with *C. trachomatis* serovar L$_2$ produces an inflammatory granulomatous protocolitis, similar to LGV rectal infections in men[203].

Laboratory animals

Rabbits and mice are susceptible to genital infection with *C. trachomatis* serovars D–K. Studies of oviductal infection and re-infection in rabbits with serovars D and F produces a self-limiting salpingitis. An initial PMN cell infiltrate occurs followed by a mononuclear cell infiltrate and deciliation with flattening of epithelial cells. Titres of chlamydial antibodies are much higher after re-infection than after primary infection[204].

Nude (athymic) and immunocompetent mice produce a PMN cell response when infected with serovar L$_2$ following progesterone treatment. Infection is self-limiting, lasting for about 60 days in both groups of animals. The nude mice do not produce serum antibodies, and these experiments indicate that T-lymphocytes and T-lymphocyte dependent antibodies are not required to eradicate infection[205]. Previously infected mice are susceptible to re-infection, but once again, this is shorter than the primary infection[206]. Transfer of spleen cells or serum to non-immune mice does not alter the duration of subsequent infection, and, therefore, the roles of humoral and cellular immune responses in shortening re-infection remain unknown[207]. Intrauterine or intrabursal infection of progesterone-treated mice with *C. trachomatis* serovar E produces infertility in C3H but not in TO mice. The oviducts of the infertile mice appear normal, and the reason for infertility appears to be a failure in the mechanism of transporting eggs to the oviduct[208].

Human cervical carcinoma has the epidemiological features of a venereal disease, and *C. trachomatis* infection may be involved in the development of this neoplasia. Repeated cervical re-infection of untreated mice with cytomegalovirus produces cervical dysplasia and cervical carcinoma in 51% and 10% of mice, respectively, compared with 3% and 0%, respectively, in mice which receive control cell culture fluid. Repeated application of inactivated L_2 EBs has no statistically significant effect on dysplasia or cervical carcinoma in mice[209].

Pneumonitis can be produced in various strains of untreated mice by intranasal infection with many strains of *C. trachomatis*. The early inflammatory response consists predominantly of PMN cells, followed by a mononuclear cell response[210]. Humoral and cellular immune responses are evoked. The decline of infection in the lungs coincides with the development of cellular immune responses which precedes the appearance of measurable antibody. These findings suggest that cellular immune responses restrict the growth of the pathogen and eliminate infection[211], unlike genital infection in progesterone-treated mice. Cortisone acetate or cyclophosphamide treatment inhibits the inflammatory response and prolongs infection, while hydrocortisone succinate treatment has no effect[212]. The differences which have been observed between the course of disease and mortality rates in different studies probably reflect differences in the numbers of EBs inoculated, the virulence of different strains and serovars of *C. trachomatis* for the mouse lung and the different strains of mice used.

Chlamydial infection in natural hosts

Guinea pigs

Guinea pig inclusion conjunctivitis (GPIC) agent is infectious for the guinea-pig conjunctiva, genital tract and rectum. Infection can be transmitted from males to females during mating and from mother to babies during birth[213-215]. Thus GPIC agent infection in guinea pigs is similar to *C. trachomatis* serovars D–K infection in humans. In females, intravaginal infection with GPIC agent evokes a mixed PMN and mononuclear cell response, while in males, urethral infection evokes a pure PMN cell response[213,214]. In females, infection lasts for about 3 weeks[213], evokes systemic and local antibodies and cellular immune responses detected by skin tests[216,217]. The number of GPIC agent inclusions starts to fall at about day seven. Chlamydial antibodies first appear in sera at this time, although they are not found in all animals until day 24[213]. In males, the infection lasts for about a week. Chlamydial antibodies appear in serum and urine and cellular immune responses are detected[214,218]. Genital GPIC agent infection in males does not always induce an immune response[218], reminiscent of men with urethritis, from *C. trachomatis* has been isolated but who lack chlamydial antibodies[29].

Some male guinea pigs have no microbiological or serological evidence of infection following urethral infection with very low doses of GPIC agent, but they are still able to transmit infection to the eyes of uninfected animals caged with them[218]. Rectal GPIC agent infection tends to last longer in males than in females, although GPIC agent can be isolated sporadically from some guinea pigs of both sexes for several weeks. Chlamydial antibodies are found in sera and in some animals, infection spreads upwards into the intestinal tract. However, there are no clinical or histopathological responses to rectal infection[215].

Treatment of guinea pigs with cyclophosphamide facilitates the spread of GPIC agent from the lower genital tract. When females are treated with cyclophosphamide to inhibit the development of humoral responses without affecting cellular immune responses, infection is prolonged and does not resolve until antibodies begin to appear[217]. When females are treated with higher levels which suppress both humoral and cellular responses, spread of infection to the upper genital tract commonly occurs[219]. When males are treated with cyclophosphamide, more of them develop cystitis[220]. These results emphasize that an intact, functioning immune response is required to terminate genital infection and prevent spread to other sites.

Treatment of females with oestradiol produces infection which lasts longer than in untreated animals and larger numbers of GPIC agent inclusions are present in cells from the vaginal wall. Infection spreads throughout the genital tract, producing endometritis, salpingitis and cystitis. The development of chlamydial antibodies in vaginal secretions is considerably delayed in treated animals, the delay depending on the dose of oestradiol, while levels of chlamydial antibodies in sera and skin-test responses are the same in both treated and untreated animals[221-223]. Treatment with a combined oral contraceptive containing mestranol and norethynodel also increases the duration of infection and delays the appearance of chlamydial antibodies in genital secretions[224]. These results demonstrate the importance of local antibodies in limiting the spread of infection within the female guinea pig genital tract, as well as the effects of hormones on their production. Progesterone does not influence the course of infection in female guinea pigs, unlike mice, and it fails to enhance the effect of oestradiol[225].

There is evidence of protection against re-infection in both sexes. Females which have already had a vaginal infection are less likely to acquire further infection from infected males than previously uninfected females. They are also resistant to experimental vaginal re-infection[216]. However, humoral responses are important in protection since females which have been treated with cyclophosphamide to suppress humoral responses and have been treated with tetracycline to cure their primary vaginal infection, remain susceptible to vaginal re-infection[226]. Males are resistant to urethral re-infection 6 weeks after infection, while the conjunctiva remains susceptible, although the duration of infection is reduced[227]. It seems likely, therefore, that immunity in the urethra is mediated by local responses. The shortened duration of conjunctival infection in animals which have had urethral GPIC agent infection, may be caused by systemic humoral and/or cellular immune responses induced by previous urethral infection.

Mice

Mice infected with mouse pneumonitis agent (MoPn), which is a strain of *C. trachomatis*, have been used as models of genital infection, pneumonitis and arthritis. Intravaginal infection of female mice produces infection lasting for about 3 weeks, evokes chlamydial IgM and IgG antibodies in sera, and renders the animals resistant to re-infection[228]. Pneumonitis caused by MoPn infection in nude mice has a high mortality rate. Larger amounts of MoPn agent can be recovered from their lungs than from the lungs of immunocompetent control mice[229]. The experiment indicates the importance of cellular immune responses and T-lymphocyte dependent antibody production in recovery from chlamydial pneumonitis caused by MoPn agent as well as human strains of *C. trachomatis*. Mice which have been immunized with MoPn agent at 6–7 weeks of age develop arthritis following injection of the MoPn agent into joints, while naive mice do not develop arthritis. Previous exposure to MoPn agent and its presence in joints is, required for the development of chlamydial arthritis in mice[230].

Other hosts

Feline keratoconjunctivitis (FKC) agent is an oculogenital strain of *C. psittaci* which infects cats. When FKC agent is inoculated into the oviducts of cats, it produces acute inflammation lasting for about 30 days, followed by chronic inflammation, fimbrial scarring and adhesions. During the acute phase, the oviductal lumens contain exudates of desquamated epithelial cells and PMN cells, while in the chronic phase there is a mixed PMN and mononuclear cell infiltration of oviduct tissues. Chlamydial antibodies can also be detected in sera and fimbrial secretions[231].

In Australia, the decreasing population of koala bears is associated with infertility following infection with a strain of *C. psittaci*. Experimental infection of the female genital tract produces ascending infection and infertility. Infection of the male genital tract produces urethritis and cystitis. This strain of *C. psittaci* also causes conjunctivitis and rhinitis in koala bears[232].

FOUR UNANSWERED QUESTIONS

There are four major questions regarding chlamydial genital infections which remain unanswered. The first question is whether or not different forms of the disease are caused by different strains or serovars. It is not known whether or not asymptomatic chlamydial urethritis and cervicitis are associated with the same strains or serovars as chlamydial epididymitis, salpingitis or perihepatitis. Until recently, typing isolates was a long and tedious operation. However, the development of monoclonal antibodies against different serovars now provides a rapid and reliable method of typing isolates, and this problem can now be tackled[233,234]. The second question concerns the role of immune responses in infection. There are indications of protective immunity following infection in humans and in animals. However, there is also evidence in animal models that previous exposure is associated with extensive tissue damage during re-exposure, indicating that immune responses can be damaging. The dual protective and damaging effects of immune responses in chlamydial genital infection appear to be similar to those in chlamydial ocular infection[58]. In addition, the roles of immune responses evoked by other chlamydial infections, such as trachoma or respiratory infections caused by *C. 207* or TWAR strains are not known. Again, cross-reactive responses could be protective and/or damaging. Immunoblotting analysis may identify those antibodies associated with protection and those associated with damage. The third question is why some people, particularly men, do not produce antibodies when they have infection. It is not known whether they also fail to produce cellular immune responses, and whether the absence of antibodies makes them prone to develop complications. The last question is what is the significance of non-specific stimulation of antibody production observed in LGV[74] and NCP[166]. This may be how *C. trachomatis* augments or depresses immune responses[235].

The answers to these questions are important for chlamydial control programmes. There may be certain strains or serovars which can only cause asymptomatic infections. If these strains were identified and if they could evoke immune responses which protect against infection by other strains and serovars, they could be used as live vaccines to prevent transmission of those strains and serovars which cause disseminated infections. If immunoblotting studies show that uncomplicated genital infection is associated with the production of antibodies against particular antigens, then these antigens could form the basis of a vaccine to prevent disseminated infections. The effects of *C. trachomatis* antigens on the regulation of immune responses must be studied in greater detail to aid vaccine development. It is not clear whether trachoma and NSGI are mutually exclusive in Iran and Gambia. If they are, then it is possible that the elimination of one form of chlamydial infection may render the population susceptible to other forms from which they were previously protected. Conversely, since exposure to ocular or respiratory chlamydial infection may also evoke immune responses associated with tissue-damage, subsequent genital infection could be accompanied by increased tissue damage with consequent effects on fertility. The aims of the immunologist must be to find answers to these questions and to develop safe and effective vaccines.

ACKNOWLEDGEMENTS

I thank everyone who has helped me in the long process of converting this chapter from a twinkle in the editor's eye to the typescript on his desk. I am grateful to the librarian and her staff at the Institute of Ophthalmology who have obtained so many references from other libraries (most of which have little to do with ophthalmology), to my colleagues with whom I have discussed many aspects of chlamydial infections, and who have read and commented on various sections of this chapter, particularly Mr R. Kirton and Drs J. Treharne and R. Woodland. I also thank Miss C. Sharp, who has converted my untidy scrawl into typescript with great accuracy and patience.

References

1. Anonymous. (1986). Sexually transmitted disease surveillance in Britain – 1984. *Br. Med. J.*, **293**, 942-3
2. Stamm, W. E. and Holmes, K. K. (1984). *Chlamydia trachomatis* infections of the adult. In Holmes, K. K., Mårdh, P.-A., Sparling, P. F. and Wiesner, P. J. (eds.). *Sexually Transmitted Diseases*, pp. 258-270. (New York: McGraw-Hill)
3. Weström, L. and Mårdh, P.-A. (1983). Chlamydial salpingitis. *Br. Med. Bull.*, **39**, 145-50
4. Stanton, S. L. (1987). Acute salpingitis. *Br. Med. J.*, **295**, 621-2
5. Anonymous. (1981). *Nongonococcal urethritis and other selected sexually transmitted diseases of public health importance*. World Health Organization Technical Report Series, 660. (Geneva: World Health Organization)
6. Tarizzo, M. L. (ed.). (1973). *Field methods for the control of trachoma*. (Geneva: World Health Organization)
7. Grayston, J. T., Kuo, C.-C., Wang, S.-P., Cooney, M. K., Altman, J., Marrie, T. J., Marshall, J. G. and Mordhorst, C. H. (1986). Clinical findings in TWAR respiratory tract infections. In Oriel, D., Ridgway, G., Schachter, J., Taylor-Robinson, D. and Ward, M. (eds.). *Chlamydial Infections*. pp. 337-340 (Cambridge: Cambridge University Press)
8. Ward, M. E. (1983). Chlamydial classification, development and structure. *Br. Med. Bull.*, **39**, 109-15
9. Todd, W. J. and Caldwell, H. D. (1985). The interaction of *Chlamydia trachomatis* with host cells: ultrastructural studies of the mechanism of release of a biovar II strain from HeLa 229 cells. *J. Infect. Dis.*, **151**, 1037-44
10. Moorman, D. R., Sixbey, J. W. and Wyrick, P. B. (1986). Interaction of *Chlamydia trachomatis* with human genital epithelium in culture. *J. Gen. Microbiol.*, **132**, 1055-67
11. Hutchinson, G. R., Taylor-Robinson, D. and Dourmashkin, R. R. (1979). Growth and effect of chlamydiae in human and bovine oviduct organ culture. *Br. J. Vener. Dis.*, **55**, 194-202
12. Swanson, J., Eschenbach, D. A., Alexander, E. R. and Holmes, K. K. (1975). Light and electron microscopic study of *Chlamydia trachomatis* infection of the uterine cervix. *J. Inf. Dis.*, **131**, 678-87
13. Allen, I. (1986). Chlamydial antigenic structure and genetics. In Oriel, D., Ridgway, G., Schachter, J., Taylor-Robinson, D. and Ward, M. (eds.). *Chlamydial Infections*. pp. 73-80 (Cambridge: Cambridge University Press)
14. Bedson, S. P. and Western, G. T. (1930). Part II Aetiology – experimental observations. In Sturdee, E. L. and Scott, W. M. (eds.). *A Disease of Parrots Communicable to Man (Psittacosis). Reports on Public Health and Medical Subjects*, **61**, 59-95.
15. Dhir, S. P., Hakomori, S., Kenny, G. E. and Grayston, J. T. (1972). Immunochemical studies on chlamydial group antigen (presence of a 2-keto-3-deoxycarbohydrate as immunodominant group). *J. Immunol.*, **109**, 116-22
16. Nurminen, M., Leinonen, M., Saikku, P. and Mäkelä, P. H. (1983). The genus-specific antigen of *Chlamydia*: resemblance to the lipopolysaccharide of enteric bacteria. *Science*, **220**, 1279-81
17. Dhir, S. P., Kenny, G. E. and Grayston, J. T. (1971). Characterization of the group antigen of *Chlamydia trachomatis*. *Infect. Immun.*, **4**, 725-30
18. Watkins, N. G., Caldwell, H. D. and Hackstadt, T. (1987). Chlamydial hemagglutinin identified as lipopolysaccharide. *J. Bacteriol.*, **169**, 3826-8
19. Caldwell, H. D. and Judd, R. C. (1982). Structural analysis of chlamydial outer membrane proteins. *Infect. Immun.*, **38**, 960-8
20. Caldwell, H. D. and Perry, L. J. (1982). Neutralization of *Chlamydia trachomatis* infectivity with antibodies to the major outer membrane protein. *Infect. Immun.*, **38**, 745-54
21. Krech, T., Gerhard-Fsadni, D., Hofmann, N. and Miller, S. M. (1985). Interference of *Staphylococcus aureus* in the detection of *Chlamydia trachomatis* by monoclonal antibodies. *Lancet*, **1**, 1161-2
22. Lipkin, E. S., Moncada, J. V., Shafer, M.-A., Wilson, T. E. and Schachter, J. (1986). Comparison of monoclonal antibody staining and culture in diagnosing cervical chlamydial infection. *J. Clin. Microbiol.*, **23**, 114-17
23. Caldwell, H. D. and Schachter, J. (1982). Antigenic analysis of the major outer membrane

protein of *Chlamydia* spp. *Infect. Immun.*, **35**, 1024–31
24. MacDonald, A. B. (1985). Antigens of *Chlamydia trachomatis*. *Rev. Infect. Dis.*, **7**, 731–5
25. Wang, S.-P., and Grayston, J. T. (1970). Immunologic relationships between genital TRIC, lymphogranuloma venereum and related organisms in a new microtitre indirect immunofluorescence test. *Am. J. Ophthalmol.*, **70**, 367–74
26. Wang, S.-P. and Grayston, J. T. (1971). Classification of TRIC and related strains with micro immunofluorescence. In Nichols, R. L. (ed.). *Trachoma and Related Disorders*, pp. 305–21 (Amsterdam, London, Princeton: Exerpta Medica)
27. Wang, S.-P. and Grayston, J. T. (1982). Micro immunofluorescence antibody responess in *Chlamydia trachomatis* infection, a review, In Mårdh, P.-A., Holmes, K. K., Oriel, J. D., Piot, P. and Schachter, J. (eds.). *Chlamydial Infections*. pp. 301–16. (Amsterdam, New York, Oxford: Elsevier Biomedical Press)
28. Forsey, T., Stainsby, K., Hoger, P. H., Ridgway, G. L., Darougar, S. and Fisher-Brugge, U. (1986). Comparison of two immunofluorescence tests for detecting antibodies to *C. trachomatis*. *Eur. J. Epidemiol.*, **2**, 163–4.
29. Treharne, J. D., Darougar, S., Simmons, P. D. and Thin, R. N. (1978). Rapid diagnosis of chlamydial infection of the cervix. *Br. J. Vener. Dis.*, **54**, 403–8
30. Richmond, S. J., Stirling, P. (1981). Localization of chlamydial group antigen in McCoy cell monolayers infected with *Chlamydia trachomatis* or *Chlamydia psittaci*. *Infect. Immun.*, **34**, 561–70
31. Reddish, M. A., Hourihan, J., Tirrell, S. and MacDonald, A. B. (1986). Characterization of a type-specific antigen of *Chlamydia trachomatis*, and associated enzymatic activity. In Oriel, D., Ridgway, G., Schachter, J., Taylor-Robinson, D., and Ward, M. (eds.). *Chlamydial Infections*. pp. 23–6. (Cambridge: Cambridge University Press)
32. Tirrell, S. M., Stuart, E. S. and MacDonald, A. B. (1986). Heterogenity among chlamydia genus specific LPS and exoglycolipid. In Oriel, D., Ridgway, G., Schachter, J., Taylor-Robinson, D. and Ward, M. (eds.). *Chlamydial Infections*. pp. 126–8. (Cambridge: Cambridge University Press)
33. Bard, J. and Levitt, D. (1986). *Chlamydia trachomatis* (L₂ serovar) binds to distinct subpopulations of human peripheral blood leukocytes. *Clin. Immunol. Immunopathol.*, **38**, 150–60
34. Mårdh, P.-A., Colleen, S. and Sylwan, J. (1980). Inhibitory effect on the formation of chlamydial inclusions in McCoy cells by seminal fluid and some of its components. *Invest Urol.* **17**, 510–13
35. Hanna, L., Keshishyan, H., Brooks, G.F., Stites, D. P. and Jawetz E. (1981). Effect of seminal plasma on *Chlamydia trachomatis* LB-1 in cell culture. *Infect. Immun.*, **32**, 404–6
36. Kondo, L. R., Hanna, L. and Keshishyan, H. (1973). Reduction in chlamydial infectivity by lysozyme. *Proc. Soc. Exp. Biol. Med.*, **142**, 131–2
37. Welch, W. D., Polek, W. and Thrupp, L. (1983). Effect of lysozyme on the *in vitro* infectivity of *Chlamydia trachomatis*. *Curr. Microbiol.*, **8**, 293–6
38. Bushell, A. C. and Hobson, D. (1978). Effect of cortisol on the growth of *Chlamydia trachomatis* in McCoy cells. *Infect. Immun.*, **21**, 946–53
39. Reed, S. I. and Hann, W. D. (1980). The effect of cortisol on glycogen and fructose-1, 6-biphosphatase in baby hamster kidney cells infected with *Chlamydia trachomatis*. *Can. J. Microbiol.*, **26**, 135–40
40. Sugarman, B. and Agbor, P. (1986). Estrogens and *Chlamydia trachomatis*. *Proc. Soc. Exp. Biol. Med.*, **183**, 125–31
41. Johnson, A. P., Osborn, M. F., Rowntree, S., Thomas, B. J. and Taylor-Robinson, D., (1983). A study of inactivation of *Chlamydia trachomatis* by normal human serum. *Br. J. Vener. Dis.*, **59**, 369–72
42. Jenkin, H. M. and Lu, Y. K. (1967). Induction of interferon by the Bour strain of trachoma in Hela 229 cells. *Am. J. Ophthalmol.*, **63**, 1110–15
43. Hanna, L., Merigan, T. C., and Jawetz, E. (1967). Effect of interferon on TRIC agents and induction of interferon by TRIC agents. *Am. J. Ophthalmol.*, **63**, 1115–19
44. Mordhorst, C. H., Reinicke, V. and Schonne, E. (1967). *In ovo* inhibition by concentrated chick interferon of the growth of TRIC agents. *Am. J. Ophthalmol.*, **63**, 1107–9
45. Kazar, J., Gillmore, J. D. and Gordon, F. B. (1971). Effect of interferon and interferon inducers on infections with a nonviral intracellular microorganism, *Chlamydia trachomatis*.

Infect. Immun., **3**, 825-32

46. Rothermel, C. D., Byrne, G. I., Havell, E. A. (1983). Effect of interferon on the growth of *Chlamydia trachomatis* in mouse fibroblasts (L cells). *Infect. Immun.*, **39**, 362-70

47. de la Maza, L. M., Peterson, E. M., Fennie, C. W., and Czarniecki, C. W. (1985). The anti-chlamydial and anti-proliferative activities of recombinant murine interferon-gamma are not dependent on tryptophan concentrations. *J. Immunol.*, **135**, 4198-200

48. Shemer, Y. and Sarov, I. (1985). Inhibition of growth of *Chlamydia trachomatis* by human gamma interferon. *Infect. Immun.*, **48**, 592-6

49. de la Maza, L. M., Plunkett, M., Peterson, E. M., and Czarniecki, C. W. (1986). Inhibition of *C. trachomatis* by recombinant Mu-IFN-gamma. In Oriel, D., Ridgway, G., Schachter, J., Taylor-Robinson, D. and Ward, M. (eds.). *Chlamydial Infections*. pp. 441-4 (Cambridge: Cambridge University Press)

50. Yong, E. C., Klebanoff, S. J. and Kuo, C.-C. (1982). Toxic effect of human polymorphonuclear leukocytes on *Chlamydia trachomatis*. *Infect. Immun.*, **37**, 422-6

51. Zvillich, M. and Sarov, I. (1985). Interaction between human polymorphonuclear leukocytes and *Chlamydia trachomatis* elementary bodies: electron microscopy and chemiluminescent response. *J. Gen. Microbiol.*, **131**, 2627-35

52. Yong, E. C., Chi, E. Y., Chen, W.-J. and Kuo, C.-C. (1986). Degradation of *Chlamydia trachomatis* in human polymorphonuclear leukocytes: an ultrastructural study of peroxidase-positive phagolysosomes. *Infect. Immun.*, **53**, 427-31

53. Söderlund, G., Dahlgren, C. and Kihlström, E. (1984). Interaction between human polymorphonuclear leukocytes and *Chlamydia trachomatis*. *FEMS Microbiol. Letts.*, **22**, 21-5

54. Hammerschlag, M. R., Suntharalingam, K. and Fikrig, S. (1985). The effect of *Chlamydia trachomatis* on luminol-dependent chemiluminescence of human polymorphonuclear leukocytes: requirements for opsonization. *J. Infect. Dis.*, **151**, 1045-51

55. Manor, E. and Sarov, I. (1986). Fate of *Chlamydia trachomatis* in human monocytes and monocyte-derived macrophages. *Infect. Immun.*, **54**, 90-5

56. Bard, J. and Levitt, D. (1984). *Chlamydia trachomatis* stimulates human peripheral blood B lymphocytes to proliferate and secrete polyclonal immunoglobulins *in vitro*. *Infect. Immun.*, **43**, 84-92

57. Barenfanger, J. and MacDonald, A. B. (1974). The role of immunoglobulin in the neutralization of trachoma infectivity. *J. Immunol.*, **113**, 1607-17

58. Monnickendam, M. A., and Pearce, J. H. (1983). Immune responses and chlamydial infections. *Br. Med. Bull.*, **39**, 187-93

59. Darougar, S., and Jones, B. R. (1983). Trachoma. *Br. Med. Bull.*, **39**, 117-22

60. Schachter, J. and Dawson, C. R. (1978). *Human Chlamydial Infections*. (Littleton: PSG Publishing)

61. Perine, P. L. and Osoba, A. O. (1984). Lymphogranuloma venereum. In: Holmes, K. K., Mårdh, P.-A., Sparling, P. F. and Wiesner, P. J. (eds.). *Sexually Transmitted Diseases*, pp. 281-91 (New York: McGraw-Hill)

62. Meheus, A., van Dyck, E., Ursi, J. P., Ballard, R. C. and Piot, P. (1983). Etiology of genital ulcerations in Swaziland. *Sex. Transm. Dis.*, **10**, 33-5

63. Plummer, F. A., D'Costa, L. J., Nsanze, H., Karasira, P., Maclean, I. W., Piot, P. and Ronald, A. R. (1985). Clinical and microbiological studies of genital ulcers in Kenyan women. *Sex. Transm. Dis.*, **12**, 193-7

64. Frei, W. (1925). Eine neue Hautreaktion bei Lymphogranuloma inguinale. *Klin. Wochenschr.*, **4**, 2148-9

65. Rake, G., McKee, C. M. and Shaffer, M. F. (1940). Agent of lymphogranuloma venereum in the yolk-sac of the developing chick embryo. *Proc. Soc. Exp. Biol. Med.*, **43**, 332-4

66. Grace, A. W., Rake, G. and Schaffer, M. F. (1940). A new material (Lygranum) for performance of the Frei test for lymphogranuloma venereum. *Proc. Soc. Exp. Biol. Med.*, **45**, 259-63

67. McKee, C. M., Rake, G. and Shaffer, M. F. (1940). Complement fixation test in lymphogranuloma venereum. *Proc. Soc. Exp. Biol. Med.*, **44**, 410-13

68. Bedson, S. P., Barwell, C. F., King, E. J. and Bishop, L. W. J. (1949). The laboratory diagnosis of lymphogranuloma venereum. *J. Clin. Pathol.*, **2**, 241-9

69. Rake, G., Eaton, M. D. and Shaffer, M. F. (1941). Similarities and possible relationships

among viruses of psittacosis meningopneumonitis, and lymphogranuloma venereum. *Proc. Soc. Exp. Biol. Med.*, **48**, 528–31

70. Hilleman, M. R., Greaves, A. B. and Werner, J. H. (1958). Group-specificity of psittacosis-lymphogranuloma venereum group skin test antigens in lymphogranuloma venereum. *J. Lab. Clin. Med.*, **52**, 53–7

71. Treharne, J. D., Forsey, T. and Thomas, B. J. (1983). Chlamydial serology. *Br. Med. Bull.*, **39**, 194–200

72. Ward, M. E., Treharne, J. D. and Murray, A. (1986). Antigenic specificity of human antibody to Chlamydia in trachoma and lymphogranuloma venereum. *J. Gen. Microbiol.*, **132**, 1599–609

73. Dan, M., Rotmensch, H. H., Eylan, E., Rubinstein, A., Ginsberg, R. and Liron, M. (1980). A case of lymphogranuloma venereum of 20 years' duration. Isolation of *Chlamydia trachomatis* from perianal lesions. *Br. J. Vener. Dis.*, **45**, 344–6

74. Lassus, A., Mustakallio, K. K. and Wager, O. (1970). Autoimmune serum factors and IgA elevation in lymphogranuloma venereum. *Ann. Clin. Res.*, **2**, 51–6

75. Barwell, C. F., Dunlop, E. M. C. and Race, J. W. (1967). Results of complement-fixation and intradermal tests for Bedsoniae in genital infection, disease of the eye and Reiter's disease. *Am. J. Ophthalmol.*, **63**, 1527–34

76. Schachter, J., Cles, L., Ray, R. and Hines, P. A. (1979). Failure of serology in diagnosing chlamydial infections of the female genital tract. *J. Clin. Microbiol.*, **10**, 647–9

77. Hanna, L., Kerlan, R., Senyk, G., Stites, D. P., Juster, R. P. and Jawetz, E. (1982). Immune responses to chlamydial antigens in humans. *Med. Microbiol. Immunol.*, **171**, 1–10

78. Tait, I. A., Rees, E., Hobson, D., Byng, R. E. and Tweedie, M. C. K. (1980). Chlamydial infection of the cervix in contacts of men with non-gonococcal urethritis. *Br. J. Vener. Dis.*, **56**, 37–45

79. Hobson, D., Karayiannis, P., Byng, R. E., Rees, E., Tait, I. A. and Davies, J. A. (1980). Quantitative aspects of chlamydial infection of the cervix. *Br. J. Vener. Dis.*, **56**. 156–62

80. Gjønnaess, H., Dalaker, K. Ånestad, G., Mårdh, P.-A., Kvile, G. and Bergan, T. (1982). Pelvic inflammatory disease: etiologic studies with emphasis on chlamydial infection. *Obstet. Gynec.*, **59**, 550–5

81. Wølner-Hanssen, P., Mårdh, P.-A., Møller, B. and Weström, L. (1982). Endometrial infection in women with chlamydial salpingitis. *Sex. Transm. Dis.*, **9**, 84–8

82. Møller, B. R., Kaspersen, P., Kristiansen, F. V. and Mårdh, P.-A. (1986). *Chlamydia trachomatis* in the upper female genital tract with negative cervical culture. *Lancet*, **2**, 390

83. Kane, J. L., Woodland, R. M., Forsey, T., Darougar, S. and Elder, M. G. (1984). Evidence of chlamydial infection in infertile women with and without fallopian tube obstruction. *Fertil. Steril.*, **42**, 843–8

84. Gump, D. W., Gibson, M. and Ashikaga, T. (1983). Evidence of prior pelvic inflammatory disease and its relationship to *Chlamydia trachomatis* antibody and intrauterine contraceptive device use in infertile women. *Am. J. Obstet. Gynecol.*, **146**, 153–9

85. Rowland, G. F., Forsey, T., Moss, T. R., Steptoe, P. C., Hewitt, J. and Darougar, S., (1985). Failure of *in vitro* fertilization and embryo replacement following infection with *Chlamydia trachomatis*. *J. in vitro Fertil. Embryo Transfer*, **2**, 151–5

86. Braley, A. E. (1938). Inclusion blennorrhea. A study of the pathologic changes in the conjunctiva and cervix. *Am. J. ophthalmol.*, **21**, 1203–7

87. Evans, B. A. (1982). Chlamydial infection of the human cervix – an ultrastructural study. *J. Infect.* **4**, 225–8

88. Paavonen, J., Vesterinen, E., Meyer, B. and Saksela, E. (1982). Colposcopic and histologic findings in cervical chlamydial infection. *Obstet. Gynecol.*, **59**, 712–15

89. Kiviat, N., Paavonen, J., Wolner-Hanssen, P., Critchlow, C., De Rouen, T., Douglas, J., Stevens, C. and Holmes, K. K. (1986). Histologic manifestations of chlamydial cervicitis. In Oriel, D., Ridgway, G., Schachter, J., Taylor-Robinson, D. and Ward, M. (eds.). *Chlamydial Infections*. pp. 209–12 (Cambridge: Cambridge University Press)

90. Hare, M. J., Toone, E., Taylor-Robinson, D., Evans, R. T., Furr, P. M., Cooper, P. and Oates, J. K., (1981). Follicular cervicitis – colposcopic appearances and association with *Chlamydia trachomatis*. *Br. J. Obstet. Gynecol.*, **88**, 174–90

91. Paavonen, J. and Purola, E. (1980). Cytologic findings in cervical chlamydial infection.

Med. Biol., **58**, 174-8
92. Kiviat, N. B., Peterson, M., Kinney-Thomas, E., Tam, M., Stamm, W. E. and Holmes, K. K. (1985). Cytologic manifestations of cervical and vaginal infections II. Confirmation of *Chlamydia trachomatis* infection by direct immunofluorescence using monoclonal antibodies. *J. Am. Med. Assoc.*, **253**, 997-1000
93. Møller, B. R., Weström, L., Ahrons, S., Ripa, K. T., Svensson, L., von Mecklenburg, C., Henrikson, H. and Mårdh, P.-A. (1979). *Chlamydia trachomatis* infection of the Fallopian tubes. Histological findings in two patients. *Br. J. Vener. Dis.*, **55**, 422-8
94. Punnonen, R., Terho, P. and Klemi, P. J. (1982). Chlamydial pelvic inflammatory disease with ascites. *Fertil. Steril.*, **37**, 270-2
95. Washington, A. E., Gove, S., Schachter, J. and Sweet, R. L. (1985). Oral contraceptives, *Chlamydia trachomatis* infection, and pelvic inflammatory disease. A word of caution about protection. *J. Am. Med. Assoc.*, **253**, 2246-50
96. Wølner-Hanssen, P. (1986). Oral contraceptive use modifies the manifestations of pelvic inflammatory disease. *Br. J. Obstet. Gynecol.*, **93**, 619-24
97. Sweet, R. L., Blankfort-Doyle, M., Robbie, M. O., Schachter, J., (1986). The occurrence of chlamydial and gonococcal salpingitis during the menstrual cycle. *J. Am. Med. Assoc.*, **255**, 2062-4
98. Rees, E., Tait, I. A., Hobson, D. and Johnson, F. W. A. (1977). Chlamydia in relation to cervical infection and pelvic inflammatory disease. In Hobson, D. and Holmes, K. K. (eds.). *Non-gonococcal Urethritis and Related Infections*, pp. 67-76 (Washington: American Society for Microbiology)
99. Qvigstad, E., Skaug, K., Jerve, F., Fylling, P. and Ulstrup, J. C. (1983). Pelvic inflammatory disease associated with *Chlamydia trachomatis* infection after therapeutic abortion. A prospective study. *Br. J. Vener. Dis.*, **59**, 189-92
100. Terho, P. and Meurman, O. (1981). Chlamydial serum IgG, IgA and local IgA antibodies in patients with genital-tract infections measured by solid-phase immunoassay. *J. Med. Microbiol.*, **14**, 77-87
101. Cevenini, R., Rumpianesi, F., Donati, M., Moroni, A., Sambri, V. and La Placa, M., (1986). Class specific immunoglobulin response to individual polypeptides of *Chlamydia trachomatis*, elementary bodies, and reticulate bodies in patients with chlamydial infection. *J. Clin. Pathol.*, **39**, 1313-16
102. Forsey, T., O'Connor, B. H., Azad, A., West, S., Darougar, S. and Adler, M. W. (1984). *Chlamydia trachomatis* infection in women with acute pelvic inflammatory disease in London, England. *Eur. J. Sex. Transm. Dis.*, **1**, 181-3
103. Treharne, J. D., Ripa, K. T., Mårdh, P.-A., Svensson, L., Weström, L. and Darougar, S., (1979). Antibodies to *Chlamydia trachomatis* in acute salpingitis. *Br. J. Vener. Dis.*, **55**, 26-9
104. Puolakkainen, M., Vesterinen, E., Purola, E., Saikku, P. and Paavonen, J. (1986). Persistence of chlamydial antibodies after pelvic inflammatory disease. *J. Clin. Microbiol.*, **23**, 924-8
105. Brunham, R. C., Martin, D. H., Kuo, C.-C., Wang, S.-P., Stevens, C. E., Hubbard, T. and Holmes, K. K. (1981). Cellular immune response during uncomplicated genital infection with *Chlamydia trachomatis* in humans. *Infect. Immun.*, **34**, 98-104
106. Brunham, R. C., Kuo, C.-C., Cles, L. and Holmes, K. K., (1983). Correlation of host immune response with quantitative recovery of *Chlamydia trachomatis* from the human endocervix. *Infect. Immun.*, **39**, 1491-4
107. Hallberg, T., Wølner-Hanssen, P. and Mårdh, P-A., (1985). Pelvic inflammatory disease in patients infected with *Chlamydia trachomatis: in vitro* cell mediated immune responses to chlamydial infections. *Genitourin. Med.*, **61**, 247-51
108. Mårdh, P.-A., Helin, I., Bobeck, S., Laurin, J. and Nilsson, T., (1980). Colonisation of pregnant and puerperal women and neonates with *Chlamydia trachomatis*. *Br. J. Vener. Dis.*, **56**, 96-100
109. Persson, K., Rönnerstam, R., Svanberg, L. and Holmberg, L., (1981). Maternal and infantile infection with Chlamydia in a Swedish population. *Acta. Paed. Scand.*, **70**, 101-5
110. Skjeldestad, F. E. and Dalen, A., (1986). The prevalence of *Chlamydia trachomatis* in the cervix of puerperal women, and its consequences for the outcome of pregnancy. *Scand. J. Primary Health Care*, **4**, 209-12

111. Martin, D. H., Pastorek, J. G. and Faro, S., (1986). Risk factors for *Chlamydia trachomatis* infection in a high risk population of pregnant women. In Oriel D., Ridgway, G., Schachter, J., Taylor-Robinson, D. and Ward, M., (eds.). *Chlamydial Infections*. pp. 189–92. (Cambridge: Cambridge University Press)

112. Spence, M. R., Barbacci, M., Kappus, E. and Quinn, T., (1986). A correlative study of Papanicolaou smear, fluorescent antibody, and culture for the diagnosis of *Chlamydia trachomatis*. *Obstet. Gynecol.*, **68**, 691–5

113. Amortegul, A. J., Meyer, M. P. and Gnatuk, C. L., (1986). Prevalence of *Chlamydia trachomatis* and other micro-organisms in women seeking abortions in Pittsburgh, Pennsylvania, United States of America, *Geniturin Med.*, **62**, 88–92

114. Stamm, W. E. and Holmes, K. K., (1984). *Chlamydia trachomatis* infections of the adult. In Holmes, K. K., Mårdh, P.-A., Sparling, P. F. and Wiesner, P. J., (eds.). *Sexually Transmitted Diseases*, pp. 258–70. (New York: McGraw-Hill)

115. Mallinson, H., Arya, O. P. and Goddard, A. D., (1982). Quantitative study of *Chlamydia trachomatis* in genital infection. *Br. J. Vener. Dis.*, **58**, 36–9

116. Gump, D. W., Storey, C. C. and Richmond, S. J., (1986). Immunoblot analysis of sera from women attending gynaecology clinics in the UK. In; Oriel, D., Ridgway, G., Schachter, J., Taylor-Robinson, D. and Ward, M., (eds.). *Chlamydial Infections*, pp. 225–8. (Cambridge: Cambridge University Press)

117. Brunham, R. C., Maclean, I., McDowell, J., Peeling, R., Persson, K. and Osser, S. (1986). *Chlamydia trachomatis* antigen specific serum antibodies among women who did and did not develop acute salpingitis following therapeutic abortion. In Oriel, D., Ridgway, G., Schachter, J., Taylor-Robinson, D. and Ward, M., (eds.). *Chlamydial Infections*, pp. 221–4. (Cambridge: Cambridge University Press)

118. Brunham, R. C., Peeling, R., Maclean, I., McDowell, J., Persson, K. and Osser, S., (1987). Postabortal *Chlamydia trachomatis* salpingitis: correlating risk with antigen-specific serological responses and with neutralization. *J. Infect. Dis.*, **155**, 759–55

119. Podgore, J. K., Holmes, K. K. and Alexander, E. R., (1982). Asymptomatic urethral infections due to *Chlamydia trachomatis* in male U.S. military personnel, *J. Infect. Dis.*, **146**, 828

120. Stamm, W. E., Koutsky, L. A., Benedetti, J. K., Jourden, J. L., Brunham, R. C. and Holmes, K. K., (1984). *Chlamydial trachomatis* urethral infections in men. Prevalence, risk factors, and clinical manifestations. *Ann. Intern. Med.*, **100**, 47–51

121. Stamm, W. E. and Cole, B., (1986). Asymptomatic *Chlamydia trachomatis* urethritis in men. *Sex. Transm. Dis.*, **13**, 163–5

122. Karam, G. H., Martin, D. H., Flotte, T. R., Bonnarens, E. O., Joseph, J. R., Mroczkowski, T. F. and Johnson, W. D., (1986). Asymptomatic *Chlamydia trachomatis* infections among sexually active men. *J. Infect. Dis.*, **154**, 900–3

123. Hawkins, D. A., Taylor-Robinson, D., Thomas, B. J., Osborn, M. F. and Harris, J. R. W., (1986). *Chlamydia trachomatis* in acute epididymitis: aspirations without aspirates. In; Oriel, D., Ridgway, G., Schachter, J., Taylor-Robinson, D. and Ward, M., (eds.). *Chlamydial Infections*. pp. 259–62 (Cambridge: Cambridge University Press)

124. Mulcahy, F. M., Bignell, C. J., Rajakumar, R., Waugh, M. A., Hetherington, J. W., Ewing, R. and Whelan, P., (1987). Prevalence of chlamydial infection in acute epididymo-orchitis. *Genitourin. Med.*, **63**, 16–18

125. Bowie, W. R., Wang, S.-P., Alexander, E. R., and Holmes, K. K., Etiology of non-gonococcal urethritis. In; Hobson, D. and Holmes, K. K., (eds.). *Nongonococcal Urethritis and Related Infections*. pp. 19–29. (Washington: American Society for Microbiology)

126. Treharne, J. D., Dines, R. J. and Darougar, S., (1977). Serological responses to chlamydial ocular and genital infections in the United Kingdom and Middle East. In Hobson, D. and Holmes, K. K., (eds.). *Nongonococcal Urethritis and Related Infections*. pp. 249–58. (Washington: American Society for Microbiology)

127. Wang, S.-P., Grayston, J. T., Kuo, C.-C., Alexander, E. R. and Holmes, K. K., (1977). Serodiagnosis of *Chlamydia trachomatis* infection with the micro-immunofluorescence test. In Hobson, D. and Holmes, K. K., (eds.). *Nongonococcal Urethritis and Related Infections*. pp. 237–48. (Washington: American Society for Microbiology)

128. Auroux, M. R., De Mouy, D. M. and Acar, J. F., (1987). Male fertility and positive chlamydial serology. A study of 61 fertile and 82 subfertile men. *J. Androl.*, **8**, 197–200

129. Suominen, J., Grönroos, M., Terho, P. and Wichmann, L., (1983). Chronic prostatitis, *Chlamydia trachomatis* and infertility. *Int. J. Androl.*, 6, 405-13
130. Cevinini, R., Rumpianesi, F., Sambri, V. and La Placa, M., (1986). Antigenic specificity of serological response in *Chlamydia trachomatis* urethritis detected by immunoblotting. *J. Clin. Pathol.*, 39, 325-7
131. Nilsson, S., Johannisson, G. and Lycke, E., (1981). Isolation of *Chlamydia trachomatis* from the urethra and from prostatic fluid in men with signs and symptoms of acute urethritis. *Acta Dermatovener. (Stockh.)*, 61, 456-9
132. Alani, M. D., Darougar, S., Burns, D. C., MacD., Thin, R. N. and Dunn, H., (1977). Isolation of *Chlamydia trachomatis* from the male urethra. *Br. J. Vener. Dis.*, 53, 88-92
133. Keat, A., Thomas, B. J. and Taylor-Robinson, D., (1983). Chlamydial infection in the aetiology of arthritis. *Br. Med. Bull.*, 39, 168-74
134. Keat, A. C., Thomas, B. J., Taylor-Robinson, D., Pegrum, G. D., Maini, R. N. and Scott, J. T., (1980). Evidence of *Chlamydia trachomatis* infection in sexually acquired reactive arthritis. *Ann. Rheum. Dis.*, 39, 431-7
135. Keat, A., Dixey, J., Sonnex, C., Thomas, B., Osborn, M., Taylor-Robinson, D., (1987). *Chlamydia trachomatis* and reactive arthritis: the missing link. *Lancet*, 1, 72-4
136. Kanerva, L., Kousa, M., Niemi, K-M., Lassus, A., Juvakoski, T. and Lauharanta, J., (1982). Ultrahistopathology of balanitis circinata. *Br. J. Vener. Dis.*, 58, 188-95
137. Martin, D. H., Pollock, S., Kuo, C-C., Wang, S-P., Brunham, R. C. and Holmes, K. K., (1984). *Chlamydia trachomatis* infections in men with Reiter's syndrome. *Ann. Intern. Med.*, 100, 207-13
138. Ford, D. K., da Roza, D. M., Shah, P. and Wenman, W. M., (1980). Cell-mediated immune responses of synovial mononuclear cells in Reiter's syndrome against ureaplasmal and chlamydial antigens. *J. Rheumatol.*, 7, 751-5
139. Moncada, J. V., Schachter, J. and Wofsy, C., (1986). Prevalence of *Chlamydia trachomatis* lung infection in patients with acquired immune deficiency syndrome. *J. Clin. Microbiol.*, 23, 986
140. Rees, E., Tait, T. A., Hobson, D. and Johnson, F. W. A., (1977). Perinatal chlamydial infection. In; Hobson, D. and Holmes, K. K., (eds.). *Nongonococcal Urethritis and Related Infections.* pp. 140-7. (Washington: American Society for Microbiology)
141. Gravett, M. G., Nelson, H. P., DeRouen, T., Critchlow, C., Eschenbach, D. A. and Holmes, K. K., (1986). Independent associations of bacterial vaginosis and *Chlamydia trachomatis* infection with adverse pregnancy outcome. *J. Am. Med. Assoc.*, 256, 1899-903
142. Berman, S. M., Harrison, H. R., Boyce, W. T., Haffner, W. J. J., Lewis, M. and Arthur, J. B., (1987). Low birth weight, prematurity, and postpartum endometritis. Association with prenatal cervical *Mycoplasma hominis* and *Chlamydia trachomatis* infections. *J. Am. Med. Assoc.*, 257, 1189-94
143. Frommell, G. T., Rothenberg, R., Wang, S. P., McIntosh, K., Wintersgill, C., Allaman, J. and Orr, I., (1979). Chlamydial infection of mothers and their infants. *J. Pediatr.*, 95, 28-32
144. Heggie, A. D., Lumicao, G. G., Stuart, L. A. and Gyves, M. T., (1981). *Chlamydia trachomatis* infection in mothers and infants. *Am. J. Dis. Child.*, 135, 507-11
145. Thompson, S., Lopez, B., Wong, K.-H., Ramsay, C., Thoas, J., Reising, G., Jenks, B., Peacock, W., Sanderson, M., Goforth, S., Zaidi, A., Miller, R. and Klein, L., (1982). A prospective study of chlamydia and mycoplasma infections during pregnancy: relation to pregnancy outcome and maternal morbidity. In Mårdh, P.-A., Holmes, K. K., Oriel, J. D., Piot, P. and Schachter, J., (eds.). *Chlamydial Infections.* pp. 155-158. (Amsterdam, New York, Oxford: Elsevier Biomedical Press)
146. Prentice, M. J., Hutchinson, G. R. and Taylor-Robinson, D., (1977). A microbiological study of neonatal conjunctivae and conjunctivitis. *Br. J. Ophthalmol.*, 61, 601-7
147. Pierce, J. M., Ward, M. E. and Seal, D. V., (1982). Ophthalmia neonatorum in the 1980s: incidence, aetiology and treatment. *Br. J. Ophthalmol.*, 66, 728-31
148. Winceslaus, J., Goh, B. T., Dunlop, E. M. C., Mantell, J., Woodland, R. M., Forsey, T. and Treharne, J. D., (1987). Diagnosis of ophthalmia neonatorum. *Br. Med. J.*, 295, 1377-9
149. Persson, K., Rönnerstam, R., Svanberg, L. and Pohla, M.-A., (1983). Neonatal chlamydial eye infection: an epidemiological and clinical study. *Br. J. Ophthalmol.*, 67, 700-4
150. Jarvis, V. N., Levine, R. and Asbell, P. H., (1987). Ophthalmia neonatorum: study of a decade of experience at the Mount Sinai Hospital. *Br. J. Ophthalmol.*, 71, 295-300

151. Rapoza, P. A., Quinn, T. C. and Taylor, H. R., (1986). Chlamydial neonatal conjunctivitis: etiology, epidemiology, diagnostic techniques and treatment. In; Oriel, D., Ridgway, G., Schachter, J., Taylor-Robinson, D. and Ward, M., (eds.). *Chlamydial Infections*. pp. 297–300. (Cambridge: Cambridge University Press)

152. Heggie, A. D., Jaffe, A. C., Stuart, L. A., Thombre, P. S. and Sorensen, R. L., (1985). Topical sulfacetamide vs oral erythromycin for neonatal chlamydial conjunctivitis. *Am. J. Dis. Child.*, **139**, 564–6

153. Harrison, H. R. and Alexander, E. R., (1984). *Chlamydia trachomatis* infection of the infant. In: Holmes, K. K., Mårdh, P.-A., Sparling, P. F. and Wiesner, P. J., (eds.). *Sexually Transmitted Diseases*. pp. 270–280. (New York: McGraw-Hill)

154. Dunlop, E. M. C., Harris, R. J., Darougar, S., Treharne, J. D. and Al-Egaily, S. S., (1980). Subclinical pneumonia due to serotypes D-K of *Chlamydia trachomatis*. Case reports of two infants. *Br. J. Vener. Dis.*, **56**, 337–40

155. Brewster, D. R., De Silva, L. M. and Henry, R. L. (1981). *Chlamydia trachomatis* and respiratory disease in children, *Med. J. Aust.*, **68**, 328–30

156. Tipple, M. A., Beem, M. O. and Saxon, E. M. (1979). Clinical characteristics of the afebrile pneumonia associated with *Chlamydia trachomatis* infection in infants less than 6 months of age. *Pediatrics*, **63**, 192–7

157. Schaefer, C., Harrison, H. R., Boyce, W. T. and Lewis, M. (1985). Illnesses in infants born to women with *Chlamydia trachomatis* infection. *Am. J. Dis. Child.*, **139**, 127–33

158. Forsey, T. (1987). Seroepidemiological studies of chlamydial infections in man. PhD Thesis, University of London

159. Hammerschlag, M. R., Anderka, M., Semine, D. Z., McComb, D. and McCormack, W. M. (1979). Prospective study of maternal and infantile infection with *Chlamydia trachomatis*. *Pediatrics*, **64**, 142–8

160. Bell. T. A., Stamm, W. E., Kuo, C.-C., Holmes, K. K. and Grayston, J. T. (1986). Chronic *Chlamydia trachomatis* infections in infants. In Oriel, J., Ridgway, G., Schachter, J., Taylor-Robinson, D. and Ward, M. (eds.). *Chlamydial Infections*. pp. 305–8 (Cambridge: Cambridge University Press)

161. Schachter, J., Grossman, M. and Azimi, P. H. (1982). Serology of *Chlamydia trachomatis* in infants. *J. Inf. Dis.*, **146**, 530–5

162. Skaug, K., Otnaess, A.-B., Ørstavik, I. and Jerve, F. (1982). Chlamydial secretory IgA antibodies in human milk. *Acta. Pathol. Microbiol. Immunol. Scand.*, Section C Immunology, **90**, 21–5

163. Chandler, J. W., Alexander, E. R., Pheiffer, T. A., Wang, S.-P., Holmes, K. K. and English, M. (1977). Ophthalmia neonatorum associated with maternal chlamydial infections. *Trans. Am. Acad. Ophthalmol. Otolaryngol.*, **83**, 302–8

164. Puolakkainen, M., Saikku, P., Leinonen, M., Nurminen, M., Väänänen, P. and Mäkelä, P. H. (1984). Chlamydial pneumonitis and its serodiagnosis in infants. *J. Infect. Dis.*, **149**, 598–604

165. Mahony, J. B., Chernesky, M. A., Bromberg, K. and Schachter, J. (1986). Accuracy of immunoglobulin M immunoassay for diagnosis of chlamydial infections in infants and adults. *J. Clin. Microbiol.*, **24**, 731–5

166. Levitt, D., Newcomb, R. W. and Beem, M. O. (1983). Excessive numbers and activity of peripheral blood B cells in infants with *Chlamydia trachomatis* pneumonia. *Clin. Immunol. Immunopathol.*, **29**, 424–32

167. Persson, K. and Bröms, M. (1986). Chlamydial respiratory infection in childhood and spurious immunoglobulin M. *Eur. J. Clin. Microbiol.*, **5**, 581–3

168. Meheus, A. Z. (1984). Practical approaches in developing nations. In Holmes, K. K., Mårdh, P.-A., Sparling, P. F. and Wiener, P. J. (eds.). *Sexually Transmitted Diseases*. pp. 998–1008. (New York: McGraw-Hill)

169. Mirza, N. B., Nsanze, H., D'Costa, L. J. and Piot, P. (1983). Microbiology of vaginal discharge in Nairobi, Kenya. *Br. J. Vener. Dis.*, **59**, 186–8

170. Mabey, D. C. W. and Whittle, H. C. (1982). Genital and neonatal chlamydial infection in a trachoma endemic area. *Lancet*, **2**, 300–1

171. Bhujwala, R. A., Seth, P., Gupta, A. and Bhargava, N. C. (1982). Non-gonococcal urethritis in males – a preliminary study. *Ind. J. Med. Res.*, **75**, 485–8

172. Lim, K. B., Lee, C. T., Thirumoorthy, T., Arora, P. N., Tan, T. and Sng, E. H., (1985). The

microbiology of non-gonococcal urethritis (NGU) in Singapore. *Ann. Acad. Med.*, **14**, 686-8

173. Darougar, S., Jones, B. R., Cornell, L., Treharne, J. D., Dwyer, R. St. C. and Aramesh, B. (1982). Chlamydial urethral infection in Teheran. A study of male patients attending an STD clinic. *Br. J. Vener. Dis.*, **58**, 374-6

174. Darougar, S., Aramesh, B., Gibson, J. A., Treharne, J. D. and Jones, B. R. (1983). Chlamydial genital infection in prostitutes in Iran. *Br. J. Vener. Dis.*, **59**, 53-5

175. Douglas, F. P., Bidawid-Woodroffe, S., McDonnell, J., Hyne, S. G. and Mathews, J. D. (1986). Genital infection with *Chlamydia trachomatis* in aboriginal women in Northern Australia. In Oriel, D., Ridgway, G., Schachter, J., Taylor-Robinson, D. and Ward, M. (eds.). *Chlamydial Infections.* pp. 237-240. (Cambridge: Cambridge University Press)

176. Harrison, H. R., Boyce, W. T., Haffner, W. H. J., Crowley, B., Weinstein, L., Lewis, M. and Alexander, E. R. (1983). The prevalence of genital *Chlamydia trachomatis* and mycoplasmal infections during pregnancy in an American Indian population. *Sex. Transm. Dis.*, **10**, 184-6

177. Bentsi, C., Klufio, C. A., Perine, P. L., Bell, T. A., Cles, L. D., Koester, C. M. and Wang, S-P. (1985). Genital infections with *Chlamydia trachomatis* and *Neisseria gonorrhoeae* in Ghanaian women. *Genitourin. Med.*, **61**, 48-50

178. Meheus, A., Ballard, R., Dlamini, M., Ursi, J. P., van Dyck, E. and Piot, P. (1980). Epidemiology and aetiology of urethritis in Swaziland. *Int. J. Epidemiol.*, **9**, 239-45

179. Mabey, D. C. W., Ogbaselassie, G., Robertson, J. N., Heckels, J. E. and Ward, M. E. (1985). Tubal infertility in the Gambia: chlamydial and gonococcal serology in women with tubal occlusion compared with pregnant controls. *Bull. WHO*, **63**, 1107-13

180. Frost, K., Collet, M., Reniers, J., Leclerc, A., Ivanoff, B. and Meheus, A. (1987). Importance of chlamydial antibodies in acute salpingitis in central Africa. *Genitourin. Med.*, **63**, 176-8

181. Meheus, A., Delgadillo, R., Widy-Wirski, R. and Piot, P. (1982). Chlamydial ophthalmia neonatorum in Central Africa. *Lancet*, **2**, 882

182. Fransen, L., Nsanze, H., Klauss, V., Van der Stuyft, P., D'Costa, L., Brunham, R. C. and Piot, P. (1986). Ophthalmia neonatorum in Nairobi, Kenya: the roles of *Neisseria gonorrhoeae* and *Chlamydia trachomatis*. *J. Infect. Dis.*, **153**, 862-9

183. Hira, S. K., Sheth, J., Bhat, S., Khosla, A., Balaji, M. and Mkandawire, O. (1986). Ophthalmia neonatorum in Zambia. *Eur. J. Sex. Transm. Dis.*, **3**, 103-6

184. Mabey, D. C. W., Forsey, T. and Treharne, J. D. (1987). Serotypes of *Chlamydia trachomatis* in The Gambia. *Lancet*, **2**, 452

185. Jones, B. R. (1975). The prevention of blindness from trachoma. *Trans. Ophthalmol Soc. UK.*, **95**, 16-33

186. Ballard, R. C. and Fehler, H. G. (1986). Chlamydial infections of the eye and genital tract in southern Africa. *S. Afr. Med. J. (Suppl.)*, 76-9

187. Duncan, M. O., Bilgeri, Y. R., Fehler, H. G. and Ballard, R. C. (1981). The diagnosis of sexually acquired genital ulcerations in black patients in Johannesburg. *S., Afr. J. Sex. Transm. Dis.*, **1**, 20-3

188. Duncan, M. O., Ballard, R. C., Bilgeri, Y. R. and Fehler, H. G. (1984). Sexually acquired genital ulcerations in urban black women. *S. Afr. J. Sex. Transm. Dis.*, **4**, 23-7

189. Jacobs, N. F., Arum, E. S. and Kraus, S. J. (1978). Experimental infection of the chimpanzee urethra and pharynx with *Chlamydia trachomatis*. *Sex. Transm. Dis.*, **5**, 132-6

190. Taylor-Robinson, D., Purcell, R. H., London, W. T., Sly, D. L., Thomas, B. J. and Evans, R. T. (1981). Microbiological, serological, and histopathological features of experimental *Chlamydia trachomatis* urethritis in chimpanzees. *Br. J. Vener. Dis.*, **57**, 36-40

191. Ripa, K. T., Møller, B. R., Mårdh, P.-A., Freundt, E. A. and Melsen, F. (1979). Experimental acute salpingitis in grivet monkeys provoked by *Chlamydia trachomatis*. *Acta Pathol. Microbiol. Scand., Section B.*, **87**, 65-70

192. Møller, B. R. and Mårdh, P.-A. (1980). Experimental salpingitis in grivet monkeys by *Chlamydia trachomatis*. Modes of spread of infection to the fallopian tubes. *Acta. Pathol. Microbiol. Scand., Section B*, **88**, 107-14

193. Johnson, A. P., Hare, M. J., Willbanks, G. D., Cooper, P., Hetherington, C. M., Al-Kurdi, M., Osborn, M. F. and Taylor-Robinson, D. (1984). A colposcopic and histological study of experimental chlamydial cervicitis in marmosets. *Br. J. Exp. Pathol.*, **65**, 59-65

194. Johnson, A. P., Hetherington, C. M., Osborn, M. F., Thomas, B. J. and Taylor-Robinson, D. (1980). Experimental infection of the marmoset genital tract with *Chlamydia trachomatis. Br. J. Exp. Pathol.*, **61**, 291-5

195. Johnson, A. P., Osborn, M. F., Thomas, B. J., Hetherington, C. M. and Taylor-Robinson, D. (1981). Immunity to reinfection of the genital tract of marmosets with *Chlamydia trachomatis. Br. J. Exp. Pathol.*, **62**, 606-13

196. Møller, B. R. (1986). The grivet monkey as animal model for inflammation of the lower genital tract caused by *Chlamydia trachomatis.* In Oriel, D., Ridgway, G., Schachter, J., Taylor-Robinson, D. and Ward, M. (eds.). *Chlamydial Infections.* pp. 375-379. (Cambridge: Cambridge University Press)

197. Patton, D. L., Halbert, S. A., Kuo, C.-C., Wang, S.-P. and Holmes, K. K. (1983). Host response to primary *Chlamydia trachomatis* infection of the fallopian tube in pig-tailed monkeys. *Fertil. Steril.*, **40**, 829-40

198. Wolner-Hanssen, P., Patton, D. L., Stamm, W. E. and Holmes, K. K. (1986). Severe salpingitis in pig-tailed macaques after repeated cervical infections followed by a single tubal inoculation with *Chlamydia trachomatis.* In Oriel, D., Ridgway, G., Schachter, J., Taylor-Robinson, D. and Ward, M. (eds.). *Chlamydial Infections.* pp. 371-4. (Cambridge: Cambridge University Press)

199. Patton, D. L., Kuo, C.-C., Wang, S.-P., Brenner, R. M., Sternfield, M. D., Morse, S. A. and Barnes, R. C. (1987). Chlamydial infection of subcutaneous fimbrial transplants in cynomolgus and rhesus monkeys. *J. Infect. Dis.*, **155**, 229-35

200. Digiacomo, R. F., Gale, J. L., Wang, S-P. and Kiviat, M. D. (1975). Chlamydial infection of the male baboon urethra. *Br. J. Vener. Dis.*, **51**, 310-13

201. Møller, B. R. and Mårdh, P.-A. (1980). Experimental epididymitis and urethritis in grivet monkeys provoked by *Chlamydia trachomatis. Fertil. Steril.*, **34**, 275-9

202. Harrison, H. R., Alexander, E. R., Chiang, W.-T., Giddens, W. E., Boyce, J. T., Benjamin, D. and Gale, J. L. (1979). Experimental nasopharyngitis and pneumonia caused by *Chlamydia trachomatis* in infant baboons: histopathologic comparison with a case in a human infant. *J. Infect. Dis.*, **139**, 141-6

203. Quinn, T. C., Kappus, E. W. and James, S. P. (1986). The immunopathogenesis of lymphogranuloma venereum rectal infection in primates. In Oriel, D., Ridgway, G., Schachter, J., Taylor-Robinson, D. and Ward, M. (eds.). *Chlamydial Infection.* pp. 404-7. (Cambridge: Cambridge University Press).

204. Patton, D. L., Halbert, S. A. and Wang, S.-P. (1982). Experimental salpingitis in rabbits provoked by *Chlamydia trachomatis. Fertil. Steril.*, **37**, 691-700

205. Tuffrey, M., Falder, P. and Taylor-Robinson, D. (1982). Genital-tract infection and disease in nude and immunologically competent mice after inoculation of a human strain of *Chlamydia trachomatis. Br. J. Exp. Pathol.*, **63**, 539-46

206. Tuffrey, M., Falder, P. and Taylor-Robinson, D. (1984). Reinfection of the mouse genital tract with *Chlamydia trachomatis*; the relationship of antibody to immunity. *Br. J. Exp. Pathol.*, **65**, 51-8

207. Tuffrey, M., Falder, P. and Taylor-Robinson, D. (1985). Effect on *Chlamydia trachomatis* infection of the murine genital tract of adoptive transfer of congenic immune cells or specific antibody. *Br. J. Exp. Pathol.*, **66**, 427-33

208. Tuffrey, M., Falder, P., Gale, J., Quinn, R. and Taylor-Robinson, D. (1986). Infertility in mice infected genitally with a human strain of *Chlamydia trachomatis. J. Reprod. Fertil.*, **78**, 251-60

209. Heggie, A. D., Wentz, W. B., Reagan, J. W. and Anthony, D. D. (1986). Roles of cytomegalovirus and *Chlamydia trachomatis* in the induction of cervical neoplasia in the mouse. *Cancer Res.*, **46**, 5211-14

210. Harrison, H. R., Lee, S. M. and Lucas, D. O. (1982). *Chlamydia trachomatis* pneumonitis in the C57BL/KsJ mouse: pathologic and immunologic features. *J. Lab. Clin. Med.*, **100**, 953-62

211. Kuo, C.-C., and Chen, W.-J. (1980). A mouse model of *Chlamydia trachomatis* pneumonitis. *J. Infect. Dis.*, **141**, 198-202

212. Stephens, R. S., Chen, W.-J. and Kuo, C.-C. (1982). Effects of corticosteroids and cyclophosphamide on a mouse model of *Chlamydia trachomatis* pneumonitis. *Infect. Immun.*, **35**, 680-4

213. Mount, D. T., Bigazzi, P. E. and Barron, A. L. (1972). Infection of genital tract and transmission of ocular infection to newborns by the agent of guinea pig inclusion conjunctivitis. *Infect. Immun.*, **5**, 921-6
214. Mount, D. T., Bigazzi, P. E. and Barron, A. L. (1973). Experimental infection of male guinea pigs with the agent of guinea pig inclusion conjunctivitis and transmission to females. *Infect. Immun.*, **8**, 925-30
215. Mount, D. T. and Barron, A. L. (1976). Intrarectal infection of guinea pigs with the agent of guinea pig inclusion conjunctivitis. *Proc. Soc. Exp. Biol. Med.*, **153**, 388-91
216. Lamont, H. C., Semine, D. Z., Leveille, C. and Nichols, R. L. (1978). Immunity to vaginal reinfection in female guinea pigs infected sexually with *Chlamydia* of guinea pig inclusion conjunctivitis. *Infect. Immun.*, **19**, 807-13
217. Rank, R. G., White, H. J. and Barron, A. L. (1979). Humoral immunity in the resolution of genital infection in female guinea pigs infected with the agent of guinea pig inclusion conjunctivitis. *Infect. Immun.*, **26**, 573-9
218. Ozanne, G. and Pearce, J. H. (1980). Inapparent chlamydial infection in the urogenital tract of guinea-pigs. *J. Gen. Microbiol.*, **119**, 351-9
219. White, H. J., Rank, R. G., Soloff, B. L. and Barron, A. L. (1979). Experimental chlamydial salpingitis in immunosuppressed guinea pigs infected in the genital tract with the agent of guinea pig inclusion conjunctivitis. *Infect. Immun.*, **26**, 728-35
220. Rank, R. G., White, H. J., Soloff, B. L. and Barron, A. L. (1981). Cystitis associated with chlamydial infection of the genital tract in male guinea pigs. *Sex. Transm. Dis.*, **8**, 203-310
221. Rank, R. G., White, H. J., Hough, A. J., Pasley, J. N. and Barron, A. L. (1982). Effect of estradiol on chlamydial genital infection of female guinea pigs. *Infect. Immun.*, **38**, 699-705
222. Rank, R. G. and Barron, A. L. (1982). Prolonged genital infection by GPIC agent associated with immunosuppression following treatment with estradiol. In Mårdh, P.-A., Holmes, K. K., Oriel, J. D., Piot, P. and Schachter, J. (eds.). *Chlamydial Infections*, pp. 391-4. (Amsterdam, New York, Oxford: Elsevier Biomedical Press)
223. Pasley, J. N., Rank, R. G., Hough, A. J., Cohen, C. and Barron, A. L. (1985). Effects of various doses of estradiol on chlamydial genital infection in ovariectomized guinea pigs. *Sex. Transm. Dis.*, **12**, 8-13
224. Pasley, J. N., Rank, R. G. and Barron, A. L. (1986). Effects of oral contraceptives on chlamydial genital infection in female guinea pigs. In Oriel, D., Ridgway, G., Schachter, J., Taylor-Robinson, D. and Ward, M. (eds.). *Chlamydial Infections*. pp. 392-395. (Cambridge: Cambridge University Press)
225. Pasley, J. N., Rank, R. G., Hough, A. J., Cohen, C. and Barron, A. L. (1985). Absence of progesterone effects on chlamydial genital infection in female guinea-pigs. *Sex. Transm. Dis.*, **12**, 155-8
226. Rank, R. G. and Barron, A. L. (1983). Humoral immune response in acquired immunity to chlamydial genital infection of female guinea pigs. *Infect. Immun.*, **39**, 463-5
227. Howard, L. V., O'Leary, M. P. and Nichols, R. L. (1976). Animal model studies of genital chlamydial infection. Immunity to reinfection with guinea pig inclusion conjunctivitis agent in the urethra and eye of male guinea pigs. *Br. J. Vener. Dis.*, **52**, 261-5
228. Barron, A. L., Rank, R. G. and Moses, E. B. (1984). Immune response in mice infected in the genital tract with mouse pneumonitis agent (*Chlamydia trachomatis* biovar). *Infect. Immun.*, **44**, 82-5
229. Williams, D. M., Schachter, J., Drutz, D. J. and Sumaya, C. V. (1981). Pneumonia due to *Chlamydia trachomatis* in the immunocompromised (nude) mouse. *J. Infect. Dis.*, **143**, 238-41
230. Rank, R. G., and Hough, A. J. (1986). Induction of arthritis in mice immunised with the agent of mouse pneumonitis (*Chlamydia trachomatis*). In Oriel, D., Ridgway, G., Schachter, J., Taylor-Robinson, D. and Ward, M. (eds.). *Chlamydial Infections*. pp. 400-3. (Cambridge: Cambridge University Press)
231. Kane, J. L., Woodland, R. M., Elder, M. G. and Darougar, S. (1985). Chlamydial pelvic infection in cats: a model for the study of human pelvic inflammatory disease. *Genitourin. Med.*, **61**, 311-18
232. Brown, A. S. and Grice, R. G. (1986). Experimental transmission of *Chlamydia psittaci* in the koala. In Oriel, D., Ridgway, G., Schachter, J., Taylor-Robinson, D. and Ward, M. (eds.). *Chlamydial Infections*. pp. 349-352. (Cambridge: Cambridge University Press)

233. Barnes, R. C., Wang, S.-P., Kuo, C.-C. and Stamm, W. E. (1985). Rapid immunotyping of *Chlamydia trachomatis* with monoclonal antibodies in a solid-phase enzyme immunoassay. *J. Clin. Microbiol.*, **22**, 609-13

234. Newhall, W. J., Terho, P., Wilde, C. E., Batteiger, B. E. and Jones, R. B. (1986). Serovar determination of *Chlamydia trachomatis* isolates by using type-specific monoclonal antibodies. *J. Clin. Microbiol.*, **23**, 333-8

235. Levitt, D. and Bard, J. (1987). The immunology of *Chlamydia*. *Immunol. Today*, **8**, 246-51

236. Nsanze, H., Waigwa, S. R. N., Mirza, N., Plummer, F., Roelants, P. and Piot, P. (1982). Chlamydial infections in selected populations in Kenya. In Mårdh, P-A., Holmes, K. K., Oriel, J. D., Piot, P. and Schachter, J. (eds.). *Chlamydial Infections* pp. 421-424. (Amsterdam: Elsevier)

237. Forsey, T., Darougar, S., Dines, R. J., Wright, D. J. M. and Friedman, P. S. (1982). Chlamydial genital infection in Addis Ababa, Ethiopia. *Br. J. Vener. Dis.*, **58**, 370-3

238. Omer, E.-F. E., Forsey, T., Darougar, S., Ali, M. H. and El-Naeem, H. A. (1985). Seroepidemiological survey of chlamydial genital infections in Khartoum, Sudan. *Genitourin. Med.*, **61**, 261-3

239. Darougar, S., Forsey, T., Osoba, A. O., Dines, R. J., Adelusi, B. and Coker, G. O. (1982). Chlamydial genital infection in Ibadan, Nigeria. A seroepidemiological survey. *Br. J. Vener. Dis.*, **58**, 366-9

7
Immunology of Genital Mycoplasmal Infections

D. TAYLOR-ROBINSON

CHARACTERISTICS OF MYCOPLASMAS

The features that distinguish mycoplasmas, the smallest free-living micro-organisms, from bacteria, chlamydiae and viruses are shown in Table 7.1

Table 7.1 Characteristics of mycoplasmas compared to those of bacteria, chlamydiae and viruses

Characteristic	Mycoplasmas	Bacteria	Chlamydiae	Viruses
Size (diameter)	$0.3\,\mu m$*	$1-2\,\mu m$	$0.3\,\mu m$	$<0.5\,\mu m$
Lack a cell wall	Yes	No	No	Yes
Contain both DNA and RNA	Yes	Yes	Yes	No
Multiplication in cell-free medium	Yes	Yes	No	No
Multiplication dependent on host cell nucleic acid	No	No	No	Yes
Usually require sterol and native protein for propagation	Yes	No	No	No
Intrinsic energy metabolism	Yes	Yes	Yes	No
Usually narrow range of host specificity	Yes	No	No	Yes
Growth inhibited by specific antibody alone	Yes	No	Yes	Yes
Resistant to cell-wall active antibiotics (e.g. penicillins)	Yes	No	No	Yes
Resistant to antibiotics which inhibit metabolism (e.g. tetracyclines)	No	No	No	Yes

*Smallest organisms capable of propagation

MYCOPLASMAS OF HUMAN ORIGIN

The mycoplasmas isolated from human subjects, together with some basic biological features, are presented in alphabetical order in Table 7.2. Twelve species are listed, the greatest proportion having been isolated from the respiratory tract. Five species have been isolated from both the oropharynx and the genito–urinary tract, probably reflecting orogenital contact. The first recovery of a mycoplasma reported in 1937[1], was from a Bartholin's gland abscess and, in retrospect, this was probably *Mycoplasma hominis*. The species most recently isolated, reported in 1981[2,3] is *M. genitalium*, recovered from men with non-gonococcal urethritis (NGU).

Mycoplasmas in the genito–urinary tract

The anatomical localization of the seven mycoplasmas that have been found in the human genito–urinary tract is shown in Table 7.3. Of the large-colony-forming mycoplasmas, *M. hominis* is most frequently and easily recovered and has been detected in various locations. T-strain mycoplasmas, or T mycoplasmas, first described by Shepard[4], because of their unique ability to metabolize urea were placed in a new genus and species, *Ureaplasma urealyticum*[5]. Trivially, they are termed ureaplasmas. Interest in mycoplasmas as causative agents of genito–urinary tract disease increased as ureaplasmas appeared a more likely cause of some cases of NGU. They are found in the human genito-urinary tract even more frequently than *M. hominis* and have been isolated from a wide range of anatomical sites. *M. genitalium*, on the other hand, has only been recovered with certainty from the male urethra[2,3] and oropharynx. *M. fermentans* was first isolated from patients with balanitis[6] and, like *M. primatum*[7], has been isolated rarely from the genito-urinary tract. *M. salivarium* and *M. pneumoniae* are primarily respiratory tract organisms and orogenital contact probably accounts for their occasional detection in the genito–urinary tract.

HUMORAL IMMUNITY

Serological tests for mycoplasmas

The various serological techniques which have been used to study mycoplasmas are listed in Table 7.4 and are also discussed elsewhere[15,24,25]. They are presented in diminishing order of sensitivity. Methods having minimal sensitivity but high specificity, for example the inhibition of colony development on agar, although of no value for the quantitative assessment of antibody, are used for the identification of mycoplasmas. For sero-epidemiological studies and for the serological diagnosis of mycoplasmal infections, it has been usual to use only those methods which have a sensitivity depicted as greater than ++ in Table 7.4. Of course, apart from sensitivity, the extent to which these tests are used, depends on their specificity, reproducibility, ease of performance, convenience and familiarity. In the case of mycoplasmas isolated from the human genito–urinary tract,

Table 7.2 The occurrence, some biological features and disease association of mycoplasmas isolated from human subjects

| Mycoplasma | Genito–urinary tract | Frequency of isolation from the: | | | | Metabolism of | Preferred atmosphere | Cause of disease |
		Respiratory tract	Rectum	Eye	Blood			
M.buccale	—*	Rare	—	—	—	Arginine	Anaerobic†	No
M.faucium	—	Rare	—	—	—	Arginine	Anaerobic	No
M.fermentans	Rare	—	—	—	—	Glucose & arginine	Anaerobic	No
M.hominis	Common	Rare	Common	Rare	Very rare	Arginine	Aerobic	Yes
M.genitalium	?	?	?	?	?	Glucose	Anaerobic	?
A.laidlawii	—	Rare	—	—	—	Glucose	Anaerobic	No
M.lipophilum	—	Rare	—	—	—	Arginine	Anaerobic	No
M.orale	—	Common	—	—	—	Arginine	Anaerobic	No
M.pneumoniae	Very rare	Rare**	—	—	—	Glucose	Aerobic	Yes
M.primatum	Rare	—	—	—	—	Arginine	Anaerobic	No
M.salivarium	Rare	Common	—	—	—	Arginine	Anaerobic	No
U.urealyticum	Common	Rare	Common	Rare	Very rare	Urea	Anaerobic	Yes

* — = no reports of isolation
** except in disease outbreaks
† 5% CO_2 and 95% N_2

Table 7.3 Localization of mycoplasmas found in the human genito–urinary tract

Mycoplasma	Urethral swab	Semen	Isolation of mycoplasma recorded from					Frequency of isolation
			Voided urine	Bladder urine	Kidney	Cervix/vagina	Fallopian tube	
M.hominis	+	+	+	+	+	+	+	Common*
U.urealyticum	+	+	+	+	+	+	+	Common*
M.genitalium	+	–	–	–	–	+	–	?
M.fermentans	+	–	+	–	–	+	–	Rare
M.primatum	+	–	–	–	–	–	–	Rare
M.salivarium	–	–	–	–	+?	+	–	Rare
M.pneumoniae	–	–	–	–	–	+	–	Very rare

*From urethra, urine and cervix and/or vagina

166

Table 7.4 The relative sensitivity and specificity of serological techniques for mycoplasmas

Serological technique	Sensitivity	Specificity	Reference
Radio-immunoprecipitation	++++	+++?	8
Complement-dependent cidal	+++±	+++?	9,10,11
Enzyme-linked immunosorbent assay	+++	+++	12,13,14
Metabolism inhibition	+++	+++	15,16
Inhibition of growth in liquid medium	+++	+++	15
Indirect haemagglutination	+++	++	15,17
Micro-immunofluorescence	+++	+++	15,18,19
Inhibition of cytopathic effect in			
tissue culture	++	+++	15
Immunofluorescence (colonies on agar)	++	+++	15,18
Single radial haemolysis	++	+++	20,21
Complement fixation	++	+	15,22
Cumulative haemagglutination inhibition	++	+?	15
Agglutination	++	+	15
Latex agglutination	++	+?	15
Haemadsorption inhibition	+	+++?	15
Colony inhibition on agar (disc method)	+	+++	15
Immunodiffusion and immunoelectrophoresis	+	++	15,23

+, ++, +++, ++++ = poor, moderate, good, excellent

quantitative measurement of antibody has been undertaken with relatively few procedures. The five most frequently employed procedures are discussed in the chronological order in which they gained prominence. The antigens used are whole organisms or disintegrated organisms and not extracted components, which accounts for some of the serological reactivity seen between different mycoplasma serotypes.

Complement fixation (CF)

CF was first used with the bovine mycoplasma, *M. mycoides*[15], and is sufficiently specific for the routine diagnosis of *M. pneumoniae* infections[22]. It has also been used to detect antibody to *M. hominis*. Thus, Lemcke and Csonka[26] found antibody to this mycoplasma more frequently in women who had salpingitis than in those without the disease. However, the relative lack of sensitivity and specificity of this test makes it unsuitable for detecting antibodies to the genital tract mycoplasmas.

Indirect haemagglutination (IHA)

This technique was reported in 1960 as being first used to study *M. mycoides*[15], and 5 years later had been used to detect rising antibody titres in the sera from volunteers who had been infected orally with *M. hominis*[27]. Later, Mårdh and Weström[28] used IHA to show that one-third of women with salpingitis from whom *M. hominis* had been isolated from the lower genital tract, developed a significant change in the titre of antibody to *M. hominis* during the course of their disease. The test is not much used as it is too complex, difficult to reproduce, and there is a tendency for cross-reactivity with heterologous mycoplasmas. Nevertheless, the method has had its advocates, and recently has been used in further attempts to detect antibody responses to both *M. hominis*[17] and *M. genitalium*[29] in women with salpingitis.

Metabolism inhibition (MI)

This term is applied specifically to those techniques in which inhibition of mycoplasmal growth by antibody results in inhibition of metabolic activity which is measured in various ways. The first application of MI techniques to the serological study of human mycoplasmas resulted from the ability of *M. pneumoniae* to reduce 2, 3, 5-triphenyltetrazolium from its colourless oxidized form to the reduced red formozan. This activity could be inhibited by specific antibody[30], and widespread use was made of the test to measure antibody in convalescent human and hyperimmune sera. The test was limited in application because *M. pneumoniae* is the only mycoplasma of human origin to reduce tetrazolium. However, soon other MI tests were developed[15,16] based on the ability of mycoplasmas to ferment glucose (e.g. *M. genitalium*) and metabolize arginine (e.g. *M. hominis*). The ureaplasmas are unique in possessing the enzyme urease and so they are able to liberate ammonia from urea, causing an increase in the pH of the medium. Such a pH change, made visible with phenol red, is inhibited by specific antibody[31].

In the human genito–urinary tract, the technique has been used to detect antibodies to *M. hominis* and the ureaplasmas on a sero-epidemiological basis[15,31]. The technique has also been used to measure antibody responses to ureaplasmas in infants and mothers with spontaneous pregnancy loss[32], as well as similar responses in male subjects infected intraurethrally with ureaplasmas after experimental inoculation[33]. The ability of most workers to find antibody responses to ureaplasmas in no more than a small proportion of men with NGU[34] is possibly a reflection of the serotype specificity of the MI procedure and the failure to use more than a few serotypes in the tests. One of the problems experienced with the MI technique is inhibition occurring as a result of antibiotics in serum, the effect mimicking that of antibody. This was demonstrated in a study of serum samples from men with sexually acquired reactive arthritis in which antibody to *M. hominis* was sought[35]. The inhibitory activity of some sera obtained sequentially coincided with tetracycline treatment of the patients. The results were different when a naturally resistant strain of *M. hominis* was used.

Enzyme-linked immunosorbent assay (ELISA)

Immune responses to a large number of mycoplasmas have been studied by ELISA techniques[12,24,25] because of their sensitivity, their ability to measure class-specific antibodies and because they can be automated. In addition, the results are not influenced by antibiotics in the samples being tested. For *U. urealyticum*, the ELISA was used first to characterize strains serologically[36]. Later, it was developed by two groups of workers[13,37] to detect antibodies. One of these groups[13] used a cell-lysate antigen and commercially available alkaline phosphatase conjugates to study ureaplasmal antibody responses in patients with NGU. A single serum dilution was used with a single serotype antigen to measure class-specific antibodies and quantitative differences between acute- and convalescent-phase sera. Significant changes in the levels of one or more antibody classes were detected in the sera of 12 (67%) of 18 NGU patients, 10 of the 12 having a change in the IgM class.

A four-layer modification of the conventional enzyme immunoassay was used to measure serum antibodies to *M. hominis* and was employed in a study of women with acute salpingitis[14]. The antigen comprised a soluble cell fraction which masked the serological diversity of different strains and allowed a single representative strain to be used. The application of heavy chain-specific second antibody followed by conjugated anti-species antibodies increased the overall sensitivity. Serological evidence of recent *M. hominis* infection, as demonstrated by a significant change in IgG antibody levels, was observed in 23% of the women with salpingitis. In addition, levels of IgG and IgA antibodies were significantly higher among women with salpingitis than among those serving as controls.

Micro-immunofluorescence (MIF)

Immunofluorescence techniques have had a long history in the study of mycoplasmal infections[15]. Techniques for staining mycoplasmas sedimented from broth cultures and fixed to glass slides were described first in 1963[38] and, in reference to the genito–urinary tract, this procedure was used first to demonstrate a serological response to *M. hominis* in a patient with febrile gynaecological disease from whose blood this mycoplasma was recovered[39]. After a long period of not being used, the procedure of indirect MIF on slides was developed for measuring antibody to *M. genitalium*[19], being rapid to perform, easy to read, reproducible and, at least with this mycoplasma, more sensitive than MI. Furthermore, differentiation between antibody classes is possible and spurious results do not occur as a consequence of antibiotics in the serum samples. The MIF test has been used to detect antibody responses to *M. genitalium* in men with NGU[40] and in women with salpingitis[41]. The procedure has also been useful in detecting antibody responses to this mycoplasma in various sub-human primates inoculated via the genito–urinary tract[42–44].

Mycoplasmal antigens recognized

Genital tract mycoplasmal antigens that are recognised by the host have been little studied. The respiratory tract mycoplasma, *M. pneumoniae*, has two major proteins, including the P1 protein involved in attachment, that are regularly recognized. Antibody to these surface protein antigens has been detected in convalescent sera and in respiratory secretions by radio-immunoprecipitation using staphylococcal protein A or by sodium dodecyl sulphate–polyacrylamide gel electrophoresis and Western blot transfer[45,46]. The Western blotting technique has also been used to study *M. genitalium* which is closely related to *M. pneumoniae*, although it does not contain the P1 protein. The detection of protein antigens of *M. genitalium* by using this procedure in the synovial fluid of a patient with inflammatory arthritis, hints at a possible aetiological involvement (J. B. Baseman, personal communication).

Unique and common protein bands among strains of *M. hominis* have been demonstrated by Western blot analysis with a specific rabbit antiserum[47], but the human response to such antigens has not been assessed. In the case of *U. urealyticum*, immunoblotting with human sera and rabbit antisera has suggested the possibility of non-protein antigens being involved in the immune response[48].

Systemic antibody response

A four-fold or greater rise in the titre of serum IHA antibody to *M. hominis* was noted from 9 to between 34 and 47 days after laparoscopy of patients with acute salpingitis[28]. In a further series, a four-fold or greater rise in the titre of antibody to *M. genitalium*, measured by MIF, was seen in 9, and a similar fall in 3, of 31 women within about one month of admission to hospital with acute salpingitis.[41] Clearly, collection of a convalescent-phase serum conventionally 2 weeks after the first may be too early to detect an antibody response, and thought should always be given to obtaining a serum specimen at 1 month or even later. This is reinforced by the finding of late antibody responses in some female monkeys developing acute upper genital tract disease after experimental inoculation of *M. genitalium*[42].

In men with acute NGU, a four-fold or greater rise or fall in the titre of antibody to ureaplasmas detected by ELISA or MI was seen in sera collected 10–35 days after the first samples[13]. An antibody response to ureaplasmas was seen during the same time interval in two subjects who had been inoculated intraurethrally with these organisms.[33] Antibody responses to *M. genitalium* were seen in 3 of 10 heterosexual men with NGU from whom a second serum was obtained 14 days after the first[40]; in one other patient, a response was noted 9 months later. Of course, this may have been unrelated to the NGU but, as in women, a similar delayed antibody response was detected in some male chimpanzees as late as 5–9 weeks after intraurethral inoculation with *M. genitalium*[43,44].

It is usual for the serum isotype response after infection to follow the course of IgM, IgG and IgA. This has been observed after infection of the respiratory tract with *M. pneumoniae* in man and in animals inoculated experimentally with this mycoplasma[49]. Whether sequential development of antibodies occurs in genital tract mycoplasmal infections for the most part can only be assumed. However, consistent with this sequence are the observations made in two studies. In the first,[50] an increase in serum IgM was noted in one-third of patients with acute salpingitis, concentrations of IgG and IgA being normal or only slightly raised; IHA antibody to *M. hominis* was found in nearly all of the patients who had an increased serum IgM concentration but in few of those with a normal IgM concentration, although IgM specifically directed against *M. hominis* was not sought. In the second study[13], men with NGU were found to have serum IgM, IgG and IgA antibody levels to ureaplasmas, measured by ELISA, greater than the normal serum standard, and 10 of 12 individuals had a change in the IgM class, suggesting an active infectious process. In some mycoplasmal infections the usual sequential development of IgM, IgG and IgA has not been observed[24]. Thus, contrary to convention was the observation that serum IgG antibody appeared first when the three classes were detected by an immunofluorescence technique following pyelonephritis associated with *M. hominis*[51].

Local antibody response

Antibody in secretions has been demonstrated in a number of mycoplasmal infections[24,25], but observations pertaining to the human genital tract are wanting. However, subjects with pyelonephritis developed antibody to *M. hominis*, measured by IHA, in urine[52]; when an immunofluorescence test was used, IgA antibody appeared shortly before IgG, while IgM was usually absent. On the other hand, female mice infected experimentally in the lower genital tract with *M. pulmonis* had IgM and IgG antibodies to this mycoplasma, measured by IMF, in vaginal washings taken about eight months later, but specific IgA antibody could not be detected (P. M. Furr and D. Taylor-Robinson, unpublished observation). Differences in animal species, mycoplasmas involved and the time of specimen collection could account for the discrepancy between the observations.

ROLE OF ANTIBODY IN RESISTANCE TO INFECTION

There is no simple direct relationship between the level of circulating antibody and resistance to mycoplasmal infections[24]. This is not surprising as local antibody plays an important role in protection at a mucosal surface. However, serum antibody can sometimes be a useful measure of immunity. In this regard there is no information of any kind relevant to the human genital tract but there are data available from a mouse model of mycoplasmal genital tract infection. Thirty-one mice of strain TO were infected vaginally with *M. pulmonis* and all of them were free of the organisms in the vagina when re-challenged 236 days later. All of the mice were resistant, whereas of 21 mice that had not been infected originally, 15 (71%) became infected after re-challenge[53]. In general mice that were resistant to re-infection possessed serum antibody, measured by MIF, unlike mice that were susceptible. A similar correlation existed with the presence or absence of local IgG antibody (P. M. Furr and D. Taylor-Robinson, unpublished data). Therefore, antibody is a key factor in protection and perhaps local antibody is the more important, serum antibody being only an indirect indicator of immunity.

MYCOPLASMAL INFECTIONS IN HYPOGAMMAGLOBULINAEMIA

The importance of antibody in immunity is underlined by the spread of mycoplasmas from their initial site of infection in patients with hypogamma-globulinaemia. Persistent urethritis, attributable to ureaplasmas has been documented[54], and dissemination of *M. hominis* and ureaplasmas has been seen on a number of occasions to cause septic arthritides, the organisms being recovered directly from the joints[35,55].

CELL-MEDIATED IMMUNITY (CMI)

Information regarding CMI relevant to genito–urinary tract mycoplasmal infections is sparse compared to that available for other mycoplasmal infections[24,25]. Lymphocyte transformation (LT) which appears to reflect the proliferative response of immune memory cells to the recognition of antigen has been observed in various mycoplasmal infections[24,25]. In relation to human genital tract mycoplasmas, blast transformation of cells from two male volunteers who had been infected experimentally with *U. urealyticum* in the genito–urinary tract was not detected[33]. However, CMI responses detectable by LT were reported in female grivet monkeys which had developed salpingitis following inoculation of *M. hominis* directly into the oviducts[56], as well as in a group of women with inflammatory pelvic disease attributed to *M. hominis*[57].

Since LT responses to antigen indicate prior *in vivo* exposure and sensitization to the antigen, the test has been used in attempts to implicate certain micro-organisms in the aetiology of disease. Thus, Ford[58] used this approach in studies of Reiter's syndrome. Mononuclear synovial cells from patients with the sexually acquired form of the disease had a greater response to ureaplasmas in an LT assay than cells from patients with enteric Reiter's syndrome or those from patients with rheumatoid arthritis. This suggests a possible role for ureaplasmas in the sexually acquired form of the arthritis. However, other than indicating previous exposure to antigens, the further significance of a positive LT test is not clear. Apart from the report of inhibition of leukocyte migration by *M. fermentans* in tests on patients with rheumatoid arthritis[59], which has not been confirmed[24], there is no information on leukocyte or macrophage migration inhibition tests or delayed hypersensitivity skin reactions with other genital tract mycoplasmas.

NON-SPECIFIC DEFENCE MECHANISMS

On gaining entry to the host, mycoplasmas encounter a variety of non-specific defences, namely inhibitory substances in secretions, complement and phagocytic cells. The role that these have in the respiratory tract against mycoplasmal infections is well understood[24,25], but there is less information about their role in the genito–urinary tract, particularly in relation to mycoplasmas. Complement may be involved in resistance early in infection before a specific immune response has been mounted, complement being activated by the alternative pathway or by cross-reacting IgM. Killing of *M. hominis* by C3a has been demonstrated[60], so that activation of the complete complement system may not always be necessary for killing to occur.

In general, the capacity of some mycoplasmas to attach to phagocytic cells in the absence of antibody, distinguishes mycoplasmas from most bacteria[24]. The attached mycoplasmas are considered to survive on the cell surface without becoming engulfed; when specific antibody of an appropriate isotype is present, namely one for which receptors exist on the phagocytic cell, phagocytosis ensues[24]. However, the results of experiments undertaken recently[61] with two genital tract mycoplasmas, *M. hominis* and *U.*

urealyticum, are only partially in keeping with the above conventional view. These micro-organisms induced the release of chemiluminescence from neutrophils in the absence of antibody. Furthermore, organisms were seen within phagocytic vacuoles by electron microscopy. Opsonization occurred either by way of receptors for the organisms on the neutrophil surface, or through the known activation of complement (C1) which then presumably enhanced binding by neutrophil complement receptors. Other studies showed that the mycoplasmas were not killed by the neutrophils in the absence or presence of complement, and confirmed that the intact organisms seen by electron microscopy were viable. Thus, particularly in the absence of antibody, as likely in hypogammaglobulinaemia, the neutrophils would seem to have little defensive role and may even aid dissemination.

PATHOGENESIS OF DISEASE

Lesions induced by several mycoplasmal infections are, at least partly, composed of infiltrating lymphocytes and in some instances these have been shown to be synthesizing specific antibodies to the mycoplasmas. Furthermore, lesions produced in T-cell-depleted animals by some mycoplasmas have been less severe than in immunologically competent animals[24,25] Thus, it appears that the immunological response of the host is capable of contributing to the pathological process. In the case of the genito–urinary tract, however, only a few observations are pertinent and no differentiation has been made between B- and T-cells. Examination of the lesions of vulvitis in cattle following infection by bovine ureaplasmas, has revealed many infiltrating lymphocytes[62]. Lymphoid follicles were also seen in the urethral submucosa of a male pig-tailed macaque after inoculation of ureaplasmas of human origin[63]. In addition, lymphocytic infiltration has been observed in the upper genital tract of female monkeys inoculated with *M. hominis* and in those given *M. genitalium*[42]. Parallel observations in man are lacking. In relation to human disease, however, the known development of autoimmunity following infection by *M. pneumoniae*[64], and the close biological similarity between this mycoplasma and *M. genitalium*, raises the possibility that autoimmune-stimulated lesions could develop in response to infection by the latter. Whether this is a valid proposition will depend to a large degree on the extent to which *M. genitalium* is found eventually to be a significant human pathogen.

CONCLUSIONS

Seven mycoplasmas have been found in the human genito–urinary tract, *M. hominis* and the ureaplasmas occurring most frequently. *M. genitalium* is the most recently discovered, but how often it occurs is unknown. Of the various serological techniques used to study mycoplasmas, indirect haemagglutination, metabolism inhibition, ELISA and immunofluorescence have been used widely for the quantitative measurement of antibody. They have been employed particularly to detect antibody responses to ureaplasmas and *M. genitalium* in men with NGU and to *M. hominis* and *M. genitalium* in women with salpingitis. Western blot analysis to define specific antigens responsible for the development of the antibodies has been little used; in the case of the ureaplasmas, immunoblotting has suggested the possibility of non-protein antigens being involved in the immune response. In general, antibody is detectable within 2–3 weeks of infection, but the possibility of late responses to infection by *M. genitalium* should be considered because these have been observed in sub-human primates infected experimentally. It seems that the serum isotype response in genital tract mycoplasmal infections follows the usual sequence of IgM, IgG and IgA. Little information is available about the development of local antibody although this has been seen in a mouse model of genital tract mycoplasmal (*M. pulmonis*) infection. This model has been used to show the importance of antibody in resistance to re-infection. The involvement of antibody in confining organisms (*M. hominis*, ureaplasmas) to the genital tract is in stark contrast to their dissemination in patients with hypogammaglobulinaemia. *M. hominis* and ureaplasmas are engulfed by neutrophils in the absence of antibody and are not killed even in the presence of complement. Thus, neutrophils, particularly in the absence of antibody, as seems likely in hypogammaglobulinaemia, appear to have little defensive role and may even aid dissemination. There are few examples of the development of cell-mediated immune responses to genital tract mycoplasmal infections, but there is little doubt that the immunological response of the host contributes to the development of genital tract lesions.

References

1. Dienes, L. and Edsall, G. (1937). Observations on the L-organism of Klieneberger. *Proc. Soc. Exp. Biol. Med.*, **36**, 740–4
2. Tully, J. G., Taylor-Robinson, D., Cole, R. M. and Rose, D. L. (1981). A newly discovered mycoplasma in the human urogenital tract. *Lancet*, **1**, 1288–91
3. Taylor-Robinson, D., Tully, J. G., Furr, P. M., Cole, R. M., Rose, D. L. and Hanna, N. F. (1981). Urogenital mycoplasma infections of man: a review with observations on a recently discovered mycoplasma. *Isr. J. Med. Sci.*, **17**, 524–30
4. Shepard, M. C. (1954). The recovery of pleuropneumonia-like organisms from Negro men with and without nongonococcal urethritis. *Am. J. Syph.*, **38**, 113–24
5. Shepard, M. C., Lunceford, C. D., Ford, D. K., Purcell, R. H., Taylor-Robinson, D., Razin, S. and Black, F. T. (1974). *Ureaplasma urealyticum* gen. nov., sp. nov.: Proposed nomenclature for the human T (T-strain) mycoplasma. *Int. J. Syst. Bact.*, **24**, 160–71
6. Ruiter, M. and Wentholt, H. M. M. (1952). The occurrence of a pleuropneumonia-like organism in fuso-spirillary infections of the human genital mucosa. *J. Invest. Dermatol.*, **18**, 313–25
7. Thomsen, A. C. (1974). The isolation of *Mycoplasma primatum* during an autopsy study of the mycoplasma flora of the human urinary tract. *Acta Path. Microbiol. Scand.*, **82B**, 653–6
8. Brunner, H. and Chanock, R. M. (1973). A radioimmunoprecipitation test for detection of *Mycoplasma pneumoniae* antibody. *Proc. Soc. Exp. Biol. Med.*, **143**, 97–105
9. Brunner, H., James, W. D., Horsewood, R. L. and Chanock, R. M. (1972). Measurement of *Mycoplasma pneumoniae* mycoplasmacidal antibody in human serum. *J. Immunol.*, **108**, 1491–8
10. Brunner, H. (1983). The mycoplasmacidal test (MCT). In Razin, S. and Tully, J. G. (eds.), *Methods in Mycoplasmology*, Vol. 1, pp. 423–430. (New York: Academic Press)
11. Lin, J. S. L. and Kass, E. H. (1975). Complement-dependent and complement-independent interactions between *Mycoplasma hominis* and antibodies *in vitro*. *J. Med. Microbiol.*, **8**, 397–404

12. Cassell, G. H. and Brown, M. B. (1983). Enzyme-linked immunosorbent assay (ELISA) for detection of anti-mycoplasmal antibody. In Razin, S. and Tully, J. G. (eds.). *Methods in Mycoplasmology*, Vol. 1, pp. 457–469. (New York: Academic Press)

13. Brown, M. B., Cassell, G. H., Taylor-Robinson, D. and Shepard, M. C. (1983). Measurement of antibody to *Ureaplasma urealyticum* by an enzyme-linked immunosorbent assay and detection of antibody responses in patients with nongonococcal urethritis. *J. Clin. Microbiol.*, **17**, 288–95

14. Miettinen, A., Paavonen, J., Jansson, E. and Leinikki, P. (1983). Enzyme immunoassay for serum antibody to *Mycoplasma hominis* in women with acute pelvic inflammatory disease. *Sex. Transm. Dis.*, **10** (Suppl.), 289–93

15. Purcell, R. H., Chanock, R. M. and Taylor-Robinson, D. (1969). Serology of the mycoplasmas of man. In Hayflick, L. (ed.). *The Mycoplasmatales and the L-phase of Bacteria*, pp. 221–264. (NY: Appleton)

16. Taylor-Robinson, D. (1983). Metabolism inhibition tests. In Razin, S. and Tully, J. G., (eds.). *Methods in Mycoplasmology*, Vol. 1, pp. 411–417. (NY: Academic Press)

17. Lind, K., Kristensen, G. B., Bollerup, A. C., Ladehoff, P., Larsen, S., Marushak, A., Rasmussen, P., Rolschau, J., Skoven, I., Sørensen, T. and Lind, I. (1985). Importance of *Mycoplasma hominis* in acute salpingitis assessed by culture and serological tests. *Genitourin. Med.*, **61**, 185–9

18. Gardella, R. S., DelGiudice, R. A. and Tully, J. G. (1983). Immunofluorescence. In Razin, S. and Tully, J. G. (eds.). *Methods in Mycoplasmology*, Vol. 1, pp. 431–39. (New York: Academic Press)

19. Furr, P. M. and Taylor-Robinson, D. (1984). Microimmunofluorescence technique for detection of antibody to *Mycoplasma genitalium*. *J. Clin. Pathol.*, **37**, 1072–4

20. Howard, C. J., Collins, J. and Gourlay, R. N. (1977). A single radial haemolysis technique for the measurement of antibody to *Mycoplasma bovis* in bovine sera. *Res. Vet. Sci.*, **23**, 128–30

21. Howard, C. J. (1983). Single radial hemolysis technique. In Razin, S. and Tully, J. G. (eds.). *Methods in Mycoplasmology*, Vol. 1, pp. 485–487. (New York: Academic Press)

22. Clyde, W. A. and Senterfit, L. B. (1983). The complement fixation test for diagnosis of *Mycoplasma pneumoniae* infection. In Tully, J. G. and Razin, S. (eds.). *Methods in Mycoplasmology*, Vol. 2, pp. 47–56. (New York: Academic Press)

23. Kenny, G. E. (1983). Agar precipitin and immunoelectrophoretic methods for detection of mycoplasmic antigens. In Razin, S. and Tully, J. G. (eds.). *Methods in Mycoplasmology*, Vol. 1, pp. 441–456. (New York: Academic Press).

24. Howard, C. J. and Taylor, G. (1985). Humoral and cell-mediated immunity. In Razin, S. and Barile, M. F. (eds.) *The Mycoplasmas*, Vol. 4, pp. 259–292. (New York: Academic Press)

25. Taylor, G. and Lemcke, R. M. (1985). Immunity to mycoplasma infections. In Gylstorff, I. (ed.). *Infektionen durch Mycoplasmatales*, pp. 116–166. (Jena: VEB Gustav Fischer Verlag)

26. Lemcke, R. M. and Csonka, G. W. (1962). Antibodies against pleuropneumonia-like organisms in patients with salpingitis. *Br. J. Vener. Dis.*, **38**, 212–17

27. Taylor-Robinson, D., Ludwig, W. M., Purcell, R. H., Mufson, M. A. and Chanock, R. M. (1965). Significance of antibody to *Mycoplasma hominis* type 1 as measured by indirect hemagglutination. *Proc. Soc. Exp. Biol. Med.*, **118**, 1073–83

28. Mårdh, P.-A. and Weström, L. (1970). Antibodies to *Mycoplasma hominis* in patients with genital infections and in healthy controls. *Br. J. Vener. Dis.*, **46**, 390–7

29. Lind, K. and Kristensen, G. B. (1987). Significance of antibodies to *Mycoplasma genitalium* in salpingitis. *Eur. J. Clin. Microbiol.*, **6**, 205–7

30. Senterfit, L. B. and Jensen, K. E. (1966). Antimetabolic antibodies to *Mycoplasma pneumoniae* measured by tetrazolium reduction inhibition. *Proc. Soc. Exp. Biol. Med.*, **122**, 786–90

31. Purcell, R. H., Taylor-Robinson, D., Wong, D. and Chanock, R. M. (1966). Color test for the measurement of antibody to T-strain mycoplasmas. *J. Bacteriol.*, **92**, 6–12

32. Quinn, P. A., Shewchuk, A. B., Shuber, J., Lie, K. I., Ryan, E., Sheu, M. and Chipman, M. L. (1983). Serologic evidence of *Ureaplasma urealyticum* infection in women with spontaneous pregnancy loss. *Am. J. Obstet. Gynecol.*, **145**, 245–50

33. Taylor-Robinson, D., Csonka, G. W. and Prentice, M. J. (1977). Human intra-urethral inoculation of ureaplasmas. *Q. J. Med.*, **46**, 309–26

34. Taylor-Robinson, D. and Csonka, G. W. (1981). Laboratory and clinical aspects of mycoplasmal infections of the human genitourinary tract. In Harris, J. R. W. (ed.). *Recent Advances in Sexually Transmitted Diseases*, No. 2, pp. 151-186. (Edinburgh: Churchill-Livingstone)

35. Taylor-Robinson, D., Thomas, B. J., Furr, P. M. and Keat, A. C. (1983). The association of *Mycoplasma hominis* with arthritis. *Sex. Transm. Dis.*, **10** (Suppl.), 341-4

36. Turunen, H., Leinikki, P. and Jansson, E. (1982). Serological characterization of *Ureaplasma urealyticum* strains by enzyme-linked immunosorbent assay (ELISA). *J. Clin. Pathol.*, **35**, 439-43

37. Wiley, C. A. and Quinn, P. A. (1984). Enzyme-linked immunosorbent assay for detection of specific antibodies to *Ureaplasma urealyticum* serotypes. *J. Clin. Microbiol.*, **19**, 421-6

38. Clark, H. W., Bailey, J. S., Fowler, R. C. and Brown, T. M. (1963). Identification of Mycoplasmataceae by the fluorescent antibody method. *J. Bacteriol.*, **85**, 111-18

39. Tully, J. G., Brown, M. S., Sheagren, J. N., Young, V. M. and Wolff, S. M. (1965). Septicemia due to *Mycoplasma hominis* type 1. *N. Engl. J. Med.*, **273**, 248-50

40. Taylor-Robinson, D., Furr, P. M. and Hanna, N. F. (1985). Microbiological and serological study of non-gonococcal urethritis with special reference to *Mycoplasma genitalium*. *Genitourin. Med.*, **61**, 319-24

41. Møller, B. R., Taylor-Robinson, D. and Furr, P. M. (1984). Serological evidence implicating *Mycoplasma genitalium* in pelvic inflammatory disease. *Lancet*, **1**, 1102-3

42. Møller, B. R., Taylor-Robinson, D., Furr, P. M. and Freundt, E. A. (1985). Acute upper genital-tract disease in female monkeys provoked experimentally by *Mycoplasma genitalium*. *Br. J. Exp. Pathol.*, **66**, 417-26

43. Taylor-Robinson, D., Tully, J. G. and Barile, M. F. (1985). Urethral infection in male chimpanzees produced experimentally by *Mycoplasma genitalium*. *Br. J. Exp. Pathol.*, **66**, 95-101

44. Tully, J. G., Taylor-Robinson, D., Rose, D. L., Furr, P. M., Graham, C. E. and Barile, M. F. (1986). Urogenital challenge of primate species with *Mycoplasma genitalium* and characterisation of infection induced in chimpanzees. *J. Infect. Dis.*, **153**, 1046-54

45. Leith, D. K., Trevino, L. B., Tully, J. G., Senterfit, L. B. and Baseman, J. B. (1983). Host discrimination of *Mycoplasma pneumoniae* proteinaceous immunogens. *J. Exp. Med.*, **157**, 502-14

46. Hu, P. C., Huang, C.-H., Collier, A. M. and Clyde, W. A. (1983). Demonstration of antibodies to *Mycoplasma pneumoniae* attachment protein in human sera and respiratory secretions. *Infect. Immun.*, **41**, 437-9

47. Brown, M. B., Minion, F. C., Davis, J. K., Pritchard, D. G., and Cassell, G. H. (1983). Antigens of *Mycoplasma hominis*. *Sex. Transm. Dis.*, **10** (Suppl.), 247-55

48. Horowitz, S. A., Duffy, L., Garrett, B., Stephens, J., Davis, J. K. and Cassell, G. H. (1986). Can group- and serovar-specific proteins be detected in *Ureaplasma urealyticum? Pediatr. Infect. Dis.*, **5** (Suppl.), 325-31

49. Fernald, G. W. (1979). Humoral and cellular immune responses to mycoplasmas. In Tully, J. G. and Whitcomb, R. F. (eds.). *The Mycoplasmas*, Vol. 2, pp. 399-423. (New York: Academic Press)

50. Mårdh, P.-A. (1970). Increased serum levels of IgM in acute salpingitis related to the occurrence of *Mycoplasma hominis*. *Acta Pathol. Microbiol. Scand.*, **78B**, 726-32

51. Erno, H. and Thomsen, A. C. (1980). Immunoglobulin classes of urinary and serum antibodies in mycoplasmal pyelonephritis. *Acta Pathol. Microbiol. Scand.*, **88C**, 237-40

52. Thomsen, A. C. and Lindskov, H. O. (1979). Diagnosis of *Mycoplasma hominis* pyelonephritis by demonstration of antibodies in urine. *J. Clin. Microbiol.*, **9**, 681-7

53. Taylor-Robinson, D. and Furr, P. M. (1986). Immunity to mycoplasmal infection of the genital tract: a mouse model. *Immunology*, **58**, 239-43

54. Taylor-Robinson, D., Furr, P. M. and Webster, A. D. B. (1985). *Ureaplasma urealyticum* causing persistent urethritis in a patient with hypogammaglobulinaemia. *Genitourin. Med.*, **61**, 404-8

55. Taylor-Robinson, D., Furr, P. M. and Webster, A. D. B. (1986). *Ureaplasma urealyticum* in the immunocompromised host. *Pediatr. Infect. Dis.*, **5** (Suppl.), 236-8

56. Møller, B. R. and Freundt, E. A. (1978). Experimental infection of the genital tract of female grivet monkeys by *Mycoplasma hominis*. *Zbl. Bakt. Parasitkde*, Abt. I. Orig. A., **241**, 218

57. Sethi, K. K. (1975). *Mycoplasma hominis* und entzündliche Erkrankungen des Beckens. In-vitro-Stimulation der Leukozyten bei Exposition gegen *M. hominis. Münch. Med. Wschr.*, **117**, 1045–6

58. Ford, D. K. (1986). Synovial lymphocyte responses show that ureaplasmas cause sexually transmitted reactive arthritis. *Pediatr. Infect. Dis.*, **5** (Suppl.), 353

59. Williams, M. H., Brostoff, J. and Roitt, I. M. (1970). Possible role of *Mycoplasma fermentans* in pathogenesis of rheumatoid arthritis. *Lancet*, **2**, 277–80

60. Taylor-Robinson, D., Schorlemmer, H. U., Furr, P. M. and Allison, A. C. (1978). Macrophage secretion and the complement cleavage product C3a in the pathogenesis of infections by mycoplasmas and L-forms of bacteria and in immunity to these organisms. *Clin. Exp. Immunol.*, **33**, 486–94

61. Webster, A. D. B., Furr, P. M., Hughes-Jones, N. C., Gorick, B. D. and Taylor-Robinson, D. (1988). Critical dependence on antibody for defence against mycoplasmas. *Clin. Exp. Immunol.*, **71**, 383–7

62. Doig, P. A., Ruhnke, H. L. and Palmer, N. C. (1980). Experimental bovine genital ureaplasmosis: 1. Granular vulvitis following vulvar inoculation. *Can. J. Comp. Med.*, **44**, 252–8

63. Gale, J. L., DiGiacomo, R. F., Kiviat, M. D., Wang, S.-P. and Bowie, W. R. (1977). Experimental nonhuman primate urethral infection with *Chlamydia trachomatis* and *Ureaplasma* (T-Mycoplasma). In Hobson, D. and Holmes, K. K. (eds.). *Nongonococcal Urethritis and Related Infections*, pp. 205–213. (Washington: Am. Soc. Microbiol.)

64. Biberfeld, G. (1985). Infection sequelae and autoimmune reactions in *Mycoplasma pneumoniae* infection. In Razin. S. and Barile, M. F. (eds.). *The Mycoplasmas*, Vol. 4, pp. 293–311. (New York: Academic Press)

8
Immunobiology of Sexually Transmitted Disease:
Herpes Simplex Virus

M. J. HALL AND D. J. JEFFRIES

INTRODUCTION

Herpes simplex is an enveloped DNA virus able to cause both acute and recurrent diseases in man. There are two types, namely HSV-1 and HSV-2, but the latter is most often associated with genital lesions. The frequency of isolation of HSV-2 from genital episodes varies between investigators and may range from over 90% to as low as 60%[1]. It is evident, therefore, that HSV-1 is also a major aetiological agent in genital herpes infections and both types will be considered in this chapter.

The normal portals of entry for genital herpes virus are the mucous membranes of the genital tract. Infection may be acquired at birth from the mother's genital infection. If not acquired at birth then the teenage years offer the greatest risk coinciding as they do with the onset of sexual activity[2]. It should be noted that herpes infection acquired at birth may be severe and can be life-threatening. Thereafter, the severity lessens in the healthy host as the immune system matures. Reference 2 provides an extensive account of these aspects of HSV infections.

Members of the Herpesviridae differ from most other viruses in their ability to establish latent infection[3]. In discussing latency, it should be noted that reactivation, recurrence and recrudescense have precise but distinct meanings. Thus, 'reactivation' implies the appearance of infectious virus at the site of latency, 'recurrence' implies the appearance of virus in peripheral tissue without the development of clinical signs, and 'recrudescence' describes the clinical lesions arising in the host tissue caused by recurrent virus[4]. In genital infections latent virus is usually located in the neurons of sensory ganglia in the lumbosacral region. This latent form is able to reactivate at intervals throughout life. Although reactivation does not always result in clinical symptoms it often causes recrudescence at the site of the primary infection. It

179

is usually contained there but may, if the immune status of the host permits, erupt at other regions within the dermatome, spread contiguously within the mucous membranes or, more rarely, give rise to CNS or generalized infections which may be fatal. The clinical sequelae which may follow an initial genital or neonatal infection are shown in Figure 8.1.

Our present knowledge of immunity in man is largely extrapolated from *in vitro* and animal studies in which individual components are often dissected out for investigation. This 'isolationist approach' may underestimate the importance of compensatory mechanisms, especially in individuals with an element of immunodeficiency. Hence, considerable uncertainty surrounds both the relevence of many of these observations to humans and the extent to which the components co-operate to control infection. A discussion of these components and their possible interaction in primary infection occupies the bulk of this chapter. This is followed by a consideration of the role of immunity in the establishment and maintenance of latency and finally by a brief discussion of the prospects for developing a successful vaccine for herpes simplex virus.

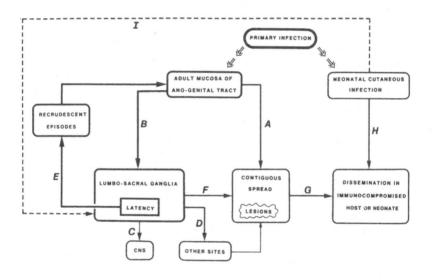

Figure 8.1 Hypothetical scheme of events following an initial genital infection in immunologically mature humans and in neonates. In the adult the primary infection most usually occurs in the mucocutaneous tissue of the anogenital region. Virus may replicate and spread to surrounding contiguous tissue (**A**) or may resolve without further sequelae. Frequently neurons in the subepithelium and subsequently lumbosacral ganglia become infected (**B**) with rare instance of dissemination to the CNS or other sites (**C,D**). Reactivation may result in the centrifugal spread of virus down the axons to give recrudescent episodes at the primary site (**E**) or in contiguous tissue (**F**). In immunodeficient or immunosuppressed adults this may be severe and result in widespread dissemination of virus (**G**). In the neonate dissemination may also occur via the bloodstream (**H**) or via infected ganglia and spinal cord (**I**) resulting in multiple organ involvement including the central nervous system (**C**)

THE IMMUNE RESPONSE IN PRIMARY HERPES INFECTION

Cellular and humoral interactions within the immune system

The response to herpes infection is complex and exhibits an interplay of non-specific with specific mechanisms which embrace both cellular and humoral immunity (Table 8.1). Non-specific mechanisms which do not require exposure to antigens may in many ways be regarded as the first line of defence. They include the multiple actions of the mononuclear phagocytic system (monocytes and macrophages), the cytolytic activity of natural killer (NK) cells and the induction of interferons. Central among these is the macrophage which exhibits non-specific actions and also plays a pivotal role in the regulation and amplification of many specific aspects of immunity. These include immune responses to T-lymphocyte dependent viral antigens, regulation up or down of T- and B-lymphocyte responses, secretion of complement components that enhance both virus neutralization and the destruction of virus infected cells and finally, participation in antibody dependent cell-mediated cytotoxicity. Many of these virus specific responses come into effect in the later stages of infection and play an important part in the limitation of primary lesions and in healing.

Table 8.1 Possible mechanisms involved in the immune response to herpes simplex virus infection

Virus non-specific mechanisms	Virus specific mechanisms
Extrinsic macrophage activities	Virus neutralization by antibody with or without complement
Intrinsic macrophage activities	Complement-mediated cellular cytotoxicity
Interferon – direct antiviral action – indirect action on immune effector cells	Antibody-dependent cellular cytotoxicity
Natural killer cell activity	Cellular immunity mediated by cytotoxic T-lymphocytes

Virus non-specific responses

The mononuclear phagocytic systems

Mononuclear phagocytes (MP), which include circulating monocytes and tissue macrophages, are widely distributed within the spleen, liver, lungs and body cavities. Their importance in non-specific resistance to viral infection was first recognized in the mid-1960s[5]. Since then, non-specific resistance has been shown to be a complex phenomenon divisible into extrinsic and intrinsic mechanisms[6]. Extrinsic resistance is defined as the ability of macrophages to inactivate extracellular virus or reduce virus production in surrounding cells that are normally permissive. Intrinsic resistance is the ability of MP to destroy virus by intracellular mechanisms following phagocytosis, or their ability to restrict virus replication by acting as non-permissive host cells.

Extrinsic effects of macrophages. Extrinsic manifestations of macrophage action are independent of the infected target cell type, are virus non-specific and can be mediated by macrophages from a range of species activated by a variety of stimuli. In HSV-infected mice extrinsic activity peaks on days 3–4 after inoculation and declines by day 7–8 before specific humoral or cell-mediated responses have developed[7]. This is consistent with the observation that mononuclear infiltrates are prominent in early viral foci where they are presumed to restrict replication before specific immune responses are induced.

Studies on the mechanisms underlying extrinsic effects[8,9] (Figure 8.2) have shown that macrophages secrete a range of products[10]. These include neutral proteinases, prostaglandins and reactive oxygen radicles[11] which have the capacity to destroy extracellular virus either by degrading viral envelope glycoproteins or by disorganizing the lipid components in the membrane. Nevertheless, attempts to demonstrate HSV inactivation by incubation of virus in cell-free media from macrophage cultures have not.been successful[7].

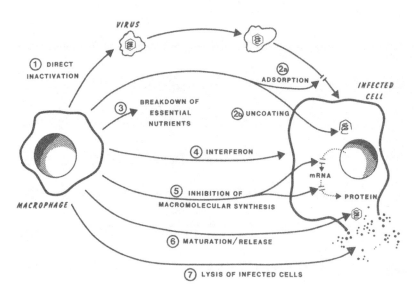

Figure 8.2 Possible mechanisms of extrinsic macrophage mediated resistance to herpes virus infection. Macrophages may secrete a range of factors such as proteases, prostaglandin-like substances or oxygen radicles which may directly inactivate virus particles (**1**). These, or other factors, may block adsorption to the cell membrane (**2a**) or, if penetration occurs' may inhibit uncoating (**2b**). New virus production may be prevented by macrophage-induced breakdown of some extracellular essential nutrient such as arginine (**3**), by interferon induction (**4**) or by other mechanisms which interfere with macromolecular synthesis at the transcriptional or translational level (**5**). If the component parts of new virions are synthesized then their assembly may not occur, thereby preventing maturation and/or release (**6**). Finally, there may be direct lysis of infected cells (**7**) in response to early viral antigen production and before the assembly of mature virions

Many prostaglandins and reactive oxygen species have but a transient existence and would be unlikely to survive in medium filtrate, and hence their significance *in vivo* remains uncertain.

The extrinsic action of macrophages has also been attributed to the induction of an antiviral state in infected target cells by interferon. However, interferon levels in differentiated macrophage cultures have generally been zero or very low, and transfer of antiviral activity in culture supernatant fluid has not been successful[8,12]. It is also notable that macrophages exhibit activity against a range of virus infected cell types, including mouse embryo, BHK 21 and monkey VERO cells: contrary to the species specificity normally associated with interferon action[8,13]. Also anti-mouse interferon antibodies failed to ablate the macrophage induced antiviral effect[8]. On present evidence, therefore, such a role for interferon seems unlikely.

Another soluble factor, arginase, has been implicated, and antiviral activity shown to correlate with its secretion[14]. Although it is difficult to determine the role of arginase *in vivo*, arginine is known to be an essential amino acid for herpes virus replication. Thus, local depletion may reduce the rate of new virus assembly.

Finally, profound effects of activated macrophages on both protein and DNA synthesis have been reported. This could account for the macrophage-induced cytostatic effects observed in various infected cell lines[8,13], but the precise points of biochemical intervention require further investigation.

Intrinsic effects of macrophages. In addition to displaying extrinsic activity, mature macrophages, but not those from human neonates or weanling animals[15], engage actively in phagocytosis of virus and may be either intrinsically non-permissive for replication or engage in intracellular destruction of engulfed virus. Macrophages may be modified in these functions by the presence of specific lymphocytes, antibody or lymphokines[8].

Certain points concerning the nature of intrinsic resistance have a direct bearing on experimental studies. Thus, some strains of inbred mouse such as C57BL/6 are more resistant to HSV infection than others such as BALB/c, DBA/2 and AKR, a factor which appears under the control of two separate genes[16]. However, while some studies have revealed a correlation between the level of intrinsic macrophage resistance and susceptibility of the animal to infection[8] others have failed to confirm this completely for HSV-1[17] and HSV-2.[18] These results imply that the restriction of HSV *in vivo* is not solely determined by intrinsic macrophage resistance but must involve other components of the immune system. It is also notable that *in vitro* there is no correlation between the presence of intrinsic and extrinsic activity within a given cell population, and macrophages lacking self-restriction of HSV may still be able to suppress replication in neighbouring cells. *In vitro* studies, however, need careful interpretation as the methods of macrophage collection, separation and culture can all have a marked effect on the level of intrinsic resistance observed[8]. It is well known that the permissiveness of macrophages increases as they 'age' or differentiate in culture.

Studies with human cells have employed both primary cultures and mononuclear phagocyte-like lines mostly from peripheral blood or peritoneal washes. In general the findings have paralleled those reported for the mouse: the same *in vitro* 'ageing' phenomenon has been observed. Few studies have been conducted on human tissue macrophages, although those from alveolar washes of adults permitted little or no HSV replication[19].

The mechanisms underlying intrinsic resistance are not entirely clear. It would appear that virus adsorption, penetration and uncoating take place equally well in permissive and non-permissive cells[20] and that at least some synthesis of viral DNA and herpes antigens occurs[21], the latter expressing at the cell surface in K562, a human granulocyte cell line[22]. The synthesis of DNA is detectable by enhanced thymidine incorporation and increased rate of phosphorylation of the nucleosides observed in HSV infected macrophages[23]. There appears, however, to be a failure in the later stages of assembly of new virions, and electron microscopy reveals the presence of many empty or defective capsids[21,24]. An alternative hypothesis would suggest that engulfed or newly assembled HSV particles are destroyed by general virucidal mechanisms[21] including low intracellular pH, cationic proteins, proteolytic enzymes, interferon-induced endonucleases or the generation of highly reactive oxygen species such as superoxide anion (O_2^-), hydrogen peroxide or the hydroxyl radical $(OH^{\bullet})$[25]. Unfortunately, most of these mechanisms have not been investigated specifically in connection with HSV infections, though arginase has been assigned a role in the restriction of

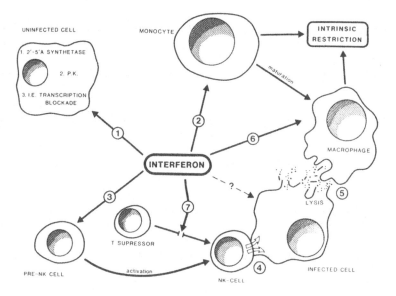

Figure 8.3 Some points of involvement of interferon in the immune response to HSV infection. Interferon induces a direct antiviral state in many cells probably in the case of HSV, by the blockade of immediate-early transcription (1). Alternatively, it may promote recruitment of monocytes to macrophages (2) or activate pre-NK cells to NK cells (3). Such activated NK cells can destroy cells expressing virus antigen (4) while the macrophages remove the resultant cellular debris (5). Interferon may further promote these actions by a direct activation of macrophages (6) or through modulation of NK cell activity by blockade of suppressor cells (7)

intrinsic replication[26]. In studies with vesicular stomatitis virus it was concluded that oxygen metabolites were involved only in extrinsic killing[11]. However, the danger of extrapolating between different viruses was evident from studies which concluded that the macrophage-mediated antiviral activity against mouse hepatitis virus was quite different to that expressed against HSV[27]. A final factor which has been shown to play a role in the intrinsic restriction of HSV replication in human monocyte cultures is interferon (IFN)[28]. Whether it does so by direct antiviral action or by inhibiting the differentiation of non-permissive monocytes to macrophages is not clear. The role of IFN in HSV infections is discussed further below.

Interferons

Interferon (IFN) was first defined as a substance made during a virus infection which was capable of converting susceptible uninfected cells into cells resistant to infection[29]. It may, therefore, limit contiguous spread during primary herpes infection before specific immune responses have been mounted. The mechanisms involved are undoubtedly complex (Figure 8.3) and the issue has been greatly complicated by the discovery of three major IFN classes (α or leukocyte, β or fibroblast and γ or immune) and at least 15 subtypes of α-IFN. It is important to note that α-IFN is produced by macrophages and other non-T-cells in response to infection with virus while γ-IFN is a product of antigen-stimulated T-lymphocytes. The α-subtypes are, therefore, the prime concern of this section, though γ-IFN will be mentioned where appropriate.

In animal models strong evidence favouring a role for IFN in controlling herpes infection has been generated. Resistance of C57BL/6 mice has been correlated with high level IFN production at the site of infection, while susceptible strains (BALB/c, DBA/2) are poor producers[30]. Thus peak levels of IFN were produced intraperitoneally in C57BL/6 mice 4 hours after infection and were maintained above 100 i.u./ml for 24 hours. Production was markedly inoculum-dependent, and only reached maximal values (1000 i.u./ml) at very high levels of infectivity ($2 \times 10^5 - 2 \times 10^7$ pfu/ml)., the mice were resistant to these high infectivity titres, but were susceptible at lower inoculum levels within the range 2×10^4 to 2×10^5 (2.5–25 LD$_{50}$) where interferon levels were reduced or absent[30]. A role for interferon is also supported by the observation that the treatment of resistant mice with potent anti-IFN serum renders them susceptible to infection with HSV-1[31]. Also notable is the protective action of killed *Corynebacterium parvum* against HSV encephalitis in C57BL/6 mice which has been attributed both to interferon induction (though *in vitro* studies suggested it resembled γ rather than the α type)[32] and to NK-cell augmentation.

In humans, there are relatively few studies on the role of endogenous interferon in genital herpes. Studies on a group of mainly homosexual males with acquired immunodeficiency syndrome have revealed an association between severe HSV infection and inability of their peripheral blood mononuclear cells to synthesise α-IFN when challenged with HSV-1[16]. In a further study of recurrent genital herpes conducted in the USSR, none of 53 patients had detectable blood levels of IFN during either relapse or remission. Furthermore, the capacity of their leukocytes to produce IFN on antigenic stimulation *in vitro* was 4–5 times lower than normal, and 88.9% were stated to have shown clinical improvement on α-interferon therapy associated with enhanced NK cell activity[33].

At least three virus non-specific mechanisms have been proposed to account for the action of IFN at the cellular level (Figure 8.3). One of these, namely its action as a component of the extrinsic and intrinsic activities of macrophages, was discussed above. In connection with this mechanism, it has been reported that human monocytes are able to support the production of infectious virus only after differentiation into macrophages. It is possible that IFN plays a role in the monocyte–macrophage transition and monocyte-mediated restriction of replication. This view is supported by the following observations: (1) IFN-like activity was demonstrated in the medium from HSV-exposed monocyte cultures (as opposed to macrophage cultures) and the level of IFN was directly proportional to multiplicity of infection and inversely proportional to virus yield, and (2) anti-α-IFN serum enhanced virus replication even in monocyte cultures with low m.o.i. in which levels of IFN in the medium were undetectable[28]. From the data, however, it was not possible to exclude that the action might involve a more direct antiviral action as discussed below.

A second possible mechanism proposes that IFN has a direct antiviral action thereby limiting the quantities of infectious virus produced. The induction of the oligo-2', 5'A-synthetase/endonuclease and protein kinase systems known to be responsible for the inhibition of growth of RNA viruses are not, however, thought to be so important in HSV infections. Recent studies have shown that IFN inhibits immediate early protein synthesis of HSV prior to or at the level of translation[34], and though relatively high levels are needed (1000–2000 i.u./ml) the *in vivo* studies discussed above show that these are achievable, at least at high infectivity levels in the C57BL/6 mouse.

The final mechanisms proposed for IFN action invoke either the augmentation of NK cell-mediated lysis or the recruitment of pre-NK cells to differentiate into mature effectors. The good evidence for these mechanisms in man and animals will be discussed more fully in the next section.

Natural killer (NK) cell activity

Natural killer cytotoxicity is defined as the ability of leukocytes to destroy virus-infected target cells in the absence of antibody. The precise nature and origin of the effector cells involved, however, is unclear but the high level of NK activity in athymic nude mice shows they are not thymus dependent. They are however, non-adherent and lack surface immunoglobin and thus are neither macrophages nor mature B-cells. Some NK cells express surface markers characteristic of T-cells and macrophages. The situation is further complicated by the demonstration of subsets of NK cells in both mice and man. For example, some NK cells obtained from man are able to lyse the erythroleukaemic cell line K562 *in vitro*, while others are able to lyse HSV-1 infected fibroblasts: notably the two types showed differences in their surface markers. These aspects of the identity and function of NK cells have been concisely reviewed by Lopez[16]. Morphologically, NK cells in man are large granular lymphocytes and make up just a few percent of peripheral blood mononuclear cells. Although they have Fc surface receptors, target cell recognition is not thought to be via specific antibody. This distinguishes them from killer (K) cells though the physical separation of these two cell types remains problematical.

Studies on the role of NK cells in non-specific resistance to HSV infection in mice identified two separately segrating genes, and showed that they were not linked to the H2 major histocompatibility locus. Ablation of the bone marrow of mice with radioactive strontium (^{89}Sr) resulted in severely depressed NK cell function, and previously resistant mice were rendered susceptible to HSV infection. Reconstitution of irradiated susceptible mice with marrow from resistant animals rectified the deficiency[35,36]. Studies using different mouse strains have also shown that genetically resistant mice had NK cell responses while most susceptible strains lacked the ability to lyse HSV-1 infected target cells by this mechanism. CBA mice, however, were an exception and had normal to high NK activity but were moderately susceptible to HSV-1 infection. These data taken together with the previous section, indicate that both interferon induction and NK cell activity correlate with genetic resistance, and it is interesting to speculate that these may be the two properties encoded by the resistance genes.

Though most of this section has dealt with intraperitoneal infections using HSV-1, very similar results have been obtained with HSV-2 and with different mouse strains infected intravaginally with HSV-1[37]. However, mice infected intraperitoneally with HSV-2 demonstrated an augmented capacity of macrophages to restrict virus replication in addition to elevated NK cell activity[18,38].

Much useful information has now been acquired on the nature and function of NK cells in humans by studying inherited immunodeficiency and other diseases. Direct evidence of NK cell heterogeneity has been obtained from patients with aplastic anaemia. The NK cells of some of these patients could lyse K562 cells normally but HSV-1 infected fibroblasts only poorly and vice versa, suggesting at least two sub-populations[16]. Patients with hypogammaglobulinaemia and classical severe combined immunodeficiency disease were found to have normal NK responses, suggesting that the cells are neither of B-cell nor T-cell lineage. By contrast, some patients with monocyte/macrophage deficiencies exhibit depressed NK function while others do not. This implies that NK cells may be of different haematopoietic lineage but may also be accounted for by compensatory mechanisms in some individuals. Wiscott–Aldrich patients usually have depressed NK function both during and between bouts of HSV infection, but their immunity is so generally impaired that it is not possible to attribute the susceptibility to HSV solely to NK deficiency. In one study on patients with recurrent genital herpes, 37.5% had depressed NK cell activity compared with only 5.1% of normal controls, a defect partly rectified by the administration of leukocyte interferon[33]. A word of caution in interpreting results on NK cell activity is necessary, however, as it is not always easy to distinguish this property from antibody-dependent cell-mediated cytotoxicity (ADCC). This was illustrated in a recent study[39] in which peripheral blood monocytes from 28 individuals were compared for ADCC and NK activity against HSV infected fibroblasts. Only those samples (20) showing positive ADCC reactions killed the fibroblasts while the remaining eight did not, though most of them killed K562 cells by NK action.

The relationship of interferon to NK cell activity was mentioned in the previous section. It is known that α-, β- and γ-interferons can augment NK activity[16,40], and evidence shows that they do so, at least in part, by the recruitment of pre-NK cells into lytic effectors[41,42] and by assisting their recycling[43] (Figure 8.3). However, NK mediated lysis of target cells does not correlate with IFN levels *in vitro* and continues when all detectable IFN is neutralized by specific antibody. Similarly, some individuals have normal NK cell action but low capacity for IFN synthesis. This suggests that, contrary to earlier notions, IFN is not essential for the actual event of target cell lysis[16].

Relatively little is known about the receptors recognized by NK cells, but recently the role of the Mac-1, LFA-1, and p150, 95 leukocyte glycoproteins have been investigated[44]. Using mononuclear cells from eight patients genetically deficient for these glycoproteins and monoclonal antibodies (MAb) directed towards them it was shown that MAb to LFA-1-alpha or -beta ablated NK cytotoxicity. Adoptive transfer models in neonatal mice, in which human interferon was used to stimulate NK activity, also showed that Mac-1-dependent cellular adhesive properties were necessary for normal NK cytotoxicity. A further study has implicated the transferrin receptor (TR) and a direct correlation was found between its expression and susceptibility to NK lysis in both virus infected and uninfected cells. NK cell lysis, however, could not be inhibited by excess iron-saturated transferrin or affinity purified TR, and it was concluded that the transferrin and NK receptors were not the same[45].

It will have become clear from the above that although considered separately, there are complex relationships between macrophages, interferons and NK cells, which are summarized in Figure 8.3. Interferon clearly has a central role as it is able to augment the functions of both cell types. This may occur via a role in monocyte transition, in monocyte restriction of HSV or by the induction of early transcriptional blockade of HSV immediate early protein synthesis in infected cells. Equally, IFN may act by increasing the efficiency of NK effector cell function or by promoting the differentiation of pre-NK into mature NK cells. Much more work is required before the relative importance of each of these actions in the limitation of HSV genital infections in man is fully understood.

Virus specific responses

Virus specific responses resemble non-specific responses in involving a range of effector molecules and cell types, participating in a co-operative and interrelated manner. These include antibodies, complement components, lymphokines and a range of effector cells. For the sake of simplicity, they are discussed separately though their interdependence is emphasized where appropriate.

Antibody responses to herpes simplex virus infection

The role of antibodies in the limitation of disease and the prevention of transmission of HSV in man remains a matter of some controversy. This is partly because of the difficulty of studying primary infection in truly naive hosts, and partly because of differences in the methods used to measure antibody levels. As with other components of the immune response, our knowledge draws substantially on animal models and the data are often controversial and conflicting[46].

Several studies have indicated that systemically administered hyperimmune rabbit serum can protect mice from death provided it is given prophylactically or within 12–24 hours of an intraperitoneal HSV inoculation. It was also shown that viral spread to and within the CNS could be prevented, and that effects were better against homologous than heterologous virus types. Protection has been correlated with antibody titre, and virus neutralization appears to occur but only in tissue compartments outside the CNS. In neonatal mice, protection with high titre anti-HSV-1 serum could be achieved up to six days post-infection.

Further indications as to the role of antibodies in the protection of animals have arisen from the investigation of various 'vaccine' preparations. It is clear from those studies which have monitored both humoral and cellular immunity that many different vaccine preparations provoke a multitude of responses, and the protective effects found are as much attributable to cell-mediated mechanisms as they are to the production of antibodies[46]. A fuller consideration of vaccines in connection with genital infections in animals and man is included in the final section of this chapter.

In human subjects, the primary response to HSV-2 is broadly similar to that for HSV-1[47]. There is an initial synthesis of complement dependent 19s neutralizing antibodies of the IgM class from days 3–8 post-infection which wanes within a month. This is supplanted by 7s IgG, from the second week onwards. The synthesis of serum IgG probably continues for life. The nature of the IgG synthesized may differ with time, and in the rabbit the early antibodies required complement in order to neutralize, whereas both complement dependent and slow-reacting neutralizing antibodies were present in late IgG[48]. More recent studies in man have shown that in adult healthy seropositives and patients with both primary and recurrent HSV-1 infections, HSV specific IgG1 and IgG3 are detectable, and occasionally IgG4[49]: an almost identical picture to that observed in babies.

Considerable difficulty attaches to studying the serum IgG antibodies in adults because by the age of 30 almost all will have been exposed to subclinical infections of HSV-1 and some to HSV-2. In a recent study of 24 patients with non-primary first episode genital herpes, seven had anti-HSV-1, eleven anti-HSV-2 and six anti-HSV-1 and HSV-2 antibodies measured by a standard microneutralization test[50]. A further study of 100 patients with anogenital herpes indicated that 17 had HSV-1 and 83 HSV-2 virus. Using an

ELISA technique, a predominance of anti-HSV-2 antibody was found in sera of 40 of these patients taken during recrudescence, invariably associated with HSV-2 infection, while a predominance of HSV-1 antibody was found in 37 patients, 11 of whom had HSV-1 and 26 HSV- 2 infection. However, there was no correlation between antibody levels and the number of recurrences although HSV-2 appeared to recur more often than HSV-1[51]. Although these studies used serum carefully adsorbed to remove cross-reacting antibodies, many other studies have not and the results may reflect the existence of type common HSV-1 and HSV-2 epitopes as well as indicating prior infection.

The nature of the epitopes provoking humoral immune responses have been the subject of much study. Many responses, but not all, are related to the surface glycoproteins. Originally these were termed gA, gB, gC, gD and gE but it is now known that gA is a precursor of gB and more recently other glycoproteins, gF and gG, have been identified. HSV-2 gF appears to be the structural homologue of HSV-1 gC. The synthesis, antigenic properties and functional role of these molecules was concisely reviewed in 1984[52]. (Table 8.2). gB and gD appear to possess type common epitopes while gC and, to some extent gE, may be type specific. It is now clear that several of these glycoproteins possess multiple antigenic domains, and the mapping of these sites and elucidation of their relevance to natural immunity are the subject of intensive investigations[46]. Already it is known that gD can stimulate a protective immune response and monoclonal antibodies to all the major glycoproteins passively protect mice from lethal challenge and may prevent viral spread to the central nervous system[53,54].

Glycoprotein gG appears to be HSV-2 specific. In a study of 134 patients with recurrent genital herpes, purified gG-2 antigen was used in a sensitive immunodot enzyme assay on nitrocellulose paper to detect HSV-2 specific antibodies. Positive results were obtained in 132 convalescent sera but in only 17% of those taken earlier than 10 days after onset of infection[55]. This raises

Table 8.2 Properties and actions of herpes virus glycoproteins

Glycoprotein	Fully glycosylated MW	Type specific epitopes	Type common epitopes	Protection of animals by monoclonals	Comments
gB	120000	Yes	Yes	Yes	involved in cell penetration after virus attachment
gC	130000	Yes	—	Yes in HSV-1	possible role in infected cell fusion C3b receptor
gD	59000	—	Yes	Yes	unknown function
gE	65–80000	Yes	Yes	—	unknown. Can bind Fc region of IgG
gF	(Structural homologue in HSV-2 of HSV-1 gC)				
gG–1	25000)	Yes	Yes	?	recently described*
gG–2	72000)				

*See McGeoch, D. J. *et al.* (1987) *J. Gen. Virol.*, **68**, 19–38

the questions as to which antigens provoke the earlier antibody responses, a question addressed in several recent investigations[56-58]. In the first[56], it was shown that patients with recurrent infection generally had high IgG titres reactive with gD and gG as well as several viral capsid proteins. By contrast, patients experiencing primary genital HSV-2 displayed marked differences, and in particular it was apparent that the earliest and strongest response was directed not towards a glycoprotein but towards the internal capsid protein, p40. A second publication from the same laboratory found very similar results for HSV-1 infections in various anatomical sites[57]. In a further study on primary first episode genital herpes (10 with HSV-1 and 37 with HSV-2), patients with HSV-1 developed, sequentially, antibodies to the nucleocapsid protein p148, then to gB and gC followed by p88 and finally seroconverted to gE and a non-glycosylated protein, p66[58]. In this same study, patients with HSV-2 infection developed antibodies to p148, gB and p88 within one week, while seroconversion to p66, gD, gC and gE occurred later, at a mean time of about 3 weeks. Notably, seroconversion within 21 days to HSV-2 gD, gE and p66 was associated with a longer time to first recurrence, suggesting a possible role for these antibodies in the maintenance of HSV-2 latency in man.

Clearly the human response to HSV antigens is complex and it is important to recognize that the T-cell status, notably OKT4 and OKT8 cell ratio, can significantly influence the extent of IgG synthesis and might explain some of the interpatient variability noted above[59].

Antibodies of the IgA and IgE classes have received much less attention than IgG. Reports on the stimulation of serum IgA have been somewhat contradictory[48] though this class has been demonstrated in individuals undergoing either primary or recrudescent episodes. A rise in titre is only evident, however, in samples taken sequentially from patients with primary disease. Laboratory-induced 'mucosal immunity' possibly attributable to IgA was induced in guinea pigs infected intravaginally with a thymidine kinase negative strain of HSV-2 which protected against lethal infection with ten times the LD_{50} of the wild type[60]. In this context, a study in women with untreated first or recurrent episodes of disease due to HSV-2, included measurement of the levels of both IgA and secretory piece IgA (sIgA) in sequential samples of cervicovaginal secretions. Levels of sIgA were found in 20/31 women from whom virus was isolated and in 4/13 who were virus negative, the peak titre occurring between days 9 and 16. Virus was not isolated from any of 130 samples in which sIgA antibody titre was equal to or greater than 1:2 compared to 98 virus positives in 259 samples where the titre was equal to or less than 1:2, suggesting that local production of antibody may influence the virus titre and duration of cervical HSV infections[61]. Very little information is available on IgE, though one study found serum IgE levels significantly higher in patients with frequent recurrences compared to those with few. Elevated IgE was only detected during periods of active disease[62].

It will be evident from the above that interaction of HSV with the host can trigger the production of specific antibodies from several immunoglobulin classes. Although many of these can be shown to neutralize virus *in vitro*, their significance in the prevention or limitation of genital HSV infections in man is speculative. It is clear though that neither neutralizing nor cytolytic antibodies alone are sufficient to prevent primary or recurrent infections, and immunosuppressed patients with high neutralising antibody levels, but depressed cellular immunity, are highly vulnerable to infection by this virus[63].

Antibody-dependent cellular cytotoxicity (ADCC)

The ADCC reaction (Figure 8.4) can be mediated in the presence of specific antibody by macrophages, PMNs or killer cells, all of which carry Fc receptors[16]. It is attractive to speculate that this is a major mechanism of resistance to HSV because the level of antibody required to arm the effectors is very low and infected cells can be lysed within 2 hours under optimal conditions, long before new virions can be assembled. Unfortunately, ADCC is much less easy to demonstrate in murine than in human systems and for that reason it has remained largely an *in vitro* phenomenon. However, Kohl has shown that ADCC could be detected in adult mice 3 days post-infection while it was not detectable in newborn mice after 5 days[64,65].

ADCC is known to be augmented by interferon *in vitro* and severely depressed by elevated levels of prostaglandin E_2 (PGE_2). However, ADCC remained constant throughout the menstrual cycle despite fluctuations in

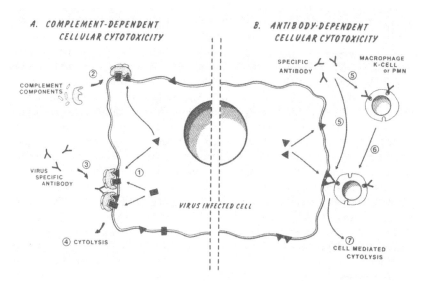

Figure 8.4 Diagramatic representation of CDC and ADCC mechanisms of cellular cytotoxicity. **A.** In CDC virus antigen and complement receptors are synthesized in the infected cell (1) and are inserted into the membrane. When sufficient density is reached complement C3b is bound, thus activating the alternate pathway (2). Virus specific Ab binds to the complement–receptor complex (3) and initiates lysis (4). **B.** In ADCC receptors are again inserted into the membrane. Specific antibody binds to effector cells carrying Fc receptors (the arming reaction) or to the cellular antigens (5). Armed cells, or those with vacant Fc receptors bind to antigens (6) and release cytotoxic mediators which bring about lysis (7)

PGE$_2$ levels[66], and naproxen, an inhibitor of prostaglandin synthetase, failed to alter ADCC in human volunteers though it did significantly increase NK activity[67]. It has also been shown that the peripheral mononuclear cells and sera of 20/28 healthy adult volunteers were capable of killing HSV infected fibroblasts by ADCC, while the material from the remaining eight could not[39]. Most recently, the leukocyte glycoproteins Mac-1, LFA-1 and p150, 95 have been implicated in ADCC in that antibodies to them abolished ADCC reactivity both *in vitro* and in an adoptive passage model in which neonatal mice were given human monocytes and antibody to protect them from HSV infection[44]. These studies give a tantalizing hint of the importance of ADCC, but further proof of its role in resistance to genital herpes in man is still needed.

Complement-dependent cellular cytotoxicity

Following the infection of cells, virus antigen is synthesized and inserted into the membrane (Figure 8.4); a process which takes from 3–6 or 7 hours, depending on the multiplicity of infection and the cell line[48]. The antigens, which may be type common or type specific are able to activate the complement cascade via the alternate pathway. Although lysis does not occur in the absence of immunoglobins of the IgG class, in their presence more complement is fixed and lysis ensues[68], resulting in complement-dependent cytotoxicity (CDC). In contrast to the ADCC reaction which requires intact immunoglobulin molecules, the CDC reaction can be initiated by divalent Fab'2 arms and does not require the presence of the Fc portion.

To a large extent CDC, like ADCC, also remains an *in vitro* phenomenon, and though it has formed the basis of a number of useful diagnostic tests its role in limiting HSV infection of the human genital tract is largely unknown. Humans and guinea pigs with complement deficiency are not more prone to HSV infection though this does not rule out a role for complement in individuals with an intact system.

An interesting recent publication[69] has shown that HSV-1, but not HSV-2, induces the C3b receptor on a range of cell lines and that this receptor is functionally related to HSV-1 gC, a type specific glycoprotein. All cell lines permissive for HSV-1 examined expressed the receptor. The equivalent receptor for HSV-2 appears to be unknown though HSV-2 infected cells certainly participate in CDC-type reactions in the presence of HSV-2 specific IgG. Some effector cells (macrophages, PMNs) carry C3 receptors and may also become involved in cytolysis *in vivo*, though this remains to be proven.

Cytotoxic T-lymphocyte responses and cell-mediated immunity

This section, which draws on the concise review of Rouse[70], is concerned with those reactions in which T-lymphocytes (T-LC) and their subsets are involved as the effector cells. In contrast to many other cell types described above, subsets of T-cells display a dual requirement for activation which involves both the foreign antigen and a self-antigen coded for by genes of the major histocompatability complex (MHC) (Figure 8.5).

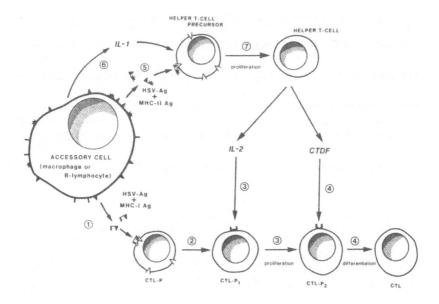

Figure 8.5 Scheme of possible interactions during induction of cytotoxic T-lymphocyte (CTL) response to viral antigens (based on Reference 70). Viral antigen can be presented by accessory cells to cytotoxic T-lymphocyte precursors (CTL-P) in association with MHC class I antigens (**1**). This initiates the expression of IL-2 receptors (**2**) which upon stimulation induce a proliferative response (**3**) and receptors for cytotoxic T-cell differentiation factor (CTDF). CTDF can then trigger complete maturation of CTLs (**4**). Viral antigen may also be presented by the accessory cells to helper T-cell precursors (**5**) probably in association with IL-1 (**6**) to induce the formation of mature T-helper cells (**7**). These in turn synthesize the IL-2 and CTDF (**3,4**) which act on the CTL-precursors (CTL-P_1 and CTL-P_2)

Several theories have been evolved to explain T-cell mediated antiviral effects. In the direct theory, cytotoxic T-lymphocytes (CTL) recognize certain MHC related glycoproteins (class I antigens) on infected cells and destroy them. In the indirect theory the MHC class II antigens, which are restricted largely to B-lymphocytes and macrophages, are recognized in conjunction with viral antigen. In this latter pathway helper and suppressor T-lymphocyte subsets are involved in positive and negative regulation, respectively. This is brought about by the release of either antigen specific or non-specific soluble mediators which modulate cellular function and may lead to an inflammatory response dominated by mononuclear cells. Should this lead to tissue damage it is often referred to as delayed-type hypersensitivity (DTH).

CTL responses have been extensively studied *in vitro* and potent responses can be obtained by secondary stimulation of T-LCs taken from animals primed with infectious virus. Such procedures have demonstrated that CTL precursors pass sequentially through a series of maturation steps before becoming fully effective (Figure 8.5), and have also demonstrated the existence of a subset of memory cells. With HSV though, as with many other viruses, it has not proved possible to induce CTL responses in unprimed cell populations, possibly due to the very low ratio of CTL-precursors (CTL-P) present. The initial stimulus for maturation of CTL-P cells is brought about by dual viral and MHC-1 antigen presentation. This antigen may be free but is more usually associated with the membranes of accessory cells such as macrophages or B-cells which, in turn, induce the expression of interleukin-2 (IL-2) receptors on the CTL-precursors. For further maturation these cells have then to be stimulated by IL-2 and then by cytotoxic T-cell differentiation factors (CTDF). The former induces clonal proliferation and the latter differentiation into fully functional cytotoxic T-lymphocytes. Notably, exogenously added IL-2 is able to induce a proliferative response to HSV antigens in cultures depleted of macrophages[71]. This would imply that macrophages may be the natural trigger of helper T-cells as they are a source of endogenously produced IL-2 (Figure 8.5). Interferon-γ is also a product of antigen stimulated T-LC and may enhance macrophage activity as described in an earlier section. IFN-γ production is itself regulated by IL-2[72].

Macrophage produced interleukin-1 (IL-1) has also been shown to be involved in the herpes virus CTL-system by promoting the maturation of helper T-cell precursors[73]. Thus Ia positive syngeneic virus-infected accessory cells could not provide accessory function following glutaraldehyde treatment, which ablates their ability to produce IL-1, but their activity could be restored by exogenously added IL-1. Finally, although not shown in Figure 8.4 suppressor cells are present *in vivo* and are probably responsible for fine tuning of this immune response.

Early work suggested that CTL reactions to HSV-1 and HSV-2 were type-specific but the consensus now favours some degree of cross-reactivity[70]. This is likely to arise from shared epitopes on viral glycoprotein components of the antigen-receptor complex expressed on HSV infected cells rather than from any variation in the HLA antigen. However, glycoprotein C in HSV-1 does not seem to be involved, because a mutant strain deficient in gC production has been shown to induce a type specific CTL response. This type of study has been extended by generating CTL clones specific for HSV-1 or HSV-2 and then analysing the viral glycoproteins they recognize on autologous HSV-infected cells[74]. Some HSV-1 specific clones were found to be directed against glycoprotein B (gB-1) and others against gD-1 or gE-1 while HSV-2 clones were directed against gC-2, gD-2, gE-2 or gG. the role of these glycoproteins as receptors for CTL-reactions was further confirmed by the observation that genetically engineered gB-1 and gD-1 were able to stimulate the proliferation of human peripheral blood lymphocytes and induce the synthesis of IL-2 in seropositive individuals, indicating the presence of gB-1 and gD-1 memory cells. Such stimulated lymphocytes were able to lyse, specifically, HSV-1 and HSV-2 infected autologous target cells. It seems probable, therefore, that these glycoproteins are part of the receptor complex in human T-cell-mediated immunity to HSV[75].

The MHC component of the receptor complex has also received some attention. It is known that viral antigen components on the target cell surface must be presented in unique association with class I MHC antigens. However, productive infection of the target cells is essential, and exposure to inactivated virus or viral components is insufficient unless they have a fusion activity[70].

Some T-cell clones for HSV-1 were found to lyse cells with which they shared no class I antigen. Analysis of these has shown that they lysed HSV-1 infected cells associated with class II MBI or class II DRI antigens, implying that the class II antigens encoded by the HLA D region may also be important in some individuals for the recognition and destruction of virus infected cells[76].

Finally, it is necessary to consider the role of CTL-responses *in vivo*. Ironically, it is much easier to demonstrate CTL responses to most viruses in the mouse than in man except in the case of HSV. Specific CTL responses first become detectable in the mouse 3–4 days post-infection, peak at days 6–8 and decline by day 21. For HSV only weak responses have been found, but they can be induced to appear *in vitro* by culturing cells for 2–3 days. It is not clear why this should be though suppressor cells might be acting in the mouse-HSV system *in vivo*[70]. Alternatively, HSV may be a poor promotor of T-helper subsets, a theory supported by the observation that differentiation of primed murine CTL *in vitro* is enhanced by IL-2. In humans the *in vivo* CTL response is also controversial, though lymphocytes from patients with HSV can abrogate lectin driven mitogenesis, which in turn can be overcome with T-cell differentiation factor[77]. Also, as noted above, CTL clones to HSV-1 and HSV-2 have now been produced from the peripheral blood lymphocytes of infected patients[75] following stimulation with gB-1 and gD-1. Thus although the evidence is still meagre, a role for the CTL response in humans seems probable.

Herpes infections in the neonate

It is over 50 years since the first demonstration of age-related susceptibility to HSV infection in mice[78]. This is known to relate to the maturation of peripheral resistance as injection of HSV directly into the brain is fatal for both adult and neonatal animals.

It is also known that in humans, resistance to herpes virus infection develops between the third and fifth week of life[79]. Consequently the newborn infant is especially vulnerable when exposed to HSV, but the nature of the specific immunodeficiencies which result in this susceptibility remain to be fully defined.

The role of humoral immunity in protection from neonatal HSV infection is unclear. Protection by passively administered antibody in animals is well established, and beneficial results can be obtained using a variety of routes of infection in mice provided the viral inoculum is not excessive[64]. Newborn mice can achieve systemic levels of antibody from maternal milk and weanlings suckling to immune mothers are protected from viral challenge compared to those with non-immune mothers. Whether this immunity is acquired transplacentally or in colostrum remains to be elucidated[64]. Active production of neutralizing antibody and ADCC in neonatal animals are delayed compared to adult animals and their role in protection in the newborn must be minimal.

In man there is a close correlation between maternal and cord blood anti-HSV IgG titres, and although amniotic fluid contains neutralizing antibody, its role in the control of infection is obscure. Unlike mice, human infants do not acquire significance antibody levels from milk, and several careful studies which investigated serum antibody levels in relation to HSV infection of neonates reached different conclusions. In one, a correlation was detected between severity of infection and the titre of antibody[80], while in another, no such correlation was seen[81]. More recently, 59 neonates with HSV infection were studied and infants with disseminated disease or onset during week 1 were less likely to have neutralizing antibodies than those developing disease from weeks 2–8[82]. In a further study which examined the IgG subclasses of 10 infants, titres were similar in both neonatal and later HSV infections, and it was concluded that antibody was not part of the selective deficiency of HSV-specific immunity following neonatal infection[83]. Clearly, this important issue has not yet been adequately resolved though the clinical use of post-exposure serum prophylaxis has been considered[84].

A number of inadequacies in neonatal cellular function have been found in the newborn. Macrophages from adult and suckling mice become equally infected with HSV but the former do not pass on the infection to other organs while the latter do[15]. This intrinsic antiviral activity of adult macrophages and their ability to protect on transfer to suckling animals has been confirmed in subsequent studies in mice and humans[64]. Lymphocyte transformation responses may also be absent or delayed in the neonate to both HSV antigen and to mitogens such as phytohaemagglutinin[64,80,82,85], but to date it has not been possible to correlate these responses with disease severity.

Killer cytotoxicity plays a more definite role in the susceptibility of the neonate, and a defect in human cord blood adherent and non-adherent mononuclear cell cytoxicity has been confirmed repeatedly[64]. NK cells may also display a reduced responsiveness to stimulation by interferon or other lymphokines such as IL-2[86], and some evidence exists that interferon levels in the neonate are, in any case, lower than in the adult[64,82]. This lack of responsiveness is further implicated by a recent observation that there are about 10-fold fewer and less effective NK cytotoxic cells directed against HSV infected fibroblasts and K562 (a granulocytic myeloid cell line) in cord blood than circulating in the blood of adults.[86]

The role of ADCC is less clear in the human neonate. Certainly the ADCC reaction, especially that mediated by macrophages, is usually low if cord blood mononuclear cells are used, but this is partly compensated for by their greater numbers. Interpretation in many earlier studies has, though, been difficult as they failed to state the method of the baby's delivery. It has now been claimed that vaginally delivered infants had ADCC levels equivalent to adults, while those delivered by Caesarean section prior to labour display lower levels[87]. This may of course reflect the fact that Caesarean delivered babies were somewhat premature compared to those delivered naturally.

In conclusion, significant defects in macrophage and NK cell function appear to be involved in neonatal susceptibility to HSV. There may also be contributory defects in antibody handling or synthesis, in ADCC reactions, in lymphocyte transformation and in production of, or response to, interferons or other lymphokines. Many areas of uncertainty remain and much more research is required before the many other components of the neonate immune system[88] are properly understood.

THE ROLE OF IMMUNITY IN LATENCY AND RECRUDESCENT INFECTIONS

The latent state

It is beyond the scope of this chapter to explore deeply the nature of latency in herpes simplex infections. However, a brief consideration of the latent state and its relationship to the various arms of the immune system is essential bearing in mind that the majority of clinical problems in adults are encountered in patients with recrudescent disease rather than primary infections. More extensive reviews of latency have been published[4].

Dynamic versus static theories of latency

These two theories[89] have been proposed to describe the state of the herpes virus during periods of latency. In the dynamic state a very slow but continuous replication of virus in infected neurons is proposed so that at any given time such cells will contain infective virus particles. In the static theory, it is proposed that DNA can remain indefinitely in the neuron without productive infection, though whether it is integrated into host chromosomes or free is unclear. Investigation has proved difficult due to the extremely low levels of virus and/or genome present and the practical difficulties which arise when ganglia are handled – a process which can reactivate virus and appears to favour the dynamic theory. The consensus of opinion at present would favour the static theory with, perhaps, partial expression of virus in some hosts, though Klein has suggested that recent data showing the detection of infectious virus, viral mRNA and viral encoded thymidine kinase in ganglia has led to a blurring between the two theories[90].

Establishment of latency following primary infection

Primary infection is followed by viral invasion of the neurons within the first few hours. Ganglia then undergo a productive infection which eventually resolves to be followed by latency. Three mechanisms have been proposed to account for the establishment of latency. In the first, called 'immune modulation', it is presumed that the ganglia are permissive for HSV and that immunity converts this from a lytic to a non-lytic response, thereby leaving intact cells harbouring virus. In the second, 'immune elimination', it is presumed that there are two populations of neurons, one permissive and one non-permissive. The former are lysed while the latter remain to harbour latent virus. Finally, it is possible that ganglionic cells are normally non-permissive but that various stimuli convert the neurons to a permissive state[91]. In the first two of these at least the immune system is presumed to play an active role in establishing latency.

An active role for immunity is supported by a number of observations[89,91]. Firstly, it is clearly more difficult to establish latency in animals previously infected or immunized. Secondly, the administration of silica to mice to produce partial reduction of macrophages and/or NK cells greatly enhances the rate of establishment of the latent state. Thirdly, immunosuppression by corticosteroids or cyclophosphamide or the administration of anti-IgM serum can enhance the latency rate. Fourthly, the viral titre in ganglia of immunocompetent mice falls progressively up to day 12 post-infection, while the titre in the ganglia of immunodeficient athymic nude mice increases over the same period and culminates in death. Further, studies in which high titres of antibody were administered to nude mice failed to prevent acute ganglionic infection, and, by inference, this implicates cell-mediated immunity in the control of this event. Despite this clear evidence for an involvement of the immune system, it is still not possible to state whether immune modulation or immune elimination is the more probable theory in animals, let alone man where experimental manipulation is almost impossible.

Maintenance of latency

It is not known whether the factors involved in establishing latency are the same as those involved in maintaining it. Explant studies have shown that neither immunoglobulin nor interferon prevent expression of virus *in vitro*, but such studies are flawed because the very process of explantation may act as a stimulus for replication. Similar criticisms apply to studies in which ganglia were explanted from one animal to another. In an attempt to resolve this problem Openshaw[91] passively immunized mice with rabbit anti-HSV serum following inoculation with HSV-1 into the lip. Serum antibody levels declined to almost undetectable levels by 4 months, but the infection was maintained in the latent state with only 14% spontaneous seroconversion over a period of 13 weeks. Traumatization of the lip by freezing produced a 90% seroconversion rate but no clinical disease. It was concluded that serum neutralizing antibodies to HSV were unnecessary for the maintenance of latent infection. Neither tolerance nor immunosuppression were evident upon rechallenge with virus.

Reactivation, recurrences and recrudescent infections

Reappearance of virus in the mucous membranes or skin implies that a series of events have already taken place, including lifting of the transcriptional block in infected neurons, viral replication and assembly, transport down the axons and spread to contiguous epidermal cells. This last step is likely to be particularly efficient in herpes due to its ability to spread from cell to cell even in the presence of a fully functional immune system.

Several model studies have attempted to mimic reactivation and recrudescence. Some involve the re-infection of previously infected hosts, but these are highly artificial and mimic human disease only poorly[89]. More relevant models rely on traumatizing the epidermal tissue of latently infected animals by scarification, application of solvents or irritants, sellotape stripping or UV-light irradiation. One of the most widely used models of this type has employed sellotape stripping of the mouse ear. This procedure traumatically depilates the epithelial tissue which results in the release of mediators, promotes thymidine incorporation in skin and ganglia and may deplete Langerhans cells which serve an important accessory function in the control of cutaneous infection[92]. Models of spontaneous genital herpes recrudescence have also been described in mice[93] and guinea pigs[94].

Mechanisms involved in the mouse ear model may include the release of PGE-2, which can markedly depress both the ADCC reaction and IL-2 production, or the loss of Langerhans cells which could allow infected foci to avoid immune elimination and permit the development of a clinical lesion. Notably, elevated PGE-2 has also been shown to depress specific T-cell stimulation by HSV antigens in the cells of human volunteers[95]. The addition of an immunosuppressive regime (cyclophosphamide) to these models has produced variable results. Some workers have found a marked rise in recrudescence[91] while others have not. Mechanistically, immunosuppression may simply amplify spontaneous reactivation, may depress cellular or humoral immune factors which may be involved in the transcriptional block that maintains the latent state or may allow a recurrence to develop into a recrudescence.

What is clear, however, is that immune responses play a major role in the limitation of recrudescent lesions and immunosuppression greatly prolongs healing time in both animals and man, but the precise factors involved remain uncertain. There is general agreement that neutralizing antibody in serum does not markedly change during active episodes of disease, and no specific defects have been found in antibody production to particular viral antigens in people suffering frequent recurrences of HSV-1[56,91]. Further, patients with hypogammaglobulinaemia do not seem to be especially prone to HSV and about 75% of renal transplant patients with high antibody titres develop lesions and shed virus within 1–2 months[96], suggesting a more important role for cellular immunity. Experimental studies on CMI, however, have produced somewhat conflicting results, though it has recently been claimed that reactivation is associated with the induction of a dialysable factor in the serum of patients undergoing recrudescent disease[97] that interferes with interferon or IL-2 mediated NK cell enhancement. This would be consistent with the observation of reduced capacity of lymphocytes to produce interferon and of reduced NK activity in patients with recurrent genital herpes[33]. Finally, patients with recurrent oral HSV-1 were reported to have increased Fc bearing T-cells and natural cytotoxic T-lymphocytes. These increased levels were maintained for months, but fell in the week preceding a recrudescent episode[98].

VACCINES AND THE IMMUNE RESPONSE TO HSV

Prospects and status for a herpes virus vaccine

This topic has recently been reviewed in detail[46] and will only briefly be considered here. The search for a herpes vaccine has gone on almost continously since immunization of rabbits was first demonstrated in 1921. The sophistication of the preparations used has improved with time, from attenuated or whole killed virus to the specific glycoproteins or synthetic peptides epitopes being used experimentally today. The results obtained have generally not improved in parallel with the technology, and no suitable preparation is yet available for use in man despite many studies in animal models which have shown good protection against primary infection and, in some cases, reduction in the frequency or severity of recrudescent lesions.

Using an attenuated strain of HSV-1 to 'vaccinate' mice intraperitoneally, protection against ganglionic infection following subsequent intravaginal challenge was observed. An HSV-2 strain failed to give similar protection. This contrasted with studies in the guinea pig in which HSV-1 produced moderation of acute HSV-2 induced vaginitis but did not affect the subsequent development of chronicity. The use of an attenuated TK⁻ strain of HSV-2 was more successful when used to immunize mice intravaginally. It replicated in the vaginal mucosa causing mild clinical disease and produced complete immunity to challenge with ten times the LD_{50} of wild type virus. The use of formaldehyde inactivated HSV-1 or HSV-2 as vaccines subcutaneously in mice gave lifelong protection against subsequent genital challenge with HSV-2, though the HSV-1 vaccine was more effective than that prepared from HSV-2.

Considerable effort has been devoted to the development of a safe subunit vaccine, and an HSV-1 preparation extracted from MRC-5 cells produced long-lasting protection in mice against intravaginal challenge with HSV-2. To avoid the presence of contaminating viral DNA, with which cervical cancer has been epidemiologically associated, an alternative preparation used the herpes glycoprotein-containing membranes of MRC-5 cells infected with HSV-2 as a vaccine in guinea pigs. Once again immunized animals developed only mild disease when challenged intravaginally, while unimmunized controls developed extensive organ involvement often leading to death.

Genetically engineered glycoproteins have also been used in a range of model systems. A series of injections of gD-1 protected mice from lethal challenge with HSV-1 but not with HSV-2 virus. gD-1 in Complete Freunds Adjuvant protected when immunization was extended over a prolonged period of time. Similarly, vaccinia virus recombinants containing the HSV-1 gD gene were claimed to protect mice from subsequent lethal challenge. Of the other gylcoproteins, gC and gB have been shown to protect against virus of the appropriate type and a combination of gC, gB and the gB precursor also protected mice against an otherwise fatal intracerebral challenge.

Further sophistication has arisen from the mapping, and subsequent synthesis, of peptides representing major antigenic sites on herpes glycoproteins. To date these have only tended to be significantly immunogenic when coupled to carrier proteins, but in this form peptides representing amino acids 1–23 and 8–23 of HSV-1 gD have been shown to protect mice against lethal infection with HSV-1 and HSV-2.

Studies in humans also have a long history, but most are open to criticism because they have been inadequately controlled. Nevertheless, claims of beneficial results have been made persistently and at least one product has been marketed in Europe (Lupidon G) but without finding general acceptance. The vaccine from MRC-5 cells referred to above has been used in open studies to determine whether it could protect uninfected consorts of HSV infected partners or reduce the rate of recrudescence. Results appear encouraging but badly need confirmation under controlled trial conditions. Similar encouraging reduction of attack rate and time to healing have also been reported for a vaccine developed at the *Institut Pasteur*.

Many animal and human studies with vaccines have attempted to monitor various components of the immune response. There is almost universal agreement that such preparations stimulate antibody production, but the titres are often low. Investigations of cellular immunity have been much more sporadic and subject to technical difficulties (different species, routes of immunization, time intervals, age of animals, methods of sample collection, methods of *in vitro* analysis) which make interpretation a problem. In humans, there are reports of long lasting complement fixing antibody and cell-mediated immune responses to whole killed virus, of stimulated lymphocyte transformation and enhanced cell-mediated immunity (CMI) in response to subunit vaccination. ADCC and long lasting CMI responses have been observed following the use of glycoprotein vaccines. Even the synthetic peptides have been shown to stimulate neutralizing antibody and enhance the IL-2 driven proliferation of antigen specific T-cells.

In conclusion, it would appear on both theoretical grounds and on the weight of evidence available that vaccination against primary genital herpes infection should be possible and successful. Whether such preparations would be socially or ethically acceptable for such a non life-threatening disease is questionable. Vaccination to influence the interval between recurrences in those already infected or to ameliorate recrudescent lesions seems, on theoretical grounds, to be less likely to succeed, though there are sufficient claims of improvement to warrant properly conducted double-blind trials of suitable preparations. Until these have been conducted the mood of scepticism is bound to continue.

CONCLUSIONS

The complexity of the immune response to genital infections by herpes simplex virus and the sketchy nature of our present knowledge, especially in man, will be clear from the above discussion, and many questions remain without adequate answers. In particular, it is impossible to say why so many individuals undergo exposure to HSV and yet do not develop clinical disease or have subsequent recurrences. It is probable that following genital exposure to the virus, early defence will be provided by the non-specific actions of NK cells and macrophages, stimulated by local production of interferon. If these processes fail to contain virus replication then secretory or systemic immunoglobulin production possibly coupled with cytotoxic T-lymphocyte-, antibody-, or complement-dependent cytotoxicity may come into play to limit widespread dissemination and CNS involvement. These same processes undoubtedly limit the severity of most recrudescent episodes, though their role in the establishment and maintenance of ganglionic latency remains more speculative. With all of these uncertainties, the prospects for developing a successful vaccine, especially against recrudescent disease, must remain questionable.

References

1. Nahmias, A. J., Dannenbarger, J., Wickliffe, C. and Muther, J. (1981). Clinical aspects of

infection with herpes simplex virus 1 and 2. In Nahmias, A. J., Dowdle, W. R. and Schinazi, R. F. (eds.). *The Human Herpesviruses. An Interdisciplininary Perspective*, pp. 3-9. (NY: Elsevier Press)

2. Rawls, W. E. and Campione-Piccardo, J. (1981). Epidemiology of herpes simplex type 1 and 2 infections. In Nahmias, A. J., Dowdle, W. R. and Schinazi, R. F. (eds.). *The Human Herpesviruses. An Interdisciplinary Perspective*, pp. 137-152. (NY: Elsevier Press)

3. Baringer, J. R. (1981). Latency of herpes simplex and varicella zoster viruses in the nervous system. In Nahmias, A. J., Dowdle, W. R. and Schinazi, R. F. (eds.). *The Human Herpesviruses. An Interdisciplinary Perspective*, pp. 202-205. (NY: Elsevier Press)

4. Wildy, P., Field, H. J. and Nash, A. A. (1982). Classical herpes latency revisited. In Mahy, B., Minson, A. C. and Darby, G. K. (eds.). *Symposium 33, Society for General Microbiology*, pp. 133-168. (NY: Cambridge University Press)

5. Mims, C. A. (1964). Aspects of the pathogenesis of viral disease. *Bacteriol. Rev.*, **28**, 30-71

6. Morahan, P. S., Kern, E. R. and Glasgow, L. A. (1977). Immunomodulator-induced resistance against herpes simplex virus. *Proc. Soc. Exp. Biol. Med.*, **154**, 615-20

7. Morahan, P. S., Morse, S. S. and McGeorge, M. E. (1980). Macrophage extrinsic antiviral activity during herpes simplex virus infection. *J. Gen. Virol.*, **46**, 291-300

8. Morahan, P. S. (1984). Interactions of herpesviruses with mononuclear phagocytes. In Rouse, B. T. and Lopez, C. (eds.). *Immunobiology of Herpes Simplex Virus Infection*, pp. 71-89. (Florida: CRC Press)

9. Morahan, P. S., Connor, J. R. and Leary, K. R. (1985). Viruses and the versatile macrophage. *Br. Med. Bull.*, **41**, 15-21

10. Bianco, C. and Edelson, P. J. (1978). Plasma membrane expression of macrophage differentiation. In Lerner, R. A. (ed.). *Molecular Basis of Cell-Cell Interaction (Birth Defects) vol. 14 (2)*, pp. 119-124. (New York: Alan R. Liss)

11. Rager-Zisman, B., Kunkel, M., Tanaka, Y. and Bloom, B. R. (1982). Role of macrophage oxidative metabolism in resistance to vesicular stomatitis virus. *Infect. Immun.*, **36**, 1229-37

12. Stohlman, S. A., Woodward, J. G. and Frelinger, J. A. (1982). Macrophage antiviral activity: extrinsic versus intrinsic activity. *Infect. Immun.*, **36**, 672-7

13. Hayashi, K., Kurata, T., Morishima, T. and Nassery, T. (1980). Analysis of the inhibitory effect of peritoneal macrophages on the spread of herpes simplex virus. *Infect. Immun.*, **28**, 350-8

14. Wildy, P., Gell, P. G. H., Rhodes, J. and Newton, A. (1982). Inhibition of herpes simplex virus multiplication by activated macrophages: a role for arginase? *Infect. Immun.*, **37**, 40-5

15. Johnson, R. T. (1965). The pathogenesis of herpes virus encephalitis II. A cellular basis for the development of resistance with age. *J. Exp. Med.*, **120**, 359-74

16. Lopez, C. (1984). Natural resistance mechanisms against herpes virus in health and disease. In Rouse, B. T. and Lopez, C. (eds.). *Immunobiology of Herpes Simplex Virus Infections*, pp. 45-70. (Florida: CRC Press)

17. Lopez, C. and Dudas, G. (1979). Replication of herpes simplex virus type 1 in macrophages from resistant and susceptible mice. *Infect. Immun.*, **23**, 432-7

18. Armerding, D., Mayer, P., Scriba, M., Hren, A. and Rossiter, H. (1981). *In-vivo* modulation of macrophage functions by herpes simplex virus type 2 in resistant and sensitive inbred mouse strains. *Immunobiology*, **160**, 217-27

19. Mintz, L., Drew, W. L., Hoo, R. and Finley, T. N. (1980). Age-dependent resistance of human alveolar macrophages to herpes simplex virus. *Infect. Immun.*, **28**, 417-20

20. Morse, S. S. and Morahan, P. S. (1981). Activated macrophages mediate interferon-independent inhibition of herpes simplex virus. *Cell. Immunol.*, **58**, 72-84

21. Stevens, J. G. and Cook, M. L. (1971). Restriction of herpes simplex virus by macrophages. An analysis of the cell-virus interaction. *J. Exp. Med.*, **133**, 19-38

22. Rinaldo, C. R., Jr., Richter, B. S., Black, P. H. and Hirsch, M. S. (1979). Persistent infection of human lymphoid and myeloid cell lines with herpes simplex virus. *Infect. Immun.*, **25**, 521-5

23. Frank, U., Schindling, B., Lindermann, J. and Falke, D. (1978). Multiplication of herpes simplex virus types 1 and 2 in macrophages of NMRI and C57/BL mice. *Acta Virol.*, **22**, 193-202

24. Daniels, C. A., Kleinerman, E. S. and Snyderman, R. (1978). Abortive and productive infections of human mononuclear phagocytes by type 1 herpes simplex virus. *Am. J. Pathol.*,

91, 119–29
25. Johnson, R. B., Jr. (1978). Oxygen metabolism and the microbicidal activity of macrophages. *Fed. Proc.*, **37**, 2759–64
26. Sethi, K. K. (1983). Contribution of macrophage arginase in the intrinsic restriction of herpes simplex virus replication in permissive macrophage cultures induced by gamma-interferon containing products of activated spleen cells. *Immunobiology*, **165**, 459–74
27. Stohlman, S. A., Woodward, J. G. and Frelinger, J. A. (1982). Macrophage antiviral activity: extrinsic versus intrinsic activity. *Infect. Immun.*, **36**, 672–7
28. Linnavuori, K. and Hovi, T. (1983). Restricted replication of herpes simplex virus in human monocyte cultures: role of interferon. *Virology*, **130**, 1–9
29. Isaacs, A. and Lindenmann, J., (1956). Virus interference. I. The interferons. *Proc. R. Soc. Lond.* (Ser. B.), **147**, 258–67
30. Zawatzky, R., Gresser, I., DeMaeyer, E. and Kirchner, H. (1982). The role of interferon in the resistance of C57BL/6 mice to various doses of herpes simplex virus type 1. *J. Infect. Dis.*, **146**, 405–10
31. Gresser, I., Tovey, M. G., Maury, C. and Bandu, M.-T. (1976). Role of interferon in the pathogenesis of virus diseases in mice as demonstrated by the use of anti-interferon serum. II. Studies with herpes simplex virus, Maloney sarcoma, vesicular stomatitis, Newcastle disease and influenza viruses. *J. Exp. Med.*, **144**, 1316–23
32. Hirt, H. M., Becker, H. and Kirchner, H. (1978). Induction of interferon production in mouse spleen cell cultures by *Corynebacterium parvum*. *Cell. Immunol.*, **38**, 168–75
33. Barinskii, I. F., Popova, O. M., Konstantinova, I. V., Grebeniuk, V. N. and Kuznetsov, V. P. (1985). Indices of alpha-interferon and of lymphocyte natural killer activity in genital herpes and the effect on them of specific vaccination therapy and interferon therapy. *Vopr. Virusol.*, **30**, 340–3
34. Panet, A., Gloger, I. and Falk, H. (1985). Mechanisms of herpes simplex virus inhibition by interferon. In Kirchner, H. and Schellekens, H. (eds.). *The Biology of the Interferon System 1984*, pp. 325–331. (Elsevier Science Publishers)
35. Haller, O. and Wigzell, H. (1977). Suppression of natural killer cell activity with radioactive strontium: effector cells are marrow dependent. *J. Immunol.*, **118**, 1503–6
36. Lopez, C. (1978). Immunological nature of genetic resistance of mice to herpes simplex virus-type 1 infection. In de The, G., Henle, W. and Rapp, F. (eds.). *Oncogenesis and Herpes Viruses*, Vol. 3, pp. 775–781. (Lyon: WHO)
37. Schneweis, K. E., Olbrick, M., Saffig, V. and Scholz, R. (1982). Effects of genetic resistance against herpes simplex virus in vaginally infected mice. *Med. Microbiol. Immunol.*, **171**, 161–9
38. Armerding, D., Simon, M. M., Hämmerling, G. J. and Rossiter, H. (1981). Function, target cell preference and cell surface characteristics of herpes simplex virus type 2 induced non-antigen specific killer cells. *Immunobiology*, **158**, 347–68
39. El-Daher, N. and Betts, R. F. (1985). New observations regarding killing of fibroblasts infected with herpes simplex virus: co-operation between elutable factor and peripheral mononuclear cells. *J. Inf. Dis.*, **152**, 1197–205
40. Rouse, B. T. and Lopez, C. (1984). Strategies for immune intervention against herpes simplex virus. In Rouse, B. T. and Lopez, C. (eds.). *Immunobiology of Herpes Simplex Virus Infections*, pp. 145–155. (Florida: CRC Press)
41. Gidlund, M. Örn, A., Wigzell, H., Senik, A. and Gresser, I. (1978). Enhanced NK cell activity in mice injected with interferon and interferon inducers. *Nature* (Lond.), **273**, 759–61
42. Djeu, J. Y., Heinbaugh, J. A., Holden, H. T. and Herberman, R. B. (1979). Augmentation of mouse natural killer cell activity by interferon inducers. *J. Immunol.*, **122**, 175–81
43. Ullberg, M. and Jondal, M. (1981). Recycling and target-binding capacity of human natural killer cells. *J. Exp. Med.*, **153**, 615–28
44. Kohl, S., Loo, L. S., Schmalstieg, F. S. and Anderson, D. C. (1986). The genetic deficiency of leukocyte surface glycoprotein Mac-1, LFA-1, p150, 95 in humans is associated with defective antibody dependent cellular cytotoxicity *in vitro* and defective protection against herpes-simplex virus infection *in vivo*. *J. Immunol.*, **137**, 1688–94
45. Borysiewicz, L. K., Graham, S. and Sissons, J. G. (1986). Human natural killer cell lysis of virus-infected cells. Relationship to expression of the transferrin receptor. *Eur. J. Immunol.*, **16**, 405–11

46. Hall, M. J. and Katrak, K. (1986). The quest for a herpes simplex virus vaccine: background and recent developments. *Vaccine*, **4**, 138–50
47. Shore, S. L. and Feorino, P. M. (1981). Immunology of primary herpes virus infections in humans. In Nahmias, A. J., Dowdle, W. R. and Schinazi, R. F. (eds.). *The Human Herpesviruses. An Interdisciplinary Perspective*, pp. 267–288. (NY: Elsevier Pres)
48. Norrild, B., Emmertsen, H., Krebs, H. J. and Pedersen, B. (1984). Antibody-dependent immune mechanisms and herpes simplex virus infections. In Rouse, B. T., and Lopez, C. (eds.). *Immunobiology of Herpes Simplex Virus Infection*, pp. 91–105. (Florida: CRC Press)
49. Sundquist, V. A., Linde, A. and Wahren, B. (1984). Virus-specific immunoglobin G subclasses in herpes simplex and varicella-zoster virus infections. *J. Clin. Microbiol.*, **20**, 94–8
50. Bernstein, D. I., Lovett, M. A. and Bryson, Y. J. (1984). Serological analysis of first-episode non-primary genital herpes simplex virus infection. Presence of type 2 antibody in acute serum samples. *Am. J. Med.*, **77**, 1055–60
51. Devillechabrolle, A., Hugnes-Dorin, F., Fortier, B., Catalan, F. and Huraux, J. M. (1985). Prevalence of serum antibodies to herpes simplex virus types 1 and 2: application of an ELISA technique to 100 cases of anogenital herpes. *Sex. Transm. Dis.*, **12**, 40–3
52. Courtney, R. J. (1984). Virus-specific components of herpes simplex virus involved in the immune response. In Rouse, B. T. and Lopez, C. (eds.). *Immunobiology of Herpes Simplex Virus Infection*, pp. 33–44. (Florida: CRC Press)
53. Balachandran, N., Bacchetti, S. and Rawls, W. E. (1982). Protection against lethal challenge of BALB/c mice by passive transfer of monoclonal antibodies to five glycoproteins of herpes simplex virus type 2. *Infect. Immun.*, **37**, 1132–7
54. Roberts, P. L., Duncan, B. E., Raybould, T. J. G. and Watson, D. H. (1985). Purification of Herpes virus glycoproteins B and C using monoclonal antibodies and their ability to protect mice against lethal challenge – hybridoma generation, monoclonal antibody production and vaccine purification. *J. Gen. Virol.*, **66**, 1073–85
55. Lee, F. K., Coleman, R. M., Pereira, L., Bailey, P. D., Tatsuno, M. and Nahmias, A. J. (1985). Detection of herpes simplex virus type 2-specific antibody with glycoprotein G. *J. Clin. Microbiol.*, **22**, 641–4
56. Eberle, R., Mou, S. W. and Zaia, J. A. (1984). Polypeptide specificity of the early antibody response following primary and recurrent genital herpes simplex virus type 2 infections. *J. Gen. Virol.*, **65**, 1839–43
57. Eberle, R., Mou, S. W. and Zaia, J. A. (1985). The immune response to herpes simplex virus: comparison of the specificity and relative titres of serum antibodies directed against viral polypeptides following primary herpes simplex type 1 infections. *J. Med. Virol.*, **16**, 147–62
58. Ashley, R., Benedetti, J. and Corey, L. (1985). Humoral immune response to HSV-1 and HSV-2 viral proteins in patients with primary genital herpes. *J. Med. Virol.*, **17**, 153–66
59. Lum, L. G., Orcutt-Thordarson, N. and Seigneuret, M. C. (1985). Regulatory roles of human OKT4/OKT8 subsets in polyclonal immunoglobulin production induced by herpes simplex type 1 virus. *Immunobiology*, **169**, 319–29
60. McDermott, M. R., Smiley, J. R., Leslie, P., Brais, J., Rudzroga, H. E. and Bienenstock, J. (1984). Immunity in the female genital tract after intravaginal vaccination of mice with an attenuated strain of herpes simplex type 2. *J. Virol.*, **51**, 747–53
61. Merriman, H., Woods, S., Winter, C., Fahnlander, A. and Corey, L. (1984). Secretory IgA antibody in cervicovaginal secretions from women with genital infection due to herpes simplex virus. *J. Inf. Dis.*, **149**, 505–10
62. Lagace-Simard, J., Portnoy, J. D. and Wainberg, M. A. (1986). High levels of IgE in patients suffering from frequent recurrent herpes simplex lesions. *J. Allergy Clin. Immunol.*, **77**, 582–5
63. Pass, R. F., Whitley, R. J., Whelchel, J. D., Diethelm, A. G., Reynolds, D. W. and Alford, C. (1980). Identification of patients with increased risk of infection with herpes simplex virus after renal transplantation. *J. Inf. Dis.*, **140**, 487–92
64. Kohl, S. (1984). The immune response of the neonate to herpes simplex virus infection. In Rouse, B. T. and Lopez, C. (eds.). *Immunobiology of Herpes Simplex Virus Infections*, pp. 121–130. (Florida: CRC Press)
65. Kohl, and Loo, L. S. (1982). Protection of neonatal mice against herpes simplex virus infection. Probable *in vivo* antibody-dependent cellular cytotoxicity. *J. Immunol.*, **129**,

370–6
66. Gonik, B., Loo, L. S., Bigelow, R. and Kohl, S. (1985). Influence of menstrual cycle variations on natural killer cytotoxicity and antibody dependent cellular cytotoxicity to cells infected with herpes simplex virus. *J. Reprod. Med.*, **30**, 493–6
67. Gonik, B., Loo, L. S., Bigelow, R. and Kohl, S. (1984). Influence of naproxen therapy on natural killer cytotoxicity and antibody-dependent cellular cytotoxicity against cells infected with herpes simplex virus. *J. Reprod. Med.*, **29**, 722–6
68. Oldstone, M. B. A. (1981). Lysis of human cells infected with a variety of RNA and DNA viruses is dependent on the alternative complement pathway and specific divalent antibody. In, Nahmias, A. J., Dowdle, W. R. and Schinazi, R. F. (eds.). *The Human Herpes Viruses. An Interdisciplinary Perspective*, pp. 326–29. (NY: Elsevier Press)
69. Smiley, M. L., Hoxie, J. A. and Friedman, H. M. (1985). Herpes simplex virus type 1 infection of endothelial, epithelial and fibroblast cells induces a receptor for C3b. *J. Immunol.*, **134**, 2673–8
70. Rouse, B. T. (1984). Cell-mediated immune mechanisms. In Rouse, B. T. and Lopez, C. (eds.). *Immunobiology of Herpes Simplex Virus Infections*, pp. 107–120. (Florida: CRC Press)
71. Schmid, D. S., Larson, H. and Rouse, B. T. (1981). The role of accessory cells and T-cell growth factor in induction of cytotoxic T-lymphocytes against herpes simplex virus antigens. *Immunology*, **44**, 755–63
72. Ferrar, W. L., Johnson, H. M. and Ferrar, J. J. (1981). Regulation of the production of immune interferon and cytotoxic T lymphocytes by interleukin 2. *J. Immunol.*, **126**, 1120–5
73. Schmid, D. S., Larsen, H. S. and Rouse, B. T. (1982). Role of Ia antigen expression and secretory function of accessory cells in induction of cytotoxic T lymphocyte responses against herpes simplex virus. *Infect. Immun.*, **37**, 1138–47
74. Yasukawa, M. and Zarling, J. M. (1985). Human cytotoxic T-cell clones directed against herpes simplex virus infected cells. III Analysis of viral glycoproteins recognised by CTL clones by using recombinant herpes simplex virus. *J. Immunol.*, **134**, 2679–82
75. Zarling, J. M., Moran, P. A., Burke, R. L., Pachl, C., Berman, P. W. and Lasky, L. A. (1986). Human cytotoxic T-cell clones directed against herpes simplex virus-infected cells. IV. Recognition and activation by cloned glycoproteins gB and gD. *J. Immunol.*, **136**, 4669–73
76. Yasukawa, M. and Zarling, J. M. (1984). Human cytotoxic T cell clones directed against herpes simplex virus-infected cells. I. Lysis restricted by HLA class II MB and DR antigens. *J. Immunol.*, **133**, 422–7
77. Wainberg, M. A., Portnoy, J. D., Clecner, B., Hubschman, S., Lagace-Simard, J., Rabinovitch, N., Remer, Z. and Mendelson, J. (1985). Viral inhibition of lymphocyte proliferation responsiveness in patients suffering from recurrent lesions caused by herpes simplex virus. *J. Inf. Dis.*, **152**, 441–8
78. Andervont, H. B. (1929). Activity of herpetic virus in mice. *J. Infect. Dis.*, **44**, 383–93
79. Nahmias, A. J. and Visintine, A. M. (1976). Herpes simplex. In Remington, J. S. and Klein, J. O. (eds.). *Infectious Diseases of the Foetus and Newborn Infant*, p. 156. (Philadelphia: W. B. Saunders)
80. Yeager, A. S., Arvin, A. M., Urbani, L. J. and Kemp, L. A. (1980). Relationship of antibody to outcome in neonatal herpes simplex virus infection. *Infect. Immun.*, **29**, 532–8
81. Whitley, R. J., Nahmias, A. J., Visintine, A. M., Fleming, C. L. and Alford, C. A. (1980). The natural history of herpes simplex virus infections of mother and newborn. *Pediatrics*, **66**, 489–94
82. Sullender, W. M., Miller, J. L., Yasukawa, L. L., Bradley, J. S., Black, S. B., Yeager, A. S., and Arvin, A. M. (1987). Humoral and cell mediated immunity in neonates with herpes simplex virus infection. *J. Inf. Dis.*, **155**, 28–37
83. Hayward, A., Herberger, M. and Corey, L. (1986). IgG subclass of anti-HSV antibodies following neonatal HSV infections. *Eur. J. Pediatr.*, **145**, 250–1
84. Baron, S., Georgiades, J. and Worthington, M. (1981). Potential for post exposure prophylaxis of neonatal herpes using passive antibody. In Nahmias, A. J., Dowdle, W. R. and Schinazi, R. F. (eds.). *The Human Herpesviruses. An Interdisciplinary Perspective*, pp. 491–495. (NY: Elsevier Press)
85. Pass, R. F., Dworsky, M. E., Whitley, R. J., August, A. M., Stagno, S. and Alford, C. A.,

Jr. (1981). Specific lymphocyte blastogenic responses in children with cytomegalovirus and herpes simplex virus infections acquired early in infancy. *Infect. Immun.*, **34**, 166–70

86. Leibson, P. J., Hunter-Laszlo, M., Douvas, G. S. and Hayward, A. R. (1986). Impaired neonatal natural killer-cell activity to herpes simplex virus: decreased inhibition of viral replication and altered response to lymphokines. *J. Clin. Immunol.*, **6**, 216–24

87. Frazier, J. P., Kohl, S., Pickering, L. K. and Loo, L. S. (1982). The effect of route of delivery on neonatal natural killer cytotoxicity and antibody-dependent cellular cytotoxicity to herpes simplex virus-infected cells. *Pediatr. Res.*, **16**, 558–60

88. Miller, M. E. (1978). *Host Defences in the Human Neonate.* (NY: Grune and Stratton)

89. Blyth, W. A. and Hill, T. J. (1984). Establishment, maintenance and control of herpes simplex virus latency. In Rouse, B. T., and Lopez, C. (eds.). *Immunobiology of Herpes Simplex Virus Infection*, pp. 10–32. (Florida: CRC Press)

90. Klein, R. J. (1985). Initiation and maintenance of latent herpes virus infections: the paradox of perpetual immobility and continuous movement. *Rev. Inf. Dis.*, **7**, 21–30

91. Openshaw, H., Tsuyoshi, S., Wohlenberg, C. and Notkins, A. L. (1981). The role of immunity in latency and reactivation of herpes simplex virus. In Nahmias, A. J., Dowdle, W. R. and Schinazi, R. F. (eds.). *The Human Herpesviruses. An Interdisciplinary Perspective*, pp. 289–296. (NY: Elsevier Press)

92. Yasumoto, S., Okabe, N. and Mori, R. (1986). Role of epidermal Langerhans cells in resistance to herpes simplex virus infection. *Arch. Virol.*, **90**, 261–71

93. Wrzos, H. and Rapp, H. (1985). Experimental model for activation of genital herpes simplex virus. *J. Inf. Dis.*, **151**, 349–54

94. Scriba, M. (1976). Recurrent genital herpes simplex virus (HSV) infection in guinea pigs. *Med. Microbiol. Immunol.*, **162**, 201–8

95. Baker, D. A. and Thomas, J. (1985). The effect of prostaglandin E$_2$ on the initial immune response to herpes simplex virus infection. *Am. J. Obstet. Gynecol.*, **151**, 586–90

96. Merigan, T. C. (1981). Immunosuppression and herpes viruses. In Nahmias, A. J., Dowdle, W. R. and Schinazi, R. F. (eds.). *The Human Herpesviruses. An Interdisciplinary Perspective*, pp. 309–316. (NY: Elsevier Press)

97. Sheridan, J. F., Beck, M., Aurelian, L. and Radowsky, M. (1985). Immunity to herpes simplex virus: virus reactivation modulates lymphokine activity. *J. Inf. Dis.*, **152**, 449–56

98. Rola-Pleszczynski, M. and Lieu, H. (1984). Natural cytotoxic cell activity linked to time of recurrence of herpes labialis. *Clin. Exp. Immunol.*, **55**, 224–8

9
Immunobiology of Genital Warts and Molluscum Contagiosum

M. A. STANLEY AND J. D. ORIEL

GENITAL WARTS

Introduction

Warts are cutaneous or mucosal proliferations induced after infection by papillomavirus – a small DNA virus. Papillomaviruses have been the subject of interest, but of relatively limited experimental investigation until recently, primarily due to the inability to infect cells in culture and to obtain vegetative viral growth. The application of molecular virological techniques (cloning and sequencing) has resulted in the demonstration of a remarkable plurality in the papillomaviruses particularly in human infections. It is now evident that multiple types of HPV exist[1,2] and that infection of different squamous epithelial surfaces, e.g. skin, cervix, penis and buccal mucosa, is associated with specific HPV types[3]. Interest in these viruses has been intensified by the evidence that HPV infection is associated with genital, oral and laryngeal cancers[4].

There are at present 51 types of HPV. These viruses are not differentiated serologically but instead the genus is divided into types depending upon the homology or cross-hybridization of their DNA. Therefore, an isolate is considered to be of an independent type if there is less than 50% homology with known papillomaviruses. There are 14 HPV types associated with lesions in the genital tract. HPV types 6 and 11 are most frequently associated with lesions of limited malignant potential – cervical, vulvar, perianal and penile condylomata and with cervical intra-epithelial neoplasia (CIN) grades I and II[5,6]. HPV types 16 and 18 have been consistently associated with invasive carcinoma of the cervix[3,7,8], and most recently with penile carcinoma[9]. HPV16 is found in cervical, vulvar and vaginal intra-epithelial lesions and furthermore the frequency with which 16 is isolated increases with the severity of the lesion[3]. HPV31 is found most frequently in North America and is associated with CIN[10], types 33, 34 and 35 have been isolated from small numbers of premalignant genital lesions and cervical carcinomas[3]. Additional new types have recently been characterized but these types are predominantly found in low grade lesions or normal epithelia (Lorincz, personal communication).

Papillomavirus genome organization

Any understanding of the immune responses to papillomaviruses depends upon a knowledge of the genomic organization of the virus and the mechanisms of virus replication and assembly.

The genome of the papillomaviruses consists of a supercoiled circular DNA molecule of 5×10^3 kD. Several papillomavirus genomes, including 6 and 11, have been sequenced completely[11]. The organization of the genomes is well conserved between the types and shows the same overall organization, Figure 9.1. There are open reading frames which can potentially code for 10 proteins, although the actual number of virally coded proteins is not known at present. The available evidence which relies heavily on data from the bovine papillomavirus, BPV[12] and the human cutaneous wart virus HPV1[13], suggests that only one strand of the papillomavirus genome is transcribed, the other strand is assumed to be non-coding. The genomes are functionally divided into two domains, early (E) and late (L), with respect to the biological properties of BPV1, the prototype papillomavirus. Thus the E region of BPV1 is a fragment comprising 69% of the genome required for *in vitro* transformation of mouse fibroblasts[14]. The corresponding region of other papillomaviruses is presumed to contain the information for virus replication and transformation[11]. Recently, the E4 open reading frame of HPV1 has been cloned and expressed in a bacterial expression system[15]. Using antibodies raised against the purified protein product of E4 it could be shown that this protein represents up to 30% of the total protein (both cellular and viral) in a plantar wart and is distributed in a diffuse granular pattern in the cytoplasm of keratinocytes in the stratum granulosum. The abundance and cellular distribution of this protein has led to the suggestion that the E4 gene product is not an early viral protein of the classical papovavirus type required for virus replication but may be involved in virus maturation and assembly. By analogy with BPV1 and from the analysis of HPV expression in tumour cell lines[16,17] the E7 and E6 regions in HPV16 and 18 code for proteins which have transforming properties. Recently[18], it has been shown that a DNA fragment

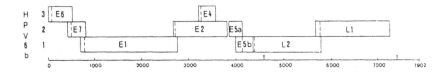

Figure 9.1 The possible open reading frames of HPV6b. The DNA has three possible reading frames which are shown on the left-hand side, the boxes represent the possible open reading frames in each of these three frames.

of HPV16 containing the early region cooperates with the vHa-ras (EJras) oncogene in transforming primary cells. The late (L) region in BPV1 contains two large open reading frames L1 and L2 which code for virion structural proteins. It is this region which has been assumed to be the most likely target for vaccines in BPV[19] and speculatively for human PVs.

Virus replication and life cycle

Papillomaviruses are strictly epitheliotropic, and virus replication and assembly appears to be absolutely dependant upon the environment provided in the normal differentiated epithelium. This interrelationship was first documented for papillomas induced by the Shope cotton-tail rabbit papilloma virus (CRPV)[20]. The basal or germinal layers of the papilloma contain a large proportion of cells in DNA synthesis, but these cells contain no virion capsid antigen or virus. Virus DNA can be detected, using *in situ* hybridization techniques, in the upper layers of the stratum spinosum and in the stratum granulosum, but viral capsid antigen and infectious virus can be detected only in the extreme superficial differentiated layers of the papilloma. This pattern of replication and the dependence upon epithelial differentiation for late gene expression is also shown in oral[21] and genital papillomas[22]. Antisera have been generated against detergent disrupted bovine papilloma-virus particles or disrupted plantar warts, and these exhibit immunospecificity against type common papillomavirus structural antigens[23]. Immunohisto-chemical studies using such antisera reveal that in genital condylomata late viral proteins are found in the nucleus. This nuclear localization is predominantly in koilocytes[24]. *In situ* hybridization of genital condylomata using both double stranded HPV DNA probes[25,26] and single stranded RNA probes[27] for specific genital HPVs shows a localization of signal to intermediate and superficial cells and to koilocytes with the strength of the signal increasing substantially with distance from the basal layer. *In situ* hybridization using double stranded DNA probes is of limited sensitivity, and the observation[22] that labelling was never seen in the basal layer or the parabasal cells suggests that these cells contain, at the most, only a very low number of viral genomes. Recent studies[28] using anti-peptide antibodies to E6 have localized the expression of the E6 protein of HPV16 to the superficial layers of CIN lesions. This observation supports the speculation that high levels of viral expression are confined to the differentiated layers of the epithelium, however, the application of anti-peptide antibodies can be criticized on the basis of possible cross-reaction with cellular sequences.

Human papilloma viruses are, therefore, exclusively intra-epithelial pathogens, and their replication cycle may represent a mechanism whereby the virus evades host defences. Virus infects the basal keratinocytes in low copy number; there is an amplification event leading eventually to cells which harbour plasmids at 100–200 copies/nucleus. High levels of vegetative replication and the production of intact viral particles occur only in terminally differentiated cells physically far removed from the host's immune forces.

Immune responses to papillomaviurses

Very little is known of host defences to papillomaviruses in general and genital HPVs in particular as a recent review has indicated[29]. The reasons for this are quite simple, there is no *in vitro* system available which supports vegetative viral growth, and, therefore, information regarding the identity and recognition of viral antigens is sparse. Thus, in this paper we shall review what is known of host immune responses to the most appropriate animal model (the cotton-tail rabbit papilloma virus CRPV), to human warts (both cutaneous and genital), and outline the current approaches and prospective developments in the investigation of the immunobiology of genital warts.

There is no doubt that immune responses are important in the pathogenesis of papilloma virus-induced lesions. Infections with HPV are one of the most frequent viral complications in immunosuppressed individuals. Thus in patients with malignant lymphoproliferative diseases cutaneous warts are found at increased frequency and growing with enhanced luxuriance[30,31]. Generalized warts have also been described in individuals with inherited immune deficiences such as the Wiskott–Aldrich syndrome[32,33] and also in common variable hypogammaglobulinaemia[34]. Individuals immunosuppressed as a consequence of renal transplantation exhibit a high frequency of cutaneous warts[35,36] and these lesions are refractory to most therapeutic strategies[37]. Immunosuppressed patients receiving renal allografts are not only at risk for benign proliferative lesions but also exhibit a higher incidence of premalignant and malignant skin lesions[38,39]. Furthermore, they have a 10-fold increase in the relative risk of developing cervical neoplasia[40–42]. The rare, frequently inherited condition, epidermodysplasia verruciformis (EV), combines immunosuppression with widespread cutaneous warts in which malignant conversion may occur. EV has been reviewed recently[43].

Rabbit papilloma virus

The most suitable animal model for cutaneous warts and genital condylomata is the cotton-tail rabbit papilloma virus (CRPV). The following observations support this assumption. In terms of tumour induction in animals there are two groups of papillomaviruses, those capable of inducing fibroblastic tumours in hamsters and capable of transforming rodent cells *in vitro* and those which do not[3]. The first group includes the bovine papilloma virus, BPV, while the second group is represented by CRPV. The bovine viruses in the natural host induce both papillomas, fibromas and fibropapillomas, whereas CRPV is exclusively an intra-epithelial pathogen inducing only papillomas or carcinomas. Computer analysis of the sequence data of the conserved regions in different papillomavirus genomes indicates that these differences in host cell specificity do reflect differences in viral evolution[11]. On this basis, the genital and cutaneous viruses (including CRPV) are more closely related to each other than to the bovine viruses, and the human cutaneous viruses HPV1 and 8 are very closely related to CRPV.

The biology of CRPV has been recently reviewed[19]. This virus induces epidermal papillomas in both domestic and wild cotton-tail rabbits. However, in wild rabbits the papillomas usually regress spontanteously, whereas the majority of domestic rabbits develop invasive metastatic carcinomas. The available evidence suggests that spontaneous regression in wild rabbits is due to immune mechanisms. Thus when regression occurs all the papillomas on the individual regress[19]. Antibody does not appear to be implicated in papilloma regression, since passive transfer of immunity from regressor to secondary host cannot be achieved with regressor sera[44]. However, prior administration of a vaccine significantly increased the frequency of papilloma regression in domestic rabbits[45]. The vaccine was derived from allogeneic minced papilloma with *Bordetella pertussis* as an adjuvant. The efficacy of this vaccine seems unlikely to have been related to presentation of virion associated antigens since domestic rabbit papillomas rarely contain viral particles and rabbits immunized with virus are not resistant to papilloma cell challenge[46]. The contribution of other mechanisms in tumour regression is implied by the observation that the vaccine was ineffective in feral rabbits[47]. In these animals non-specific immune stimulation by inoculation of the indigenous microbial flora of mucosal surfaces enhanced regression. Overall the evidence from the animal model suggests that humoral immunity does not play a significant role in defence against virus-induced papilloma formation, and that cellular immunity possibly against tumour or cell-associated rather than viral antigens and non-specific defence mechanisms such as macrophages and interferon, are of major importance.

Immunological studies of patients with warts

Humoral immunity

Serum antibodies to both HPV and wart cellular antigens have been detected[48-50]. Antibodies against wart cellular antigens occur in individuals with no recalled history of the lesion. Thus, antibody in one study[51] was found in 37% of control subjects. The controls in this work were healthy subjects with no warts at the time of investigation. Fifty per cent of those controls with a detectable antibody had no recalled history of warts. More recently however, Baird[52] used a sensitive solid phase ELISA assay for IgG directed against the type common papillomavirus antigen obtained by disruption and extraction of BPV particles; this antigen cross-reacts with HPV. He tested sera from patients with genital condylomata, CIN and cervical carcinoma and control groups of adults and children. Significant antibody levels compared to controls were found in the sera of patients who had genital condylomata. Patients who had had skin or genital warts during the past 5 years were negative or exhibited low antibody levels. Patients with CIN had antibody, but since many had evidence of co-existing HPV infection this was not a surprising result. However, patients with cervical carcinoma had the highest antibody levels of all subjects, but no clinical evidence of condylomata. This latter observation is surprising since the type common antigen has been assumed to be a late viral protein and papillomavirus late gene expression is not observed in carcinomas. It is possible that infected cell antigens rather than the type common virion structural antigens were detected in these studies since the target antigen was derived from BPV infected cells, but further studies are needed to clarify these results. The common antigenic determinant is presumed to be the major capsid protein, the L1 gene product. In a recent study (Browne, Minson and Stanley, unpublished observations) it was shown that the L1 polypeptide of HPV16 is not recognized in a Western blot by commercial antiserum raised against detergent disrupted BPV2 particles. Other workers (Firzlaff, personal communication) however, have shown that the L1 polypeptide of HPV6 is recognized in a Western blot by this antiserum which is generally considered to recognize the type common antigen. Furthermore, in immunohistochemical studies (Firzlaff, personal communication) it has been shown that antisera raised against the L1 polypeptide of HPV16 stains the superficial cells and koilocytes of HPV16 positive CIN, whereas these lesions are negative when stained by the commercial antiserum. These observations explain, to some extent, the fact that in immunohistochemical studies positive staining with commercial antiserum is found in only a proportion of genital HPV infections.

At the present time many groups are using molecular cloning and sequencing techniques to identify and characterize genital papillomaviral proteins in order to study host responses to these viruses. Using these techniques the major polypeptides of HPV6 and 16 in particular, identified as open reading frames (Figure 9.1) from published DNA sequence analyses are expressed in bacterial expression systems. The resulting fusion proteins are purified and inoculated into animals for the production of polyclonal and monoclonal antibodies. Preliminary studies using these reagents do indicate that patients with genital warts mount an immune response to HPV polypeptides. Thus antibodies directed against the L2 protein of HPV6b have been identified by Western blotting in the serum of five patients with genital warts[53]. In another study antibodies directed against the L1 protein of HPV6b have been identified in the sera of a test group of adult patients attending a colposcopy clinic, but not in the sera of a group of children under 5 years of age. Whether this reactivity represents past infection with HPV6 or cross-reactivity with other HPV types is not known, but these initial studies give hope that serological diagnosis of specific HPV infections will be possible.

However, the relationship between antibody level and papilloma presence and regression is not clear. It has been reported that regressing cutaneous warts always contain virus and are associated with the presence of wart specific antibody[50]. A correlation has been found between regression and the appearance of complement-fixing antibody[55]. However, re-infection can occur in the presence of circulating antibody[56], and some workers consider that humoral antibodies are not important in wart regression[51]. This opinion seems to be supported by the results of a recent study[57] in which the cell-mediated and humoral responses to HPV were tested in patients with CIN using a sensitive ELISA for antibody and purified HPV 1 and 2 virions as antigen. Positive antibody responses corresponded with a history of past or present cutaneous warts rather than CIN. Furthermore, a significant number of patients with warts or a previous history had no detectable antibody, and 50% of patients with no history of warts had antibody levels of comparable magnitude to those with existing warts.

Cellular immunity of papillomaviruses

Relatively little is known of the cell-mediated immune response (CMI) to HPV since there are no *in vitro* infected cells to act as targets in an immune response. In older studies CMI was assessed by *in vivo* skin testing, but *in vitro* techniques which rely on the recognition of specific antigen by primed lymphocytes are generally used at the present time. Basically there are three types of reaction:

(1) Measurement of immune cytolysis by the release of ^{51}Cr bound to the infected cell. This measures lymphocyte cytotoxicity.
(2) Measurement of lymphocyte proliferation by the incorporation of radiolabelled nucleotides after exposure of lymphocytes to viral antigens. This is a measure of T-cell memory.
(3) Measurement of lymphokine production by immune activated lymphocytes after exposure to target antigen in infected cells.

No lymphocyte cytotoxicity responses to HPV have been described. *In vitro* lymphocyte stimulation by semi-purified HPV virions has been examined using leukocyte cultures from patients with acute cutaneous wart infections compared to controls. In patients showing spontaneous remission some evidence of reactivity was found[58]. In another study[59] individuals bearing warts of less than one year's duration showed evidence of lymphoproliferation in response to wart antigen, whereas those with warts of longer duration did not. However, the responses in these studies were small and not convincing. In another study[51] a positive response in the leukocyte migration test could be measured in patients at the time of resolution of cutaneous warts. However, the immunity was transitory and the sensitivity and specificity of the test questionable.

The best evidence that cellular immunity is important in wart regression comes from studies on the involution of flat cutaneous warts. Flat warts (which are caused by HPV 3 infection) regress with a noticeable histological reaction dominated by an influx into the lesion of mononuclear cells[60], resembling that seen in delayed type hypersensitivity responses[61]. The regression of these lesions shows striking parallels to the regression of rabbit papillomas since, as shown by Aiba and his colleagues[62], the involution of one wart is accompanied by the simultaneous inflammation and involution of all other flat warts on that individual[62]. Tagami and his co-workers[63] have provided good evidence that regression in these lesions is mediated via a T-cell response. In an immunohistological study[63] using specific markers they showed that the mononuclear dermal infiltrate around the regressing lesion consisted primarily of T-helper-cells (CD4+) intermingled with large dendritic cells positive for the OKT6 marker and presumably antigen presenting cells. The epidermis in the regressing wart was infiltrated by equal numbers of helper/inducer T-cells (CD4+) and cytotoxic T-cells (CD8+). Class II MHC antigen expression (HLA-DR) was not confined to Langerhan's cells within the epidermis, but was also displayed by keratinocytes in the wart indicating the local release of lymphokines such as IFN-γ by activated T-cells. These studies certainly suggest that a T-cell-mediated response utilizing both cytotoxic T-cells and activated macrophages is the principal mechanism involved in flat wart regression. Tagami *et al.*[63] further suggest that the immune response is not directed against cells in which late viral protein is expressed, but instead is directed against an infected basal cell antigen. The evidence for this is that mononuclear attack is directed against basal cells and not superficial cells in which virus and viral capsid antigens would be expressed. Furthermore, viral structural antigen identified by immuno-staining with commercial antiserum could not be identified in regressing flat warts but was detected in 63% of ordinary flat warts[63].

The important question of course is why does the host permit proliferation of infected cells, why is the virus not recognized and cleared? There are no answers to this at the present time, but it is worth considering some aspects of host defence to intra-epithelial pathogens. The first immunologically relevant cell to encounter a virus such as a PV, (which is exclusively intra-epithelial) will be the Langerhans cell, the antigen presenting cell (APC) of skin and other stratified squamous epithelia. Langerhans cells (LC) are dendritic cells of bone marrow origin identifiable using a range of markers including HLA-DR, membrane bound ATPase and S 100 protein[64,65]. It might be supposed that viral antigen would be processed by these APC and displayed on the cell surface in association with Class II MHC in the classical manner. Antigen would then be presented to T-cells in the local lymph node, with the subsequent initiation of the cascade of reactions resulting in lymphocyte populations with specific antiviral properties. The time course of these events is not known since relatively little is known of the kinetics of LC, and of course the development of a wart implies that these events are disrupted in some way. The LC is a crucial cell in the defence against intra-epithelial pathogens, and it is interesting to note that HPV infection in the genital tract appears to result in a diminution of LC[66]. In a recent immunohistological study[67] using a range of markers to LC, it was shown that HPV infected cervical lesions and CIN showed a 60% decrease in the numbers of LC/unit sectional area of epithelium compared to normal cervical epithelium. Furthermore, LC identified by S100 staining were almost totally absent from 20% of HPV and 50% of CIN lesions. S100 positive LC may represent a histogenetically distinct subpopulation of cells, although this is speculative. In association with this depletion of LC there was a reduction in intra-epithelial lymphocytes with the T-helper subset in particular diminished[68]. Further-more, no activated lymphocytes (Tac antigen positive) were present within the epithelium compared to the underlying stroma. These observations suggest that a consequence of HPV infection is a local intra-epithelial immunologically privileged site in which foreign antigen is not recognized because of the absence or reduction in APC. Confirmation and extension of these studies will be awaited with interest.

Prospects

Although productive vegetative viral growth is not obtainable the application of molecular techniques is providing purified viral proteins which can then be used to examine host responses. Thus serological studies are already underway in some centres using the L1 and L2 proteins of genital HPVs generated as fusion proteins in bacterial expression systems. Efforts are being made to identify type common and type specific antigens in the structural proteins using monoclonal antibodies and synthetic peptides so that serological diagnosis of infection by specific HPV types will be possible in those patients in whom an antibody response is made. The assessment of T-cell responses require infected cells as tragets. Again molecular techniques can be applied. Thus viral genes can be introduced into cells using eukaryotic expression systems such as retroviral or vaccinia virus vectors. Viral proteins are synthesized by such a cell which then represents an infected cell target for the T-cell. The use of these and other approaches is dramatically altering the investigation of papilloma-virus host interactions, and the results of these studies are anticipated with intense interest.

MOLLUSCUM CONTAGIOSUM

Introduction

Molluscum contagiosum is a dermatosis characterized by the appearance of small, pink, papular lesions, many of which have an umbilicated appearance. The epidemiology is biphasic, with peaks occurring in children, when the lesions affect the face, trunk and extremities, and in young adults, in whom the genitals are predominantly affected. Genital molluscum contagiosum is believed to be a sexually transmitted disease, although it is difficult to find lesions in sex partners of index cases[68]. The disease is often seen in men and women attending clinics for sexually transmitted diseases, and in England the number of cases reported has doubled in the last decade[69,70].

Virology

Molluscum contagiosum virus is a member of the family *Poxviridae*. Negative staining shows a brick-shaped particle whose outer tubular structures are arranged spirally, giving a 'ball of yarn' appearance. The virus has not yet been propagated *in vitro*.

Pathology

The base of the molluscum papule is composed of lobules of acanthotic prickle cells. As these move towards its centre they become distorted owing to the cytoplasmic accumulation first of islets of DNA and later of clumps of mature viral particles. Eventually, the nucleus disappears completely and a large structure is formed, the 'molluscum contagiosum body', which is in effect a 'sack of virus particles'[71]. The core of the lesion is composed of these bodies and cell debris.

Blank[72] pointed out that there was a fundamental difference between the tumours induced by the viruses of molluscum contagiosum and of HPV. In the former, proliferation is followed by the necrosis of infected cells, and the papule represents the reparative efforts of the epithelium (acanthosis) in response to its gradual destruction. In warts, on the other hand, there is enduring cellular proliferation.

Immunology

Circulating antibodies against viral antigen extracted from human molluscum lesions can be detected by complement fixation, neutralization, immunofluorescence and gel agar diffusion techniques[73-77]. The specificity and comparability of these tests have not been well evaluated. However, Epstein et al.[78] detected antibodies in 58% of patients withf molluscum contagiosum and in 13.5% of controls by gel diffusion; using immunofluorescence, they found antibodies to be present in 87% of patients. The role, if any, of these antibodies in the cure of the disease is not known. Material from human molluscum lesions elicits an antibody response in guinea pigs and rabbits[74,76].

It has been suggested that the release of antigenic material into the dermis, either spontanteously or by trauma, may provoke a cell-mediated immune response[79,80]. Such a response might explain the eczematous reaction which can be seen in some patients with molluscum contagiosum, and the observation that many lesions are cured by simple pin-prick trauma[80,81].

ACKNOWLEDGEMENTS

We are grateful to Dr J. Firzlaff and Dr. D. Galloway, F. Hutchinson, Cancer Research Center, Seattle, USA for permission to describe unpublished work.

References

1. Gissmann, L., Pfister, H. and zur Hausen, H. (1977). Human papilloma viruses (HPV): characterisation of 4 different isolates. *Virology*, **76**, 569–80
2. Orth, G., Favre, M. and Croissant, O. (1977). Characterisation of a new type of human papillomavirus that causes skin warts. *J. Virol.*, **24**, 108–20
3. McCance, D. J. (1986). Human papillomaviruses and cancer. *Biochim. Biophys. Acta*, **823**, 195–205
4. zur Hausen, H. (1986). Papillomaviruses in human genital cancer: established results and prospects for the future. In Peto, R. and zur Hausen, H. (eds.). *Viral Etiology of Cervical Cancer, Banbury Report*, **21**, pp. 327–323. (Cold Spring Harbor Laboratory)
5. Gissmann, L., de Villiers, E-M. and zur Hausen, H. (1982). Analysis of human genital warts (condylomata acuminata) and other genital tumours for human papillomavirus type 6 DNA. *Int. J. Cancer*, **29**, 143–6
6. Gissmann, L., Wolnik, L., Ikenburg, H., Koldovsky, W., Schnurch, H. and zur Hausen, H. (1983). Human papillomavirus types 6 and 11 DNA sequences in genital and laryngeal papillomas and in some cervical cancers. *Proc. Natl. Acad. Sci. USA*, **80**, 560–3
7. Durst, M., Gissmann, L., Ikenberg, H. and zur Hausen, H. (1983). A new type of papillomavirus DNA from a cervical carcinoma and its prevalence in genital cancer biopsies from different geographic regions. *Proc. Natl. Acad. Sci. USA*, **80**, 3812–15
8. Boshart, M. L., Gissmann, H., Ikenberg, W., Scheurlen, A., Kleinheinz, A. and zur Hausen, H. (1984). A new type of papillomavirus DNA, its presence in genital cancer biopsies and in cell lines derived from cervical cancer. *EMBO J.*, **3**, 1151–7
9. McCance, D. J., Kalache, K., Ashdown, K., Andrade-Menezes, F., Smith, P. and Doll, R. (1986). Human papillomavirus types 16 and 18 in carcinomas of the penis from Brazil. *Int. J. Cancer*, **37**, 55–60
10. Lorincz, A. T., Lancaster, W. D., Kurman, R. J., Jenson, A. B. and Temple, G. F. (1986). Characterisation of human papillomaviruses in cervical neoplasms and their detection in

routine clinical screening. In Peto, R. and zur Hausen, H. (eds.). *Viral Etiology of Cervical Cancer, Banbury Report*, **21**, pp. 225–37. (Cold Spring Harbor Laboratory).

11. Giri, I. and Danos, O. (1986). Structure of Papillomavirus genomes from sequence data to biological properties. *Trends Genet.*, **2**, 221–4

12. Chen, E. Y., Howley, P. M., Levinson, A. D. and Seeburg, P. H. (1982). The primary structure and genetic organisation of the bovine papillomavirus type 1 genome. *Nature*, **229**, 529–34

13. Danos, O., Katinka, M. and Yaniv, M. (1982). Human papillomavirus 1a complete DNA sequence: a novel type of genome organisation among papovaviridiae, *EMBO J.*, **1**, 231–6

14. Lowy, D. R., Dvoretzky, I., Shober, R., Law, M. F., Engel, L. and Howley, P. M. (1980). *In vitro* tumorigenic transformation by a defined subgenomic fragment of bovine papillomavirus DNA. *Nature*, **287**, 72–5

15. Doorbar, J., Campbells, D., Grand, R. J. A. and Gallimore, P. H. (1986). Identification of the human papillomavirus-1a E4 gene products. *EMBO J.*, **5**, 355–62

16. Schwarz, E., Freese, U.K., Gissmann, L., Mayer, W., Roggenbuck, B., Stramlau, A. and zur Hausen, H. (1985). Structure and transcription of human papillomavirus sequences in cervical carcinoma cells. *Nature*, **314**, 111–14

17. Yee, C., Krishnan-Hewlett, I., Baker, C. C., Schlegel, R. and Howley, P. M. (1985). Presence and expression of human papillomavirus sequences in human cervical carcinoma lines. *Am. J. Pathol.*, **119**, 361–6

18. Matlashewski, G., Schneider, J., Banks, L., Jones, N., Murray, A. and Crawford, L. (1987). Human papillomavirus type 16 DNA co-operates with activated ras in transforming primary cells *EMBO J.*, **6**, 1741–6

19. Pilacinski, W. P., Glassmann, D. L., Glassmann, K. F., Reed, D. E., Lum, M. A., Marshall, R. F., Muscoplat, C. C. and Faras, A. J. (1986). Immunisation against BPV infection. *CIBA Foundation Symposium*, **120**, 136–48

20. Kreider, J. W. and Bartlett, G. L. (1981). The Shope Papilloma-carcinoma complex of rabbits: a model system of neoplastic progression and spontaneous regression. *Adv. Cancer Res.*, **35**, 81–110

21. Jenson, A. B., Lancaster, W. D., Hartmann, D. P. and Shaffer, E. L. (1982). Frequency and distribution of papillomavirus structural antigens in verrucae, multiple papillomas and condylomata of the oral cavity. *Am. J. Pathol.*, **107**, 212–18

22. Grussendorf-Conen, E. (1986). *In situ* hybridisation with papillomavirus DNA in genital lesions. In Peto, R. and zur Hausen, H. (eds.). *Viral Etiology of Cervical Cancer. Banbury Report* **21**, pp. 239–46. (Cold Spring Harbor Laboratory)

23. Jenson, A. B., Rosenthal, J. D., Olson, C., Pass, F., Lancaster, W. D. and Shah, K. (1980). Immunological relatedness of papillomaviruses from different species. *J. Natl. Cancer Inst.*, **64**, 495–500

24. Dyson, J. L., Walker, P. G. and Singer, A. (1984). Human papillomavirus infection of the uterine cervix: histological appearance in 28 cases identified by immunohistochemical techniques. *J. Clin. Pathol.*, **37**, 126–30

25. Gupta, J., Gendelman, H. E., Naghasnfar, Z., Gupta, P., Rosensheim, N., Sawada, E., Woodruff, J. D. and Shah, K. V. (1985). Specific identification of human papillomavirus type in cervical smears and paraffin sections by *in situ* hybridisation with radioactive probes: a preliminary communication. *Int. J. Gynecol. Pathol.*, **4**, 211

26. Beckman, A. M., Myerson, D., Daline, J. R., Kiviat, N. B., Fenoglio, C. M. and McDougall, J. K. (1985). Detection of human papillomavirus DNA in carcinomas by *in situ* hybridisation with biotinylated probes. *J. Med. Virol.*, **16**, 265–73

27. Stoler, M. H. and Broker, T. R. (1986). *In situ* hybridisation detection of human papillomavirus DNAs and messenger RNAs in genital condylomas and a cervical carcinoma. *Human Pathol.*, **17**, 1250–8

28. Palefsky, J., Winkler, B., Nizet, V., Kidd, J. L. and Schoolnik, G. K. (1986). Detection of HPV proteins, the synthetic peptide approach in Steinberg, B. M., Brandsma, J. and Taichman, L. (eds.). *Papillomaviruses Cancer Cells*, Vol. 5, pp. 101–103. (Cold Spring Harbor)

29. Kirchner, H. (1986). Immunobiology of human papillomavirus infection. *Progr. Med. Virol.*, **33**, 1–41

30. Morison, W. L. (1975). Viral warts, herpes simplex and herpes zoster in patients with

secondary immune deficiences and neoplasms. *Br. J. Dermatol.*, **92**, 625–30
31. Perry, T. L. and Hartmann, L. (1974). Warts in diseases with immune defects. *Cutis*, **13**, 359–62
32. Zinu, K-H., Belohradsky, H. (1977). Wiscott–Aldrich Syndrome mit Verrucae vulgares. *Hautarzt*, **28**, 664–97
33. Ormerod, A. D., Finlay, A. Y., Knight, A. G., Matthews, N., Stark, J. M. and Gough, J. (1983). Immune deficiency and multiple viral warts; possible variant of the Wiskott–Aldrich syndrome. *Br. J. Dermatol.*, **108**, 211–15
34. Reid, T. M. S., Fraser, N. G. and Kernohan, I. R. (1976). Generalised warts and immune deficiency. *Br. J. Dermatol.*, **95**, 559–64
35. Koranda, F. C., Dehmel, E. M., Kahn, G. and Penn, I. (1974). Cutaneous complications in immunosuppressed renal homograft recipients. *J. Am. Med. Assoc.*, **229**, 419–24
36. Spencer, E. S. and Andersen, H. K. (1970). Clinically evident non-terminal infections with herpes virus and the wart virus in immunosuppressed renal allograft recipients. *Br. Med. J.*, **1**, 251–4
37. Ingelfinger, J. R., Grupe, W. E., Topor, M. and Levey, R. H. (1977). Warts in pediatric renal transplant population. *Dermatologica*, **155**, 7–12
38. Marshall, V. (1974). Premalignant and malignant skin tumours in immunosuppressed patients. *Transplantation*, **17**, 272–5
39. Mullen, D. L., Silverberg, S. G., Penn, I. and Hammond, W. S. (1976). Squamous cell carcinoma of the skin and lip in renal homograft recipients. *Cancer*, **37**, 729–34
40. Hoover, R. and Fraumeri, J. F. (1973). Risk of cancer in renal transplant patients. *Lancet*, **2**, 55
41. Porreco, R., Penn, I., Droegemuller, W., Greer, B. and Makowski, M. (1975). Gynaecologic malignancies in immunosuppressed organ homograft recipients. *Obstet. Gynecol.*, **45**, 359–64
42. Shokri-Tabibzadeh, S., Koss, L. G., Molnar, J. and Romney, S. (1981). Association of human papillomavirus with neoplastic processes in the genital tract of 4 women with impaired immunity. *Gynaecol. Oncol.*, **12**, 129–40
43. Orth, G. and Favrre, M. (1985). *Clin. Dermatol.*, **3**, 27–42
44. Evans, C. A., Weiser, R. S. and Ito, Y. (1962). Antiviral and antitumor immunologic mechanisms operative in the Shope Papilloma–Carcinoma system. *Cold Spring Harbor, Symp. Quant. Biol.*, **27**, 453–62
45. Evans, C. A., Gorman, L. R., Ito, Y. and R. S., Weiser. (1962). Antitumor immunity in the Shope papilloma–carcinoma complex of rabbits. I. Papilloma regression induced by homologous and autologous tissue vaccines. *J. Natl. Cancer Inst.*, **29**, 277–86
46. Kreider, J. W. (1963). Studies on the mechanism responsible for the spontaneous regression of the Shope rabbit papilloma. *Cancer Res.*, **23**, 1593–9
47. Evans, C. A. and Thomsen, J. J. (1969). Antitumor immunity in the Shope-Papilloma–Carcinoma complex. IV. Search for a transmissible factor increasing the frequency of tumor regression. *J. Natl. Cancer Inst.*, **42**, 477–84
48. Almeida, J. D. and Goffe, A. P. (1965). Antibody to wart virus in human sera demonstrated by electron microscopy and precipitin tests. *Lancet*, **2**, 1205
49. Ogilvie, M. M. (1970). Serological studies with human (papova) wart virus. *J. Hyg.*, **68**, 479–90
50. Matthews, R. S. and Shirodaria, P. V. (1973). Study of regressing warts by immunofluorescence. *Lancet*, **1**, 689–91
51. Morison, W. L. (1975). *In vitro* assay of immunity to wart antigen. *Br. J. Dermatol.*, **93**, 545–52
52. Baird, P. J. (1983). Serological evidence for the association of papillomavirus and cervical neoplasia. *Lancet*, **2**, 17–18
53. Firzlaff, J. M., Hsia, C. N., Halbert, C. and Galloway, D. A. (1986). Polyclonal antibodies of Human papillomavirus 6b and 16: bacterially derived fusion proteins. In Steinberg, B. M., Brandsma, J. and Taichman, L. (eds.). *Papillomaviruses, Cancer Cells*, Vol. 5, pp. 105–11 (Cold Spring Harbor)
54. Li, C. C. H., Shah, K., Seth, A. and Gilden, R. V. (1987). Identification of the human papillomavirus type 6b L1 open reading frame protein in condylomas and corresponding antibodies in human sera. *J. Virol.*, **61**, 2684–90

55. Pyrhonen, S. and Johansson, E. (1975). Regression of warts. An immunological study. *Lancet*, **1**, 592-5
56. Cubie, H. A. (1972). Serological studies in a student population prone to infection with human papilloma virus. *J. Hyg.*, **70**, 677-90
57. Cubie, H. A. and Norval, M. (1987). Human and cellular immunity to papillomavirus in patients with cervical dysplasia. *J. Gen. Virol.* (In press)
58. Invanyi, L. and Morison, W. L. (1976). *In vitro* lymphocyte stimulation by wart antigen in man. *Br. J. Dermatol.*, **94**, 523-7
59. Lee, A. K. Y. and Eisinger, M. (1976). Cell mediated immunity (CMI) to human wart virus and wart associated tissue antigens. *Clin. Exp. Immunol.*, **26**, 419-24
60. Tagami, H., Ogino, A., Takigawa, M., Imamura, S. and Ofuji, S. (1974). Regression of plane warts following spontaneous inflammation: a histopathological study. *Br. J. Dermatol.*, **90**, 147-54
61. Berman, A. and Winkelman, R. K. (1977). Flat warts undergoing involution. *Arch. Dermatol.*, **113**, 1219-21
62. Aiba, S., Rokugo, M. and Tagami, H. (1986). Immunohistologic analysis of the phenomenon of spontaneous regression of numerous flat warts. *Cancer*, **58**, 1246-51
63. Tagami, H., Oguchi, M. and Ofuji, S. (1980). The phenomenon of spontaneous regression of numerous flat warts. Immunohistological studies. *Cancer*, **45**, 2557-63
64. Choi, K. L. and Sauder, D. N. (1986). The role of Langerhan's cells and keratinocytes in epidermal immunity. *J. Leuk. Biol.*, **39**, 343-58
65. Morris, H. H. B., Gatter, K. C., Stein, H. and Mason, D. Y. (1983). Langerhan's cells in human cervical epithelium: an immunohistological study. *Br. J. Obstet. Gynaecol.*, **90**, 400-11
66. Tay, S. K., Jenkins, D., Maddox, P., Campion, M. and Singer, A. (1987). Subpopulations of Langerhan's cells in cervical neoplasia. *Br. J. Obstet. Gynaecol.*, **94**, 10-15
67. Tay, S. K., Jenkins, Maddox, P. and Singer, A. (1987). Lymphocyte phenotypes in cervical intra-epithelial neoplasia and human papillomavirus infection. *Br. J. Obstet. Gynaecol.*, **94**, 16-21
68. Wilkin, J. K. (1977). Molluscum contagiosum venereum in a women's out-patient clinic. *Am. J. Obstet. Gynecol.*, **128**, 531-5
69. Sexually transmitted diseases. (1973). Extracts from the annual report of the Chief Medical Officer to the Department of Health and Social Security 1971. *Br. J. Vener. Dis.*, **49**, 89-95
70. Sexually transmitted diseases. (1983). Extracts from the annual report of the Chief Medical Officer to the Department of Health and Social Security 1980. *Br. J. Vener. Dis.*, **59**, 134-7
71. Blank, H. and Rake, H. (1955). Viral and rickettsial diseases of the skin, eye and mucous membranes of man. 182-192, *London, J. and A. Churchill*
72. Blank, H. (1952). Virus induced tumours of human skin (warts, molluscum contagiosum). *Ann. NY Acad. Sci.*, **54**, 1226
73. Mitchell, J. C. (1953). Observations on the virus of molluscum contagiosum. *Br. J. Exp. Pathol.*, **34**, 44-9
74. Neva, F. A. (1962). Studies on molluscum contagiosum. Observations on the cytopathic effect of molluscum suspensions in vitro. *Arch. Int. Med.*, **110**, 720-5
75. Raskin, J. (1963). Molluscum contagiosum: tissue culture and serologic study. *Arch. Dermatol.*, **87**, 552-9
76. Epstein, W. L., Senecal, I. P. and Massing, A. M. (1961). An antigen in lesions of molluscum contagiosum. *Nature*, **191**, 509
77. Shirodaria, P. V. and Matthews, R. S. (1977). Observations on the antibody responses in molluscum contagiosum. *Br. J. Dermatol.*, **96**, 29-37
78. Epstein, W. L., Conant, M. A. and Krasnobrod, H. (1966). Moluscum contagiosum. Normal and virus infected epidermal cell kinetics. *J. Invest. Dermatol.*, **46**, 91-9
79. Postlethwaite, R. (1970). Molluscum contagiosum: a review. *Arch. Environ. Health*, **21**, 432-52
80. Brown, S. T., Nailey, J. F. and Kraus, S. J. (1981). Molluscum contagiosum. *Sex. Transm. Dis.*, **8**, 227-34
81. Felman, Y. M. and Nikitas, J. A. (1983). Sexually transmitted molluscum contagiosum. Symposium on sexually transmitted diseases. *Dermatol. Clin.*, **1**, 103-10

10
Scabies and Selected Non-venereal Dermatoses

S. M. BREATHNACH AND J. ASHWORTH

INTRODUCTION

The differential diagnosis of venereal diseases affecting the external genitalia includes a variety of common and not so common dermatological diseases. This chapter will review what is known about the immunological mechanisms underlying the pathogenesis of some of these disorders, with particular emphasis on scabies.

SCABIES

Epidemiology

Scabies is a common skin disease with a worldwide distribution, which is caused by infestation with the mite *Sarcoptes scabei*. Scabies is usually transmitted by close personal contact, the importance of promiscuity being emphasized by the very similar age and seasonal incidence of scabies and venereal disease[1]. Scabies is not, however, exclusively transmitted by sexual contact, since overcrowding and poor hygiene are important factors in its spread. Epidemics of scabies throughout the world appear to occur in cycles of about 15 years in length for reasons which are not fully understood. Infestation involves the transfer of fertilized female mites or nymphs which do not survive for more than a few days away from the skin. The fertilized female excavates a burrow by cytolysis through the stratum corneum, granular and spinous layers of the epidermis at a rate of 2 mm per day, and deposits up to 25 ova in the burrow before dying. Larvae emerge from the eggs within 3–4 days, migrate to the skin surface and establish themselves in shallow pockets in the stratum corneum of the original or a new host, where they reach maturity in 14–17 days. Following fertilization, female mites excavate fresh burrows while the males rapidly die. The number of female mites and burrows in an infested individual is usually less than 50, and on average as little as 11.

Overwhelming infestation may, however, occur in so-called Norwegian or crusted scabies.

Clinical features

Following infestation, volunteers initially remain itch-free and asymptomatic apart from a faint erythematous rash, despite the presence of burrows containing mites; the typical rash associated with intense itching does not develop until about a month later[2,3]. By contrast, re-infestation of volunteers previously cured of scabies leads to development of itching and a rash within a few days. The occurrence of a latent period on initial infestation, and an accelerated response in a previously exposed individual, strongly suggests the importance of immunological mechanisms in the pathogenesis of the pruritus and skin eruption.

Whilst intense pruritus is the cardinal symptom, the burrow is the pathognomonic physical sign[1]. Burrows consists of curved or S-shaped, slightly raised ridges 5–15 mm long which occur most frequently on the sides of the fingers, interdigital webs, ulnar border of the hand, and anterior aspects of the wrists. Other sites which are often involved include the elbows, anterior axillary folds, peri-areolar region and natal cleft; penile lesions are present in over 30% of men with scabies (Figure 10.1). Secondary lesions of scabies include widespread small urticarial papules and excoriations, which may lead to an eczematous appearance. Infection may result in pustulation and areas of impetigo. Intensely itchy, indurated nodules up to 1 cm in diameter ocurring on the chest, axillae, abdomen, groins, scrotum or penis are also characteristic, and may persist for months following successful therapy for scabies. The diagnosis is reached by scraping a burrow and identifying mites or ova under light miscroscopy. Adult female mites measure 0.4×0.3 mm, possess a rounded body without a distinct head and four pairs of short legs.

Norwegian (crusted) scabies, in which patients are infested with large numbers of mites, presents with erythema and scaling which may progress to erythroderma, and is usually associated with considerable hyperkeratosis and crusting of the palms and soles. Itching is often absent in this form of scabies. Norwegian scabies is particularly common in patients with a mental deficiency such as mongolism, and it has been suggested that its development may be favoured by reduced or absent itching, leading to failure to eliminate infestation by removing mites by excoriation. However, this cannot be the only mechanism involved, since crusted scabies also occurs at a higher frequency in immunosuppressed patients, including those with renal transplants and the acquired immunodeficiency syndrome, and even in patients using topical corticosteroids[4-9]. An intact immunological system may, therefore, be important in the control or elimination of scabies.

Immunological features

The evidence for involvement of both humoral and cell-mediated immune mechanisms in the pathogenesis of scabies has been extensively reviewed[2]. A

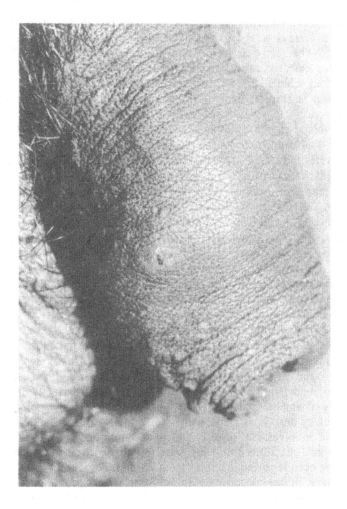

Figure 10.1 Excoriated burrow on shaft of penis

study reporting major histocompatibility complex (MHC) linkage of scabies, in that infested patients had an increased frequency of HLA-A11[10], has yet to be confirmed. A number of reports suggest the importance of a humoral IgE response to the scabies mite, as in patients with helminthic infections. IgE antibody levels are often raised in infested patients[11,12], especially in those with Norwegian scabies[13]. Antibody levels tend to fall after successful therapy[14]. Radio-allergosorbent (RAST) testing using crude scabies antigens reveals that antigen specific serum IgE is raised[11]. There may be cross-reactivity between IgE antibodies to the scabies mite and to *Dermatophagoides pteronyssinus*, the house dust mite, and *Dermatophagoides farinae*.[15,16] IgE deposits have been demonstrated in upper dermal blood vessel walls in some patients with scabies[17], and immunoperoxidase typing of dermal inflammatory cell infiltrates in scabies patients revealed that most of the plasma cells present were IgE positive[18]. Scabies may produce generalized urticaria[19,20]. The fact that intracutaneous testing with extracts of female scabies mites leads to immediate wheal reactions in a proportion of patients who have had scabies, but not in normal volunteers[15,21], and that skin test reactivity may be transferred by a serum factor, as in the classical Prausnitz–Kustner reaction[13,15,19], would also suggest that scabies-specific IgE antibody may be involved in the pathogenesis of pruritus and lesion formation in scabies. This is supported by the finding that serum from a patient with crusted scabies induced histamine release during a basophil degranulation test[22]. Increased levels of IgG and IgM, and decreased levels of IgA, antibody have been reported in scabies[23,24], but it is unknown whether these occur in response to the scabies infestation or as a result of secondary infection. Deposition of IgM and C3 at the dermo–epidermal junction in scabies[17,25,26] may similarly occur as a non-specific reaction to cutaneous inflammation.

Circulating immune complexes have been reported in patients with scabies[27,28]; but the nature of the antigen in these complexes is unknown. Scabies has been associated with generalized cutaneous vasculitis. Histopathology of lesions may show vasculitis with vessel wall necrosis, and intravascular deposition of IgM, IgA and C3 has been reported in scabies lesions[17,25,26]. Part of the cutaneous damage in scabies may, therefore, occur as a result of a local Arthus reaction or immune complex vasculitis.

The histopathology of a scabies papule is indistinguishable from that of other arthropod bites, and is characterized by a superficial and deep perivascular mixed inflammatory cell infiltrate, composed of lymphocytes, the majority of which are of T-cell type[29], histiocytes and eosinophils, oedema of the papillary dermis and epidermal spongiosis. This histological pattern suggests the involvement of a cell-mediated immune response. Delayed hypersensitivity reactions following intradermal injection of crude scabies antigen have been reported in some[2,13] but not in other studies[15].

In summary, initial infestation with *Sarcoptes scabei* provokes little in the way of any dermatitis, and the majority of the skin eruption in scabies probably occurs as a result of the host immune response, both cellular and humoral. The immune response may limit the degree of infestation by eliminiting mites either as a result of toxic products generated during immunological reactions, or by provoking scratching[2]. Absolute natural immunity does not, however, develop, since previously infested individuals may become re-infested. The nature of the antigen(s) on the scabies mite responsible for the induction of an immunological response is currently unknown; study of the immunological aspects of scabies infestation is to some extent hampered by the lack of adequate culture techniques for the mites.

FUNGAL INFECTIONS

Clinical features

Tinea cruris is caused by one of a variety of dermatophyte fungi, usually *Epidermophyton floccosum* or *Trichophyton rubrum*, or less commonly

Trichophyton interdigitale; genital candidiasis is caused by the yeast-like fungus *Candida albicans*[30,31]. Both tinea cruris and genital candidiasis are associated with pruritus. Dermatophyte infections cause erythema and scaling extending from the groin onto the thighs with an annular margin (Figure 10.2). There may be dermal nodules scattered within the affected area producing a beaded appearance along the margin, and occasionally pustules may be seen. Spread to the scrotum, penis and buttocks may also occur. *Candida balanitis* produces small papules which develop as pustules or vesicles which then produce shallow ulcers. Vulvovaginal candidiasis results in a beefy erythema of vaginal mucosa and vulval skin associated with a curdy-white discharge. In males and females there may be spread to the groins and perineum, with characteristic satellite papules and pustules, and an irregular scaling margin with pustulation.

Immunological features

Immunological aspects of dermatophyte infection and of mucocutaneous candidiasis have been extensively reviewed[30-34]. It is thought that cell-mediated immune reactions play the major part in the eradication of acute superficial infections. Fungal antigens are presented to sensitized T-lymphocytes by resident intra-epidermal macrophage-like Langerhans cells[35]. Inflammatory mediators and lymphokines produced by these cells result in abrogation of the epidermal barrier, with consequent leakage into the stratum

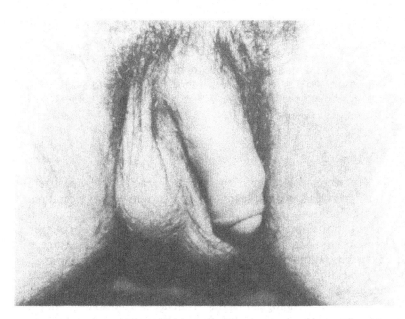

Figure 10.2 Tinea cruris of the groins, showing areas of erythema and scaling with an annular margin

corneum of serum containing a fungistatic substance termed 'serum inhibitory factor (SIF). Patients generally develop delayed hypersensitivity responses to an intradermal injection of trichophytin. Although agglutinins, precipitins and complement-fixing IgG antibodies against dermatophytes develop in most patients, they are usually short-term and disappear following resolution of the fungal infection. By contrast in chronic infections which are resistant to therapy, there is generally absent delayed hypersensitivity (but sometimes immediate hypersensitivity) to trichophytin, poor *in vitro* assessed cell-mediated immunity to fungal antigens, and antidermatophyte antibodies tend to persist. Dermatophyte infections are commoner in atopic individuals in whom a variety of defects in cell-mediated immunity have been recorded[35]. The relative importance of cell-mediated immune mechanisms in protection against Candida infection is demonstrated by experience with chronic mucocutaneous candidiasis, where defective cell-mediated immunity leads to extensive superficial candidiasis despite normal or even exaggerated humoral defences[31,34].

PSORIASIS

Clinical features

Psoriasis vulgaris may affect the glans, prepuce or shaft of the penis. Usually, typical lesions elsewhere enable the diagnosis to be made easily, but on occasion lesions may be confined to the glans. At this site, single or multiple red plaques with well-demarcated borders and a dull granular surface are seen (Figure 10.3).

Immunological features

Although a variety of immunological abnormalities have been reported in psoriasis[36], and psoriasis has recently been reported to respond well to the immunomodulatory drug cyclosporin A, a primary role for immune events remains unproven.

BEHÇET'S DISEASE

Behçet's disease is a complex multisystem disease characterized by recurrent oral ulceration and at least two of the following: recurrent genital ulceration, uveitis, synovitis, cutaneous pustular vasculitis (pathergy) and meningoencephalitis occurring in the absence of inflammatory bowel disease or collagen vascular disease. Behçet's disease is frequent in Japan and Mediterranean countries, between latitudes 30° and 45° N in Asian and Eurasian populations, coinciding with the ancient Silk Route. There is a female predominance in east Asia, while males predominate in west Asia and the Middle East. Suggested aetiological factors in Behçet's syndrome include a genetic factor, herpes virus infection, delayed hypersensitivity to streptococci, a toxic response to organic chemicals and autoimmunity.

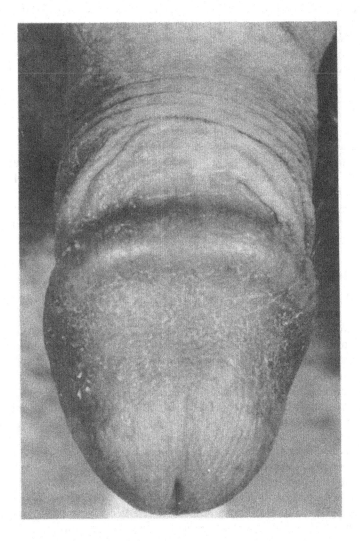

Figure 10.3 Scaling and dull erythema in psoriasis of the glans penis

The spectrum of clinical manifestations in Behçet's disease is divisible into two groups: group 1 comprises the ocular and arthritic types, and group 2 comprises the neurological and mucocutaneous types[37]. There is a high incidence of the class I MHC gene product HLA-B51, and a raised incidence of DRw52 is common to all ethnic groups studied[38], which suggests that Behçet's disease is MHC restricted. HLA-B51 is found predominantly in the ocular type, and DRw52 or DR7 may be significantly associated with the neurological type[37]. A decrease in the proportion and proliferative responses of T4 helper/inducer T-cells, and an increase in the proliferative response of

T8 suppressor/cytotoxic cells, to Herpes simplex virus type 1 (HSV1) is found mostly in group 1 patients; similarly, *in situ* hybridization studies with HSV1-DNA detected significant complementary RNA in mononuclear cells, but only in patients with the ocular or arthritic type of Behçet's disease[37]. Circulating immune complexes, some of which contain IgG anti-HSV1 antibodies, and non-specific antibodies to mucosal tissue have been demonstrated. However, neither immunoglobulin nor complement components are usually found in the orogenital lesions of Behçet's, which are, therefore, unlikely to be the result of immune complex disease[39]. Skin lesions are characterized histologically by acute inflammation with intense infiltration by polymorphonuclear leukocytes (PMNL), and in this regard it is of interest that increased chemotaxis and random motility of PMNL have been reported[40]. However, an immunohistological study of recurrent oral ulcers demonstrated that the infiltrate consisted almost exclusively of mononuclear cells with a significant proportion of T-cells, suggesting the importance of a cell-mediated immune mechanism[41].

LICHEN PLANUS

Lichen planus is a benign self-limiting skin disorder which manifests as an eruption of violaceous, lichenoid, flat-topped polygonal papules. Lichen planus can affect any part of the body, but the classical sites of involvement are the front of the wrists, the lumbar region, around the ankles and on the buccal mucosa. On the female genitalia, lichen planus may appear as bluish-white papules or delicate lace-like striae (Figure 10.4); on the glans, the papules may coalesce to produce annular lesions.

Lichen planus is thought to occur as a result of a cell-mediated immune attack on the epidermis, which is no longer recognized as 'self' following alteration of cell surface antigens by viral infection or drug therapy[35]. In this regard it is of interest that early chronic cutaneous graft-versus-host disease mimics idiopathic lichen planus very closely in terms of clinical appearance and histological and immunofluorescence findings. The histology of lichen planus is characterized by the band-like T-lymphocytic infiltrate hugging the dermo–epidermal junction, with epidermal cell necrosis and colloid body formation. The majority of T-cells in the dermal infiltrate are of helper/inducer phenotype, with up to 35% being of suppressor/cytotoxic phenotype; 90% of intraepidermal T-cells in this condition are of suppressor/cytotoxic phenotype. The deposition of immunoreactants (particularly IgM) on colloid bodies and along the dermo–epidermal junction, which is commonly observed in lichen planus, is thought to occur as a secondary phenomenon. On the basis of studies of the alteration in the number of epidermal Langerhans cells in various stages of the evolution of the condition, it has been proposed that lichen planus involves an initial phase of antigen presentation and Langerhans cell-T-helper lymphocyte inter-action, followed by a lymphocytotoxic phase. In common with a number of other lymphocyte-mediated skin disease, lichen planus is associated with the phenomenon of aberrant expression of class II MHC (HLA-DR) antigen by keratinocytes.

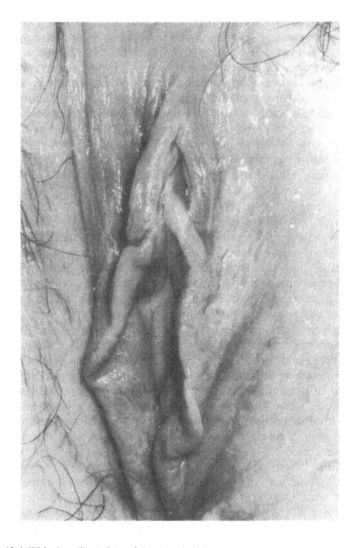

Figure 10.4 White lace-like lesions of the vulva in lichen planus

FIXED DRUG ERUPTIONS

Fixed drug eruptions can occur anywhere on the skin and mucous membranes, but the genitalia are a site of predilection[44]. In a recent series of 29 cases, genital lesions were usually single and associated with itching or burning, and the glans penis was most commonly affected[43]. Lesions were often well demarcated and oedematous, with or without vesicles and superficial erosions, and surrounded by an erythematous halo. Less commonly patients presented with superficial erosions following evanescent superficial flaccid bullae. Residual hyperpigmentation persists after the acute episode has subsided. The list of drugs implicated in the aetiology of fixed drug eruption is extensive, but amongst the best known are tetracyclines, barbiturates, sulphonamides and phenolphthalein[42]. In the majority of patients, a single drug is responsible, but there are some patients in whom fixed drug eruption occurs after ingestion of multiple drugs. Sometimes this 'polysensitivity' is a cross-reactivity, as when sulphonamides induce an exacerbation of fixed drug eruption in patients sensitive to dapsone. The offending drug can usually be identified by provocation testing; symptoms occur on re-exposure from 30 minutes to 8 hours later. However, in some patients there may be a refractory period of up to several months following each drug-induced exacerbation. Attempts to reproduce the eruption by application of the drug epicutaneously in patch testing, or by scratch or intradermal testing have yielded negative results in uninvolved skin and inconsistent results in lesional skin.

Histological changes in fixed drug eruption include dermal oedema, perivascular lymphohistiocytic infiltration, exocytosis with intra- and inter-cellular oedema, individual dyskeratotic cells within the epidermis, and hydropic change of epidermal basal cells resulting in pigmentary incontinence. These are indicative of a cell-mediated immune process. Immunofluorescence microscopic studies have revealed only non-specific epidermal intercellular deposition of IgG and C3, or deposition of fibrin along the dermo–epidermal junction. Intradermal injection of serum obtained during an acute episode of fixed drug eruption into the same patient during remission produced an inflammatory response only at previously involved sites, and not in normal skin, suggesting a role for a serum factor in the production of the lesions[44]. Incubation of the causative drug with the patient's lymphocytes produced no blast transformation in 21 patients with fixed drug eruption.[45] However, autologous serum alone did induce blast transformation, which was considerably increased on addition of the offending drug. It is unclear why the lesions should remain so localized. Autotransplantation studies, in which patients have been challenged with the causative drug following exchange of skin grafts from lesional and uninvolved sites, have been inconclusive. Small numbers of antigen-specific T-cells may be retained in previous sites of contact sensitivity for prolonged periods, resulting in local specific immunological memory which may be important in retest or flare-up reactivity[46]. It is possible that a similar mechanism may occur in fixed drug eruption.

ERYTHEMA MULTIFORME AND STEVENS–JOHNSON SYNDROME

Erythema multiforme is an inflammatory skin disorder characterized by erythematous papules, plaques, target-like annular lesions, vesicles and bullae, with or without mouth and genital ulcers, and conjunctival involvement[47,48]. The Stevens–Johnson syndrome refers to cases with marked mucosal involvement. The most frequent precipitating causes include herpes simplex infection, other infections and drugs. Although the exact mechanism is unclear, there is evidence for involvement of the immune system.

Circulating antigen–antibody immune complexes, some of which contain herpes simplex antigen, and complement activation have been reported in the blood and skin lesions of some patients. However, the histology is more in keeping with a cell-mediated immune attack upon the epidermis than an immune complex vasculitis disease[49].

MISCELLANEOUS

Cicatricial pemphigoid is a chronic scarring bullous disease primarily involving mucous membranes, including those of the genital area, and less commonly the skin[50,51]. Most patients have *in vivo* bound immunoglobulins and/or complement along the basement membrane of affected tissues. Although the frequency of patients who also have a circulating anti-basement membrane zone autoantibody is much less than in bullous pemphigoid, it is thought that, as in bullous pemphigoid, the antibody plays a major role in the generation of the mucosal lesions.

Lichen sclerosus et atrophicus is a relatively uncommon condition which may affect any area of the skin, and classically presents as ivory coloured papules with follicular plugging and hyperkeratosis. There is a predilection for the female genitalia; sheets of ivory-white atrophic skin may progress to narrowing of the introitus, and there may be fissures, erosions and lichenification. Lichen sclerosus may also affect the glans penis, with ivory-white macules becoming confluent (Figure 10.5); atrophy around the meatus

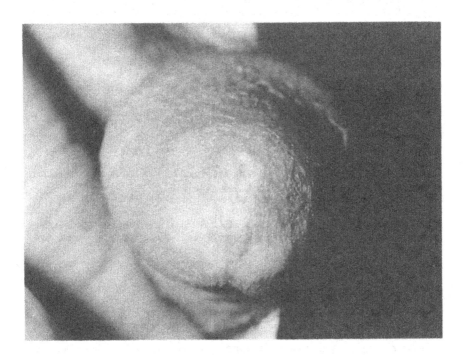

Figure 10.5 White atrophic area around the urinary meatus ian lichen sclerosus et atrophicus

(balanitis xerotica obliterans) may lead to difficulty with micturition, and involvement of the preputial area may cause phimosis. The histology is characterized by a lymphoid cell infiltrate in the mid-dermis, associated with atrophy and hydropic change of the overlying epidermis, and oedema and homogenization of the intervening collagen. There is an increased frequency of HLA-B40. Patients with lichen sclerosus have an increased incidence of autoantibodies, and a significantly higher incidence of autoimmunity[52].

In the papulonecrotic variety of tuberculide, recurrent crops of necrotizing papules occur on the extremities over months or years. Papulonecrotic ulcerative lesions of the glans penis have been recorded, and may rarely occur in the absence of other skin lesions. Tuberculides are thought to occur as a result of haematogenous dissemination of bacilli in patients with a high degree of immunity to the tubercle bacillus. Histological changes suggest an initial Arthus reaction with later transition to a delayed hypersensitivity reaction; evidence of circulating immune complexes has been found in some cases[53,54].

References

1. Rook, A. (1986). Scabies. In Rook, A., Wilkinson, D. S., Ebling, F. J. G., Champion, R.H. and Burton, J. L. (eds.). *Textbook of Dermatology*. pp. 1060-6. (Oxford: Blackwell Scientific Publications)
2. Dahl, M. V. (1983). The immunology of scabies. *Ann. Allergy*, **51**, 560-4
3. Mallanby, K. (1972). *Scabies*. 2nd Edn. (London: E. W. Classey)
4. Espy, P. D. and Jolly, H. W., Jr. (1976). Norwegian scabies: Occurrence in a patient undergoing immunosuppression. *Arch. Dermatol.*, **112**, 193-6
5. Paterson, W. D., Allen, B. R. and Beveridge, G. W. (1973). Norwegian scabies during immunosuppressive therapy. *Br. Med. J.*, **4**, 211-12
6. Youshock, E. and Glazer, S. D. (1981). Norwegian scabies in a renal transplant patient. *J. Am. Med. Assoc.*, **246**, 2608-9
7. Clayton, R. and Farrow, S. (1975). Norwegian scabies following topical steroid therapy. *Postgrad. Med. J.*, **51**, 657-9
8. Barnes, L., McCallister, R. E. and Lucky, A. W. (1987). Crusted (Norwegian) scabies. Occurrence in a child undergoing a bone marrow transplant. *Arch. Dermatol.*, **123**, 95-7
9. Glover, R., Young, L. and Goltz, R. W. (1987). Norwegian scabies in acquired immunodeficiency syndrome: Report of a case resulting in death from associated sepsis. *J. Am. Acad. Dermatol.*, **16**, 396-8
10. Falk, E. S. and Thorsby, E. (1981). HLA antigens in patients with scabies. *Br. J. Dermatol.*, **104**, 317-20
11. Rantanen, T., Bjorksten, F., Reunala, T. and Salo, O. P. (1981). Serum IgE antibodies to scabies mite. *Acta Dermatovener.*, **61**, 358-60
12. Chevrant-Breton, J., Desruies, E., Auvray, E., Giiguen, C. and De Certaines, J. (1981). Serum IgE values in human scabies: study of 79 cases. *Ann. Dermatol. Venereol.*, **108**, 979-83
13. Burks, J. W., Jung, R. and George, W. M. (1956). Norwegian scabies. *Arch. Dermatol.*, **74**, 131-40
14. Falk, E. S. (1981). Serum IgE before and after treatment for scabies. *Allergy*, **36**, 167-74
15. Falk, E. S. and Bolle, R. (1980). *In vitro* demonstration of specific immunological hypersensitivity to scabies mite. *Br. J. Dermatol.*, **103**, 367-73
16. Falk, E. S. and Bolle, R. (1980). IgE antibodies to house dust mite in patients with scabies. *Br. J. Dermatol.*, **102**, 283-8
17. Frentz, G., Veien, N. K. and Eriksen, K. (1977). Immunofluorescence studies in scabies. *J. Cutan. Pathol.*, **4**, 191-3

18. Reunala, T., Ranki, A., Rantanen, T. and Salo, O. P. (1984). Inflammatory cells in skin lesions of scabies. *Clin. Exp. Dermatol.*, **9**, 70–7
19. Chapel, T. A., Krugel, L., Chapel, J. and Segal, A. (1981). Scabies presenting as urticaria. *J. Am. Med. Assoc.*, **246**, 1440–1
20. Witkowski, J. A. and Parish, L. C. (1984). Scabies: a cause of generalised urticaria. *Cutis*, **33**, 277–9
21. Prakken, J. R. and van Vloten, T. J. (1949). Allergy in scabies. *Dermatologica*, **99**, 124–31
22. Van Neste, D. (1981). Immunologic studies in scabies. *Int. J. Dermatol.*, **20**, 264–9
23. Falk, E. S. (1980). Serum immunoglobulin values in patients with scabies. *Br. J. Dermatol.*, **102**, 57–61
24. Hancock, B. W. and Milford, W. A. (1974). Serum immunoglobulin in scabies. *J. Invest. Dermatol.*, **63**, 482–4
25. Salo, O. P., Reunala, T., Kalimo, K. and Rantanen, T. (1982). Immunoglobulin and complement deposits in the skin and circulating immune complexes in scabies. *Acta Dermatol.*, **62**, 73–6
26. Hoefling, K. K. and Schroeter, A. L. (1980). Dermatoimmunopathology of scabies. *J. Am. Acad. Dermatol.*, **3**, 237–40
27. Van Neste, D. and Salmon, J. (1978). Circulating antigen antibody complexes in scabies. *Dermatologica*, **157**, 221–4
28. Van Neste, D. and Salmon, J. (1980). Immune complexes in scabies: *in vitro* study of the serum. Ciq fixation in the presence of mite and unparasited human scale extracts. *Dermatologica*, **160**, 131–4
29. Falk, E. S. and Matre, R. (1982). *In situ* characterisation of cell infiltrates in the dermis of human scabies. *Am. J. Dermatopathol.*, **4**, 9–15
30. Roberts, S. O. B. and MacKenzie, D. W. R. (1986). Mycology. In Rook, A., Wilkinson, D. S., ebling, F. J. G., Champion, R. H. and Burton, J. L. (eds.). *Textbook of Dermatology.*, pp. 885–986. (Oxford: Blackwell Scientific Publications)
31. Goslen, J. B. and Kobayashi, G. S. (1987). Mycologic infections. In Fitzpatrick, T. B., Eisen, A. Z., Wolff, K., Freedberg, I. W. and Austen, K. F. (eds.). *Dermatology in General Medicine*, pp. 2193–248. (New York: McGraw-Hill)
32. Ahmed, A. R. (1982). Immunology of human dermatophyte infections. *Arch. Dermatol.*, **118**, 521–5
33. Hay, R. J. and Shennan, G. (1982). Chronic dermatophyte infections II. Antibody and cell-mediated immune responses. *Br. J. Derrmatol.*, **106**, 191–8
34. Jorizzo, J. L. (1982). Chronic mucocutaneous candidosis: An update. *Arch. Dermatol.*, **118**, 963–5
35. Breathnach, S. M. and Katz, S. I. (1986). Cell-mediated immunity in cutaneous disease. *Hum. Pathol.*, **17**, 161–7
36. Baker, H. (1986). Psoriasis. In Rook, A., Wilkinson, D. S., Ebling, F. J. G., Champion, R. H. and Burton, J. L. (eds.). *Textbook of Dermatology.*, pp. 1469–532. (Oxford: Blackwell Scientific Publications)
37. Lehner, T. (1986). The role of a disorder in immunoregulation, associated with herpes simplex virus type 1 in Behçet's disease. In Lehner, T. and Barnes, C. G. (eds.). *Recent Advances in Behçet's Disease.*, pp. 33–6. (London: Royal Society of Medicine Services)
38. Welsh, K. I. and Kerr, L. A. The immunogenetics of Behçet's disease – do they give an indication to the likely mechanism for the disease? In Lehner, T. and Barnes, C. G. (eds.). *Recent Advances in Behçet's Disease.* pp. 3–9. (London: Royal Society of Medicine Services)
39. Mowbray, J. F. (1986). Immune complexes in Behçet's disease. In Lehner, T. and Barnes, C. G. (eds.). *Recent Advances in Behçet's disease.* pp. 61–5. (London: Royal Society of Medicine Services)
40. Mizushima, Y. (1986). Chemotaxis and phagocytosis of leukocytes in Behçet's disease: an overview. In Lehner, T. and Barnes, C. G. (eds.). *Recent Advances in Behçet's Disease.*, pp. 85–87. (London: Royal Society of Medicine Services)
41. Poulter, L. W., Lehner, T. and Duke, O. (1986). Immunohistological investigation of recurrent oral ulcers and Behçet's disease. In Lehner, T. and Barnes, C. G. (eds.). *Recent Advances in Behçet's Disease.*, pp. 123–128. (London: Royal Society of Medicine Services)
42. Wyatt, E., Greaves, M. and Sondergaard, J. (1972). Fixed drug eruption (phenolphthalein).

Arch. Dermatol., **106**, 671–3

43. Sehgal, V. H. and Gangwani, O. P. (1986). Genital fixed drug eruptions. *Genitourin. Med.*, **62**, 56–8
44. Korkij, W. and Soltani, K. (1984). Fixed drug eruption. A brief review. *Arch. Dermatol.*, **120**, 520–4
45. Gimenez-Camarasa, J. M., Garcia-Calderon, P. and DeMoragas, J. M. (1975). Lymphocyte transformation test in fixed drug eruption. *N. Engl. J. Med.*, **292**, 819–21
46. Scheper, R. J., von Blomberg, M., Boerrigter, G. H., Bruynzeel, D., van Dinther, A. and Vos, A. (1983). Induction of immunological memory in the skin. Role of local T cell retention. *Clin. Exp. Immunol.*, **51**, 141–8
47. Nethercott, J. R. and Choi, B. C. K. (1985). Erythema multiforme (Stevens–Johnson syndrome) – chart review of 123 hospitalized patients. *Dermatologica*, **171**, 383–96
48. Elias, P. M. and Fritsch, P. O. (1987). Erythema multiforme. In Fitzpatrick, T. B., Eisen, A. Z., Wolff, K., Freedberg, I. W. and Austen, K. F. (eds.). *Dermatology in General Medicine.*, pp. 555–63. (New York: McGraw-Hill)
49. Howland, W. W., Golitz, L. E., Weston, W. L. and Huff, J. C. (1984). Erythema multiforme: clinical, histopathologic, and immunologic study. *J. Am. Acad. Dermatol.*, **10**, 438–46
50. Jordon, R. E. (1987). Bullous pemphigoid, cicatricial pemphigoid, and chronic bullous dermatosis of childhood. In Fitzpatrick, T. B., Eisen, A. Z., Wolff, K., Freedberg, I. W. and Austen, K. F. (eds.). *Dermatology in General Medicine*, pp. 580–586 (New York: McGraw-Hill)
51. Fine, J.-D., Neises, G. R. and Katz, S. I. (1984). Immunofluorescence and immunoelectron microscopic studies in cicatricial pemphigoid. *J. Invest. Dermatol.*, **82**, 39–43
52. Meyrick Thomas, R. H., Ridley, C. M. and Black, M. M. (1983). The association of lichen sclerosus et atrophicus and autoimmune related disease in males. *Br. J. Dermatol.*, **109**, 661–4
53. Morrison, J. G. L. and Fourie, E. D. (1974). The papulonecrotic tuberculide. From Arthus reaction to lupus vulgaris. *Br. J. Dermatol.*, **91**, 263–70
54. Nishigori, C., Taniguchi, S., Hayakawa, M. and Imamura, S. (1986). Penis tuberculides: papulonecrotic tuberculides on the glans penis. *Dermatologica*, **172**, 93–7

11
Allergic Reactions to Drugs

P. W. EWAN AND J. F. ACKROYD

INTRODUCTION

Although allergic reactions account for only a minority of adverse reactions to drugs, they are common. They may result in a wide variety of clinical presentations. In sexually-transmitted diseases the drugs which most commonly cause reactions are the penicillins, co-trimoxazole and the tetracyclines. There are considerable gaps in our understanding of the mechanisms of many drug reactions. This means there are often no diagnostic tests or that these tests may be unreliable. Furthermore, substantial numbers of supposed drug reactions do not recur when the drug is re-administered. These reactions, therefore, pose a difficult problem for the clinician. In this chapter, mechanisms of drug reactions and clinical presentation will be discussed, and an approach to diagnosis and management suggested.

THE PATHOGENESIS OF THE ALLERGIC REACTION

The mechanism of drug reactions is a difficult subject. Although some have been shown to have an immunological basis, in many the mechanism is obscure. The immunological reactions which may be involved in adverse drug reactions are the immediate hypersensitivity reaction, cytotoxic reactions, antigen-antibody (immune-complex) reactions and delayed hypersensitivity. These are described below, but have been more full reviewed by Ackroyd[1,2,3] Immediate hypersensitivity is responsible for the classical acute allergic reaction, which may cause anaphylaxis, but this accounts for only a minority of drug reactions.

Immediate hypersensitivity

Mast cells and basophils bear specific receptors for IgE, and the interaction of antigen with cell-bound IgE antibodies activates the mast cell leading to release of a variety of mediators, including histamine and leukotrienes. Mast

237

cells will also release these mediators in response to non-specific or non-immunological stimuli. These mediators are responsible for the patho-physiology of allergic disorders.

The type I (immediate hypersensitivity) allergic reaction involves the release of mediators from mast cells which have been sensitized by IgE antibodies. IgE antibodies are generated in response to exposure to antigen, and fix through their Fc piece to receptors on the mast cell surface. These Fc receptors on the mast cell (Fc$_\epsilon$ R1) have a high affinity for IgE antibodies. When antigen interacts with two adjacent IgE antibody molecules on the mast cell surface, the mast cell is activated. A series of biochemical events then takes place, including increased phosphatidylinositol turnover and intracel-lular calcium, leading to mediator release.

Mediators may be released from the mast cell in two ways: as preformed mediators or as newly synthesized mediators. Preformed mediators are stored in granules, and are released by exocytosis on activation of the mast cell. Synthesis of newly generated mediators is also initiated, and these are derived from metabolism of arachidonic acid in the cell membrane.

Non-specific stimuli may activate mast cells, causing mediator release (Table 11.1). It appears that different stimuli trigger different mast cells preferentially, e.g. broncho-alveolar mast cells are readily triggered by the calcium ionophore A23187 or hyperosmolar agents, while skin mast cells, but not lung mast cells, respond to basic polyamines, compound 48/80 and substance P.

Table 11.1 Agents activating mast cells

Immunological
  Antigen-IgE

Non-specific
  Cold, heat
  Osmolality
  Vibration
  Exercise
  Trauma
  Calcium ionophore A23187
  Basic agents, e.g. 48/80
  Peptides, e.g. substance P
                  bradykinin
  Anaphylatoxins: C3a, C5a
  Adenosine
  Opiates, e.g. codeine, morphine
  Other drugs

A large number of mediators may be released from mast cells; the major ones are listed in Table 11.2. Histamine was the original mediator to be studied, its main effects being to cause increased vascular permeability capillary dilatation and smooth muscle contraction. These effects are responsible for the classic wheal and flare reaction seen when histamine is injected into human skin and contribute to the tissue oedema, increased

Table 11.2 Mast cell mediators

Preformed
  Histamine
  Neutrophil chemotactic factor (NCA)
  Eosinophil chemotactic factor (ECA)
  Platelet activating factor (PAF)

Newly generated
  Prostaglandins, e.g. PGD_2, PGF_2
  Leukotrienes, e.g. LTB_4, LTV_4, LTD_4, LTE_4
  Thromboxane TXA_2

secretions and bronchoconstriction. A rise in plasma histamine has been demonstrated in allergic reactions in man – in acute asthma, in the early and late phases of bronchoconstriction induced by antigen challenge and in exercise-induced asthma.

More recent studies have emphasized the importance of other mediators, many of which have effects in common with histamine. Leukotrienes are generated by arachidonic acid metabolism through the 5-lipoxygenase pathway. The leukotrienes LTC_4, D_4 and E_4 are responsible for the activity of what was known as slow reacting substance of anaphylaxis (SRS-A). They are potent constrictors of smooth muscle, 100–300 times as potent as inhaled histamine, and, therefore, likely to be important in asthma. They also cause increased vascular permeability (oedema) and mucus secretion. Leukotreine B4 (LTB_4) is a chemotactic factor, with effects on both neutrophils and eosinopohils and is important in the genesis of inflammation. Prostaglandins are the other main group of newly formed mediators, also derived from arachidonic acid metabolism but through the cyclo-oxygenase pathway. Prostaglandin D_2 is a potent bronchoconstrictor, as is its metabolite 9α, 11β PGF_2.

The preformed mediators, neutrophil and eosinophil chemotactic factors, attract inflammatory cells to the site of the reaction, and are thought to play an important role in the late phase of asthma and in bronchial hyperreactivity. Platelet activating factor (PAF) has chemotactic activity, and increases vascular permeability. PAF causes platelet aggregation and release of 5-hydroxytryptamine (serotonin) from platelets.

This is a simplified account of the effects of some of the major mast cell mediators. Events *in vivo* are likely to be much more complex, in part because certain mediators have a secondary effect in potentiating each other and because of the heterogeneity of mast cells.

Mast cell heterogeneity

Studies in the rat have demonstrated two distinct mast cell phenotypes. These were first recognized because of their different staining characteristics, and are termed mucosal mast cells (MMC) and connective tissue mast cells (CTMC). The rat intestinal mucosa contains large numbers of MMC, whereas the classical CTMC is found in other sites such as the skin. CTMC can be stained after fixation in most solutions, whereas MMC can only be stained after fixation in Carnoy's solution. The staining pattern also differs: only CTMC stain with berberine. In the rat, MMC and CTMC differ in their histamine content (less in the MMC), granular proteins (rat mast cell protease I in the CTMC, and rat mast cell protease II in the MMC) and response to mast cell triggering agents. Although much less is known about mast cells at different sites in man there is probably considerable heterogeneity. Human lung mast cells differ from both the rat MMC and CTMC, but have more features in common with the mucosal mast cell.

Other cells with receptors for IgE

A variety of other cells also have receptors for the Fc piece of the IgE antibody, (Fc$_\epsilon$ R2) but these are of lower affinity than those on mast cells. Fc$_\epsilon$ R2 are found on neutrophils, eosinophils, monocytes and platelets. The receptor on eosinophils has been much studied. There is increased expression of Fc$_\epsilon$R2 on a subpopulation of eosinophils of low density, the so-called hypodense or activated cells. Eosinophils purified from patients with parasitic infections and bearing surface IgE, when stimulated with the appropriate parasite antigen release specific mediators such as eosinophil peroxidase or major basic protein which are important in paraside killing. In contrast a different mediator, eosinophil cationic protein, is released after an IgG dependent stimulus. Thus the mediators released depends on the antibody stimulus (IgE or IgG). How these IgE dependent reactions relate to immediate-hypersensitivity remains to be seen.

Eosinophilia is seen in helminth infections and atopic disorders, but not in all drug hypersensitivity reactions – possibly because only a small proportion of the latter are type I reactions. In allergic asthma, a number of observations suggest a role for the eosinophil in the pathogenesis of the disease. The blood eosinophil count has been shown to be related to the degree of airflow obstruction, and raised levels of eosinophil products, e.g. major basic protein, have been found in asthmatics when compared with controls. Release of eosinophil products also seem to be related to the late phase of the asthmatic reaction, and to the state of hyperreactivity which may follow an acute asthmatic reaction.

Diseases due to immediate hypersensitivity reactions

Asthma, rhinitis and conjunctivitis (e.g. hay-fever) are the commonest disorders due to immediate hypersensitivity reactions. Some forms of eczema almost certainly have an immediate hypersensitivity component. Urticaria and angioedema may also occur. Anaphylaxis results from a systemic type I reaction and may be fatal; certain drug reactions, including the true anaphylactic reactions, are caused in this way, e.g. penicillin. Because little is known of the mechanism of reactions to other antibiotics, it is not clear whether they cause type I reactions, but this would seem likely.

In immediate hypersensitivity drug reactions, an increased incidence of atopy has not been proved.

Serum sickness (acute immune-complex disease)

In this reaction (type III hypersensitivity), the binding of circulating antigen with antibody (usually IgG), leads to the formation of circulating antigen–antibody (immune) complexes. Deposition of these complexes in the walls of blood vessels at a variety of sites results in complement activation and vasculitis. Serum sickness originally attained prominence following the injection of antitoxic antisera in patients with bacterial infections, but antibiotics such as penicillin and the sulphonamides may also produce a serum-sickness-like reaction. The mechanisms is discussed below. In immune complex disorders, the antigen is commonly an infectious agent although in many instances it is unidentified. Clinical features include fever, rashes, urticaria, arthralgia and nephritis.

The immune cytopenias

The drugs in common use in venereology which can cause immune cytopenias and the mechanisms by which these reactions are produced are considered below.

Contact hypersensitivity

Contact sensitivity is a variant of delayed hypersensitivity, cell-mediated hypersensitivity or type IV reaction. These responses are mediated by T-cells, are independent of antibody and are delayed in onset. The best example in man, is an eczematous reaction at the site of contact with the allergen (contact dermatitis).

Small haptens induce contact sensitivity, but first enter the skin and become conjugated to proteins before they become immunogenic. The subject becomes sensitized to this conjugate, and T-cells are generated specific for the hapten–carrier conjugate. The antigen-presenting cell for contact hypersensitivity is the Langerhans cell. This carries class II major histocompatibility antigens (HLA-D) and presents the hapten–carrier conjugate to helper T-cells. Interleukin-2 and other T cell lymphokines are produced leading to macrophage activation. Histologically, the skin shows dilatation of small blood vessels and lymphatics in the dermis with associated oedema and infiltration mainly with mononuclear cells. This infiltrate extends into the epidermis which shows focal oedema and breakdown of epidermal cells to produce vesicles which in severe cases may coalesce to form blisters. Macroscopically the appearances vary. The mildest lesions show only a slightly raised erythema. More severe reactions will show macules and vesicles and even blistering. The predominant symptom is itching.

ALLERGIC AND PSEUDO-ALLERGIC OR ANAPHYLACTOID REACTIONS

Although adverse drug reactions are often described as 'allergic', many cannot be shown to have an immunological mechanism and strictly, therefore, should not be described as allergic. Such reactions are sometimes referred to as pseudo-allergic or anaphylactoid.

In anaphylactoid reactions, a variety of mechanisms may be responsible, but IgE antibodies are not involved. Mediator release may occur by a direct action of the drug on the mast cell. In many drug reactions the mechanism is not known. Anaphylactoid reactions often occur in response to the first dose of a drug, and not infrequently they fail to recurr when the drus is re-administered.

The antibody in allergic reactions to drugs is generally thought to be developed against an antigen formed by union of the drug with a macromolecular bodily constituent: usually a protein, although such an antigen has seldom been demonstrated. Because the antibody takes time to develop, allergic reactions do not normally occur in response to the initial dose of the drug. However, the initial dose of a drug may cause an allergic reaction, if the patient has already developed an antibody to a chemically similar drug and this antibody cross-reacts with the antigen formed by the drug now taken for the first time.

If a patient has a drug-dependent antibody in sufficiently high titre, he will develop a reaction whenever the drug is taken. Some drug-dependent antibodies disappear quite rapidly, and if the antibody titre has fallen to a sufficiently low level when the drug is taken again, the reaction may not recur in response to the first dose re-administered, although the antigenic stimulus provided by further re-administration of the drug may be expected to increase the antibody titre and cause recurrence of symptoms. Even if a drug-dependent antibody can be demonstrated, and this can be done only in a small minority of drug reactions, the demonstration of such an antibody does not necessarily prove that the patient is allergic to the drug. Haemagglutinating antibodies to penicillin, for instance, can be demonstrated in a very high proportion of healthy individuals without a history of penicillin allergy, if a sufficiently sensitive technique is used. It may be very difficult, therefore, not only to differentiate between allergic and anaphylactoid reactions, but also to prove that a reaction occurring during drug therapy was caused by one of the drugs being taken.

In terms of practical management, drug reactions are only of importance if the patient who is thought to have developed a reaction to a drug needs further treatment with that drug. The problem then arises whether the reaction will recur if the drug is re-administered. If the patient needs further treatment, and an alternative and equipotent drug, which is not chemically related, is available, this should be given. Otherwise an attempt must be made to assess the potential benefit of treatment against the risk of inducing a reaction. These problems are discussed in the section on diagnosis.

MECHANISMS OF DRUG REACTIONS IN VENEREOLOGICAL PRACTICE

Many drugs can cause immediate (type I) reactions. Penicillin is the drug most commonly involved and is the commonest cause of anaphylaxis. This is mediated by IgE antibodies. This type of reaction is considered in detail below.

Of the drug-induced cytopenias, thrombocytopenia has been the most extensively investigated. In a small number of cases an antibody can be demonstrated which causes platelet lysis in the presence of the drug and complement. Two hypotheses have been much discussed [1-5]; whether the drug combines with the platelet membrane to form an antigen whic undergoes lysis in the presence of antibody and complement, or whether the drug forms an immune complex with the antibody which activates complement on the platelet surface to cause platelet lysis. The controversy seems now to be resolved. In two different types of experiment [6,7] it has been shown that in the presence of the drug the F(ab) or F(ab)₂ components of the antibody react with the platelet membrane but that the Fc portion takes no part in this reaction, thus clearly demonstrating that the antigen must be on the platelet membrane and is presumably formed by interaction of the membrane with the drug. Co-trimoxazole can cause immune thrombocytopenia, which can be due to the sulphonamide or the trimethoprim component Penicillin given in high doses intravenously can cause haemolytic anaemia. The drug becomes covalently attached to the red cells forming an antigen which undergoes lysis in the presence of antibody and complement. This is clearly an example of the mechanism just referred to. Occasionally sulphonamides appear to cause haemolytic anaemia by a mechanism which does not involve covalent binding to red cells. Penicillin, particularly semisynthetic penicillins can cause granulocytopenia. This has usually occurred when the drug has been given in large doses intravenously. It appears most commonly to be due to marrow depression, but an immune mechanism of the type described above as causing thrombocytopenia seems occasionally to be involved.

Experimental serum sickness produced by the injection of purified proteins, usually into rabbits, is the most extensively investigated type III reaction, and the lesions produced have been convincingly shown to be due to immune complexes. However, the serum sickness-like reaction due to penicillin in man appears to be due to a somewhat different mechanism. Levine[8] has reported that the condition was associated with skin sensitizing and IgG antibodies of benzyl penicilloyl specificity. He concluded that the condition was initiated by skin sensitizing antibodies, and that during the 7-day-period following the onset of symptoms there was a sharp rise in the IgG antibody titre (100-fold or more) which coincided with the cessation of symptoms. It is interesting to speculate whether this rise in IgG antibodies was responsible for the disappearance of the symptoms.

Contact dermatitis is a type IV reaction, of which penicillin is a well-documented but not a common cause. It is of interest that delayed type reactions to penicillin injected intradermally were observed in 24 of 114 patients who had not recently received penicillin therapy and in 6 of 10 patients who had recently suffered accelerated or late urticarial reactions. Although the lesions caused by intradermal penicillin had the gross and histological appearances of the tuberculin reaction, the great majority of patients with this type of sensitivity to penicillin do not develop adverse reactions to penicillin therapy.

REACTIONS TO ANTIBIOTICS COMMONLY USED IN THE TREATMENT OF SEXUALLY TRANSMITTED DISEASES

Only the more common reactions and those which are thought to have an immunological basis are considered below.

Penicillins

Penicillins account for a large number of drug reactions and an enormous variety of adverse reactions may be seen (Table 11.3), but the most common are skin reactions. Other syndromes, such as haematological or renal disorders, are rare and are usually associated with high dose parenteral therapy. Levine's classical paper[8] give some idea of the complexity of mechanisms involved in different reactions.

Table 11.3 Adverse reactions to penicillin

Common
  Maculo-papular rashes
  Urticaria
  Angioedema
  Pruritus
  Generalized allergic reactions,
      including erythema, angioedema and asthma

Rare
  Anaphylaxis
  Serum sickness type of reaction
  Haemolytic anaemia
  Agranulocytosis
  Nephritis
  Hepatitis

Skin reactions

Exanthematic rashes. These vary greatly in morphology, from a simple erythema to a combination of macules and papules simulating an acute exanthem. They are probably the commonest reactions attributed to drugs, however, the mechanisms responsible are not known. Skin tests and tests for penicilloyl specific IgE are usually negative[9].

Pruritus. Although pruritus is a feature of many drug reactions, it may occur alone.

Urticaria. This is common and is indistinguishable from idiopathic urticaria. If the drug is withdrawn, the urticaria usually subsides in a few days, but occasionally persists for weeks. It is a major feature of the serum sickness type of reaction.

Angioedema

Angioedema is a common feature of drug reactions, particularly penicillin. It may occur at any site, but the face is frequently involved. Glottal and laryngeal oedema may cause severe airway obstruction, and can be fatal. Urticaria may also be present.

Serum sickness type of reaction

This closely resembles serum sickness caused by xenogeneic anti-sera, with fever, joint pains and urticaria. It usually occurs a few days after a course of treatment has been completed.

Anaphylactic reactions

These usually occur within minutes of administration of the drug and almost always in under an hour. If the patient does not die within the first few minutes, erythema, rashes, urticaria, angioedema and wheezing may develop, and it is essential to look for these as they are important in distinguishing this condition from other causes of acute collapse. Gastro-intestinal manifestations include nausea, vomiting, abdominal pain and diarrhoea. Other features include laryngeal oedema, hypotension, arrhythmias and shock. These reactions are caused by specific IgE antibodies probably directed in the main against the minor penicillin antigenic determinants[8].

Haemolytic anaemia

This occurs occasionally in patients taking very large doses per day, usually intavenously. The patient's red cells become coated with penicillin, the combination forming the antigen, and the Coombs' test is positive. However, only a very small proportion of patients with antibodies to penicillin-coated red cells develop haemolytic anaemia. Recovery occurs on withdrawal of the drug.

Agranulocytosis

This occurs in patients taking very large doses, usually of semisynthetic penicillins. Withdrawl of the drug results in recovery. Most cases are thought to be due to bone marrow suppression, although in some, an immunological mechanism may be involved.

Aplastic anaemia

This is a very rare complication.

Nephritis and Hepatitis

Nephritis is rare, and usually occurs when high doses are being given. Hepatitis has been recorded.

Cephalosporins

Reactions to these drugs closely resemble those due to the penicillins.

Tetracyclines

Reactions to these drugs occur less than half as commonly as do reactions to the penicillins.

Skin reactions

Apart from pruritus and exanthematic rashes, the following may occur but all are rare.

Erythema multiforme. Erythematous papules, often with central bullae, develop on the extensor surfaces of the extremities. Fever is common and there may be joint and abdominal pain.

Stevens–Johnson syndrome. This is a bullous variant of erythema-multiforme with severe involvement of the ocular, oral and genital mucosae.

Epidermal necrolysis. Also called the scalded skin syndrome, because the erythematous plaques become bullous and vast areas of necrotic skin are shed. Death may occur if a large proportion of the total body skin is involved.

Photosensitisation and oncholysis. Both have been reported.

Hepatic and renal involvement

In a few rare instances hepatic and renal reactions have been noted.

Blood dyscrasias

Severe leukopenia, thrombocytopenia, haemolytic anaemia and aplastic anaemia all occur, but very rarely. Mild reversible leukopenia, however, is not uncommon.

Doxycycline (Vibramycin)

This tetracycline is commonly used in STD clinics. It produces similar side effects to other tetracyclines, but these have only rarely been reported.

Co-trimoxazole (Trimethoprim-sulphamethoxazole)

Adverse reactions resemble those due to the sulphonamides, but may also be caused by the trimethoprim component. Reactions to co-trimoxazole are discussed below.

Metronidazole

Various rashes may occur, but adverse reactions to this drug are uncommon. There may be mild reversible leukopenia.

Erythromycin

Adverse reactions to erythromycin are relatively uncommon. Skin involvement includes pruritus, maculopapular rashes and urticaria. Anaphylaxis has been reported. Cholestatic jaundice is a well recognized side-effect of eyrthromycin estolate, but does occur with other formulations of erythromycin.

DIAGNOSIS

The diagnosis of drug hypersensitivity is difficult. The first step is to take a detailed history which may help to distinguish side-effects of the drug from a putative allergic reaction, or may reveal that the reaction was a feature of the disorder being treated. *In vitro* and *in vivo* tests have been developed, but even in the case of penicillin, which is the drug most widely studied, these tests are difficult to interpret and of doubtful value to the clinician. The most definite answer can be obtained from drug challenge, but this procedure is potentially dangerous. These issues will be discussed below, mainly using penicillin as an example, since this is the only drug for which there is extensive published work on tests for hypersensitivity.

History

It is important to obtain an accurate history of the reaction, including its timing in relation to the start of drug therapy and to establish the dose and route of administration of the drug. The disease being treated may be relevant: some drugs cause reactions in a particular disease – ampicillin frequently causes a rash when given in the early phase of infectious mononucleosis; or the reaction may be a feature of the disease – maculopapular rashes are common in viral upper respiratory infections, even when antibiotics are not given. The reaction may be a side-effect rather than a hypersensitivity reaction. Diarrhoea or nausea are common side-effects during antibiotic therapy, or candidiasis may occur in susceptiable subjects.

It should be established whether the patient has had previous exposure to the drug or drugs of similar chemical structure. The cross-allergenicity between penicillins and cephalosporins is well-documented (see below), but the exact incidence is not known. An antibody-mediated hypersensitivity reaction requires previous exposure to the drug in order to stimulate the formation of antibodies.

The time between drug administration and the occurrence of symptoms is important. In patients taking a drug for the first time, sensitization and the consequent development of symptoms does not usually occur for 7–10 days unless the patient has previously been sensitized to a chemically related, cross-reacting drug. The drug can sometimes be taken for long periods before sensilisation occurs. If the drug forms a depot, symptoms may develop after the first 10 days or at any time thereafter when the drug is being released. Unfortunately anaphylaxis often occurs without warning. Less than half the cases of anaphylaxis due to penicillin were known to have a history of a previous adverse reaction[10]. Anaphylaxis has also been reported to have occurred midway through a course of daily treatment with penicillin[11].

Recovery on withdrawal of the drug and recurrence if the drug has been re-administered provides strong evidence, but does not prove, that the drug has caused the reaction, unless one or other of these phenomena has been observed on more than one occasion.

If, after taking a history, it seems possible that the drug caused the reaction, the most sensible approach is to try to find a suitable alternative drug. Advice from a clinical microbiologist can be most helpful. If an alternative drug cannot be found, and immediate treatment is necessary, the following options are available: *in vivo* tests (skin tests or patch tests); *in vitro* tests (tests for specific IgE or other drug-dependent antibodies) or drug challenge. Intradermal skin tests and most *in vitro* tests will only detect IgE antibodies, and if the hypersensitivity reaction has occurred through some other mechanism, such as direct histamine release from mast cells, these tests are of no value. Even when the reaction is IgE-mediated, *in vivo* and *in vitro* tests are difficult to interpret and of doubtful clinical value. For antibiotics other than penicillin, there are either no tests or they are in the early stages of development and remain to be evaluated in relation to the history and to the results of drug challenge. Assays for specific antibodies to trimethoprim have recently been developed[12,13], but their clinical application needs to be established.

Skin tests

Skin tests are used to detect specific IgE antibodies. The principle is that when antigen is injected into the skin, it will combine with specific IgE antibodies bound to cutaneous mast cells and trigger local mediator release, resulting clinically in a wheal and flare. Skin tests can either be performed as prick tests scratch tests or intradermal tests. In prick tests tiny quantities of allergen (approximately 3×10^{-6} ml) are pricked through a drop of an aqueous solution of the allergen extract into the skin. These are the standard tests used in conventional allergy diagnosis, for example to inhalant and food allergens, and are extremely safe. Intradermal skin tests involve injection of larger quantities of allergen (up to 0.05 ml) into the skin, are potentially dangerous (they may cause anaphylactic reactions) and have been abandoned in the United Kingdom for diagnosis of inhalant and food allergies. Almost all of the literature on immediate skin tests for penicillin describes intradermal injection of the drug, a technique which requires practice.

Because skin tests with benzyl penicillin are often unhelpful, a great deal of effort has been put into developing reagents with different penicillin determinants in the hope of improving the specificity of skin testing. These are referred to as the major and minor determinants. The major determinant, penicilloyl, is used for skin testing as benzyl penicilloyl polylysine and can be obtained commercially (Pre-pen)*. The minor determinants are available only in research centres. For routine diagnostic use, most workers use either benzyl penicilloyl polylysine alone or both this and benzyl penicillin. The solvent is used as a control. Benzyl penicilloyl polylysine is used at a concentration of 6×10^{-5} mol/l, benzyl penicillin is used as freshly prepared solutions containing 10000 and 100u/ml. However, there are two major problems with these skin tests: safety and interpretation.

Fatal reactions to intradermal skin tests with benzyl penicillin, although rare, have been reported[10,14,15]. A fatal reaction to scratch testing with penicillin has also be reported[16]. It has been suggested, however, that benzyl penicillin should be included as a skin test reagent, because some cases of unequivocal anaphylaxis have been shown on subsequent skin testing to be negative to benzyl penicolloyl polylysine and positive to benzyl penicillin[17]. Benzyl penicilloyl polylysine seems to be remarkably safe. However several generalized non-fatal allergic reactions to this reagent have been reported[18,19,20]

The interpretation of penicillin skin tests is difficult, and a positive skin test appears to have little predictive value. In published studies much larger numbers of skin test negative patients than positive have been challenged or treated with penicillin. Heaton et al.[20] carried out penicilloyl polylysine skin tests in 3935 patients attending a venerology clinic, 3509 of whom were later treated with penicillin. Positive skin tests were seen in 102 of these patients while 34 showed indeterminate skin tests. None reacted to treatment. The remainder (3373) had negative skin tests and 5 (0.15%) had an adverse reaction to treatment. In a study using a battery of nine penicillin-derived reagents[21] four of eight patients (50%) with positive skin tests and 12 (4%) of 290 with negative skin tests reacted to challenge. Adkinson et al.[22] used two skin test reagents. Of 54 patients with histories of reactions to penicillin, but with negative skin tests, who were challenged none (possibly one) reacted adversely; of 16 with positive skin tests, the only one who was challenged developed a mild urticarial reaction. One of the largest series[19] involved over 13000 patients who were skin tested with penicilloyl polylysine and then treated with penicillin. Of 418 with a positive skin test, 30 (7%) reacted to treatment. Ten (1.3%) of 782 with equivocal skin tests, and 63 (0.5%) of 13530 with negative skin tests also reacted to penicillin therapy. Whilst most studies show that relatively small numbers with negative skin tests subsequently react to penicillin (0.15%, 4.0%, 0.0% [?2.0%] and 0.5% in the series quoted above); for an individual patient, a negative skin test cannot be relied on to mean that the patient will not react to the drug. Skin testing is, therefore, of little practical help to the practising physician.

Intradermal skin testing is not easy unless the operator is practised. In most published series, a number of uninterpretable skin test reactions has been found, and this number is likely to be high if the person performing the tests is inexperienced. This was shown in a study of 16239 patients[19]: when skin tests were carried out on 8603 patients by one experienced operator there were

*From: Kremers Urban Co., 5600 West County Line Road, PO Box 2038, Milwaukee, Wisc., 53201 USA

only 1% ambiguous reactions, but when 7636 patients were tested by several technicians at other clinics this figure rose to 10.3%s. Although some workers take an equivocal skin test to be negative, the incidence of reactions to penicillin in patients with equivocal skin tests in the large series just mentioned[19] was almost three times that in patients with negative skin tests.

IgE antibodies can disappear if patients are no longer exposed to the antigen. This is seen in bee sting allergy, and it also applies to penicillin allergy. Although penicillin antibodies have been shown to disappear in as short a period as 30 days[23], in some patients they persist for years. In one study of 32 patients, five had lost their antibody one year after last exposure and ten had no demonstrable antibody after five years[23]. It is possible that if a patient with negative skin tests was given penicillin he might be re-sensitized: 51 of 614 skin test negative subjects became skin test positive after a single therapeutic injection of benzathine penicillin, but none of these racted to a second injection of the same substance[24]. It is not clear whether skin testing could also re-sensitize a skin test negative patient, but this possibility has been put forward in defence of *in vitro* tests for IgE antibodies. However, none of 17 individuals with a history of penicillin sensitivity who were initially skin test negative with penicilloyl polylysine reacted positively when re-tested 5 weeks later with the same reagent[24].

The demonstration of specific IgE by taking blood from a patient and injecting it intradermally into a normal subject and locally challenging with antigen (Prausnitz-Küstner reaction) is virtually obsolete as it carries the risk of transmitting hepatitis or AIDS. The alternative use of monkeys instead of man is prohibitively expensive.

Patch tests may be diagnostic in contact dermatitis. Contact sensitivity to antibiotics is commonly seen with neomycin, and occasionally with penicillin. Patients sensitive to neomycin often show cross-reactivity with kanamycin, gentamicin and framycetin.

In vitro tests

A number of *in vitro* tests has been devised most of which have been designed to demonstrate antibodies to penicillin (see review by Assem,[25]). They are not generally available in routine laboratories, and none is entirely satisfactory. The most widely used and the only commercially available test, is the RAST (radio-allergo-sorbent test), which is used to measure IgE antibodies, specific for penicillin antigens. The results parallel those of skin testing[26-28], and the same shortcomings apply in their interpretation with both false positive and false negative results being found. The difficulty with the RAST possibly arises because of the definition of penicillin allergic (and non-allergic) subjects, used by the manufacturer as positives (and controls) to establish the normal range in the test. For this purpose patients were defined as penicillin allergic on the basis of the history alone. These subjects are likely to be a mixed population, and not all of these would react when re-exposed to penicillin. Patients defined as positive and negative on RAST will, therefore, not necessarily have a corresponding response to drug challenge.

The RAST is expensive and time-consuming and requires the appropriate laboratory facilities, whereas the skin test is cheap and quick. However, the RAST does eliminate the minimal risk inherent in skin testing.

Measurement of total IgE is of no value, as clinically significant levels of specific IgE may occur without a concomitant rise in total serum IgE.

Challenge tests

A history of a severe reaction is normally considered to be an absolute contra-indication to further treatment with the offending drug. If a mild or moderate reaction has occurred, and treatment with the drug is considered essential, challenge tests may be indicated, but the risks of test dosing cannot be overemphasized. The challenge test should only be done in a unit with facilities for resuscitation, preferably by a clinical allergist with experience of drug hypersensitivity. An anaesthetist should be available and intravenous access should be established before the test is started. The initial dose of the drug should be extremely small, since a severe reaction has followed the intradermal injection of 3×10^{-6} of a unit of procaine penicillin[29]. Increasing doses are given at intervals, the size of the increments and the timing depending on the severity and nature of the previous reaction. To minimise the risk, if the drug is usually administered parenterally, the initial dose may be given orally and parenteral administration started only if oral doses are tolerated. The dose is gradually increased until a single therapeutic dose is given. If no reaction occurs, a therapeutic course should be given since reactions may occur after several doses or several days treatment. For this reason, challenge tests should only be performed if it is necessary to start treatment immediately. If any reaction occurs the test is stopped immediately and the appropriate treatment is given. Adrenaline must be given immediately an anaphylactic reaction occurs (see below).

With some drugs, e.g. vaccines or radiological contrast media, when the quantity administered has been slowly increased to a full therapeutic dose, no more can be given. In this circumstance a negative reaction to a challenge test means only that the patient is not sensitive to the drug *at that time*. Challenge may stimulate a rise in antibody titre in a previously sensitized subject, so that treatment with the same drug at a later stage could still cause an adverse reaction.

CROSS-REACTIVITY BETWEEN PENICILLINS AND CEPHALOSPORINS

It is often said that cephalosporins can safely be given to patients who have reacted adversely to penicillins. This belief is based on the fact that although both groups of drugs contain the β-lactam ring, the five membered thiazolidine ring of penicillin is replaced in cephalosporins by the six membered dihydrothiazine ring and that they also have different side chains (Figure 11.1). It was, therefore, argued that cross-reactivity would be unlikely. Initially, this belief appeared to be supported by the observation that three patients with strongly positive skin tests with benzyl penicillin did not show

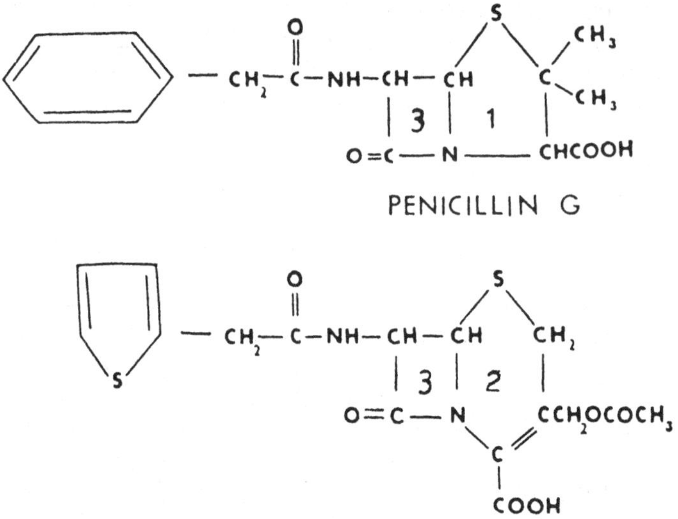

PENICILLIN G

CEPHALOTHIN

Figure 11.1 Chemical structures of penicillin G and cephalothin. 1 = thiazolidine ring; 2 = dihydrothiazine 3 = β-lactam ring

any reaction on skin testing with cephalosporin C. Furthermore, a number of reports appeared describing patients believed to be sensitive to penicillin who did not develop any adverse reaction when treated with a cephalosporin[30,31]. However, case reports soon appeared of patients thought to be sensitive to penicillins, who developed severe reactions including anaphylactic shock when given a cephalosporin[32-34].

The unpredictability of the reactions of patients to these two groups of drugs led to extensive studies of their immunogenicity in animals. Drugs which cause adverse reactions by an immunological mechanism – that is allergic reactions – can do so only if they combine with a macromolecule – almost always a protein – to form a complete antigen. It was soon found that penicillins and cephalosporins which had reacted with protein were immunogenic and could produce antibodies which could be demonstrated by techniques such as haemagglutination of red cells coated with the appropriate drug, precipitation of the corresponding drug protein conjugate and passive cutaneous anaphylaxis. Cross-reactivity could be demonstrated between penicillin and cephalosporin antibodies in these systems. Thus, for instance cephalosporin antibodies agglutinate not only red cells coated with a cephalosporin but also red cells coated with penicillin. However, the haemagglutination titres were higher with cells coated with the drug used to stimulate the formation of the antibody than when cells coated with the other antibiotic were used. Furthermore, the degree of cross-reactivity differed greatly from one serum to another. The reason for this heterogeneity is obscure. Some guinea pigs sensitized with penicillin developed such powerfully cross-reacting antibodies that they developed anaphylaxis when challenged intravenously with a cephalooridine-polylysine, conjugate[35].

The techniques used to stimulate the formation of drug-specific antibodies in experimental animals are of course very different from the mechanisms that cause the spontaneous development of such antibodies in man. However, the animal experiments do show that protein conjugates of these drugs stimulate the formation of drug specific antibodies, and very interestingly that some animals develop antibodies which are much more cross-reactive than those developed by other animals of the same species.

How far do these observations help in assessing the risk of treating with a cephalosporin a patient thought to have had an adverse reaction to penicillin? As with so many problems concerned with allergic reactions to antibiotics, apart from drug challenge, there is no way of telling with certainty that a patient's reaction was due to the suspected drug. However, there can be no doubt that cross-reactions do occur. According to Green[36] nearly 50% of patients with a history of a reaction to penicillin and a positive skin test with penicilloyl polylysine, developed an adverse reaction to cephalothin. Levine[37] has concluded that there is cross-reactivity between penicillins and cephalosporins, but that the probable clinical outcome of therapy with a cephalosporin in a patient who is allergic to penicillin differs in different individuals. In view of the impossibility at present of predicting which patients will develop strongly cross-reacting antibodies, Moellering and Swartz[38] concluded that '... all cephalosporins probably should be avoided in patients with a past history of anaphylaxis (or immediate type hypersensitivity) to any of the penicillins'. This statement is probably too sweeping for it should be remembered that many reactions attributed to penicillin are either co-incidental and not due to the drug, or if due to the drug are not immunologically mediated and, therefore that the patient may not have an antibody that could cross-react with a cephalosporin. Consequently in many cases this drug will be tolerated.

CO-TRIMOXAZOLE

Co-trimoxazole is, in general, remarkably well tolerated and seldom produces serious side-effects. Of these the most important are: neutropenia ($<1000/mm^3$), thrombocytopenia ($<50000/mm^3$), impaired hepatic and renal function and severe cutaneous reactions including erythema multiforme, Lyell's syndrome and the Stevens–Johnson syndrome. Of the minor reactions macropapular rashes are common as are minor degrees of neutropenia and thrombocytopenia. Biochemical evidence of abnormal hepatic and renal function is also not uncommon. Reactions caused by co-trimoxazole are usually attributed to the sulphonamide constituent of the drug, but this has rarely been proved.

Granulocytopenia is thought mostly to be due to marrow depression, but sulphonamides have been associated with a drug-dependent immune mechanism. Mild reversible neutropenia may occur in as many as 10% of patients.

Sulphonamide-induced thrombocytopenia due to an immune mechanism is well documented, but trimethoprim may be responsible[13].

253

Pancytopenia occurs rarely and has probably been caused by the sulphonamide component.

Sulphonamides may cause acute haemolysis in patients who are deficient in the enzyme glucose 6-phosphate dehydrogenase (G6-PD) and sulphamethoxazole – the sulphonamide component of co-trimoxazole – has been documented as a cause.

Although the severe reactions listed above rarely occur, it is important to note that deaths from co-trimoxazole increase strikingly with the age of the patient. Thus, up to 40 years of age, deaths per million prescriptions were rare; between the ages of 40 and 65 deaths numbered just over 1 per million prescriptions, but at ages 65 and over this figure rose to more than 4 deaths per million prescriptions[39].

Because severe reactions are rare the rest of this review will be concerned only with the much commoner dermatological reactions. The incidence of rashes in patients given co-trimoxazole in conventional doses for general medical and surgical conditions is usually low. In two large series including over 3000 patients the incidence was between 2% and 4%[40,41].

Rashes associated with co-trimoxazole are of particular interest in genitourinary medicine because they occur so frequently in patients with the acquired immunodeficiency syndrome (AIDS) treated with co-trimoxazole for *Pneumocystis carinii* pneumonia (PCP). In many reported series the incidence of rashes has been of the order of 50% or more [40–42].

When PCP in patients with AIDS has been treated with co-trimoxazole, the drug has usually been given in high dosage intravenously, and it has often been suggested that this may explain the high incidence of rashes. However, when PCP in non-AIDS patients has been treated with high doses of co-trimoxazole intravenously or orally the incidence of rashes has been low[45,46]. This suggests that neither administration of co-trimoxazole by the intravenous route nor the administration of high doses of the drug are the cause of the high incidence of rashes seen in patients with AIDS associated with PCP.

A third possibility to be considered is that the high incidence of rashes in patients with AIDS associated with PCP who are treated with co-trimoxazole is in some way due to the immunosuppression caused by infection with the human immunodeficiency virus (HIV). However, when non-AIDS patients with PCP who were receiving immunosuppressive therapy, usually for malignant diseases, were treated with co-trimoxazole the incidence of rashes was low[45–47]. These observations clearly emphasise the importance of infection with HIV in causing these rashes and although they, perhaps, suggest that these rashes are not due to immunosuppression it is not impossible that these rashes result from some special characteristic of the immunosuppression caused by HIV. That these rashes are due to some effect of infection with the human immunodeficiency virus itself is also suggested by the observation that 8 of 10 patients with AIDS who were given co-trimoxazole as a prophylaxis against the development PCP developed a rash[43].

Practically nothing is known about the mechanism causing rashes in AIDS patients given co-trimoxazole. They disappear if the drug is withdrawn and may even disappear during the course of uninterrupted treatment[42]. They may recur if the drug is re-administered, but do not always do so[42,44,48]. These observations suggest that more than one mechanism may be involved. Lowen and colleagues[49] have pointed out that Septrin (co-trimoxazole) dispersible tablets contain the azo dye sunset yellow, and they thought the rashes in three of their patients might have been due to an immune reaction to this substance. However, they did not challenge their patients with sunset yellow and, therefore, the possibility that some rashes occurring during treatment with co-trimoxazole may not be due to the drug but to an excipient, remains unproved.

PROPHYLACTIC STEROID THERAPY

Assem[50] has listed a number of considerations which might lead one to expect that pretreatment with corticosteroids might reduce the incidence and severity of immediate type hypersensitivity reactions. To these could be added the observation that although pretreatment with steroids does not block the immediate phase of the type I reaction induced by bronchial challenge with allergen it does inhibit the late phase reaction. However, Assem[50] concluded that 'The effect of corticosteroids on immediate type allergy is surrounded by a lot of confusion'! A major problem in assessing efficacy is that anaphylaxis may not recur when a drug believed to have caused it is again administered[51]. Certain observations in man make any significant benefit seem unlikely. The first is that patients given up to 30 mg of prednisolone daily for up to 30 days did not show any reduction in whealing in response to skin testing with pollen extracts, nor did patients treated with 1% prednisolone ointment three times a day onto the same area of skin for periods up to 6 months show any reduction in wheal formation in the treated area[52]. Furthermore two patients have been described who developed anaphylaxis penicillin after pretreatment with steroids: one after pretreatment with a single dose of 15 mg prednisone[53] and the other who had been treated with 15 mg prednisolone daily for a year before the penicillin was given[54]. This patient had been given penicillin several times previously without trouble. It has been argued that larger doses of steroids might have conferred benefit, but these findings suggest that pretreatment with steroids would be unlikely to ameliorate type I anaphylactic reactions.

DESENSITIZATION

There has been a large number of publications on desensitization for hypersensitivity to antibiotics. Although much of this literature has claimed that desensitization is successful, this has not usually been proven. The problem with the majority of these studies is that the patient has not been proven to be allergic to the drug before desensitization was begun. This is illustrated by a recent study on desensitization to penicillin[55]. The 'allergic' patients had a history of penicillin hypersensitivity and a positive skin test. Small increasing doses of penicillin were given orally followed by larger doses subcutaneously and then intramuscularly and finally intravenously. Of 30 patients treated in this way, 21 did not develop any reaction; nine developed urticaria which responded to antihistamines and one developed nephritis in the third week of therapy. All completed a full course of antibiotic therapy. The authors interpreted this as successful desensitization. In support of this they noted that when the skin tests of these patients were repeated after they had been given small but increasing doses and at a time when they were receiving full therapeutic doses intravenously, the tests had become negative or less intensely positive. The significance of this observation is uncertain. It has been interestingly discussed by Sullivan[56] who was one of the authors of the original report. As Sullivan[56] pointed out, intravenous penicillin therapy results in very high concentrations of penicillin (hapten) in the body fluids, and one possible explanation for the reduced skin sensitivity is that it was due to hapten inhibition. If this was so, it could equally well happen in patients with positive skin tests who do not react to treatment even when not 'desensitized'. In fact, the observations interpreted as evidence of successful desensitization could, in the absence of proof of sensitivity by drug challenge, equally well be interpreted as negative reactions to drug challenge.

However, there are some publications which appear to show that desensitization may be effective in patients where the diagnosis of drug allergy was established. Finegold[57] for instance reported a patient with AIDS and *Pneumocystis carinii* pneumonia, who was treated with intravenous co-trimoxazole on three separate occasions, each time developing fever, rash and wheezing. An attempt was made to desensitize him, starting with an oral dose of co-trimoxazole containing $0.01\,\mu g$ sulphamethoxazole followed by incremental doses. He developed cutaneous tingling, but the dose was gradually increased. On the third day intravenous doses were given, starting with 1 ml of the intravenous preparation and increasing to a therapeutic dose of 19 ml. This dose was then given intravenously every six hours. The patient developed mild fever and arthralgia which subsided by the fourth day. It was possible to continue the course of treatment with co-trimoxazole intravenously. This appears to have been an example of successful desensitization. However, in a patient who has had a severe reaction to a drug, desensitization is hazardous[59], and at least one death which was probably due to this procedure has been reported[59].

TREATMENT OF DRUG REACTIONS

Whenever a drug reaction is suspected, the drug should be stopped. If the symptoms subside, this suggests that the suspect drug was the cause, although it must be remembered that the symptoms may have been due to an unrelated, self-limited, condition. Symptoms may persist if the drug was given in depot form, from which it was slowly released.

Anaphylaxis

The immediate treatment of anaphylactic shock is the subcutaneous injection of adrenaline. The usual recommended dose in an adult is 0.5 ml of 1 in 1000 dilution. Intramuscular adrenaline may be better absorbed if there is poor peripheral circulation. Time should not be wasted setting up an intravenous line until this has been given. A further dose of adrenaline may be given in 5 minutes if there is no improvement. Chlorpheniramine maleate (Piriton) 10 mg may be given intravenously or intramuscularly. Hydrocortisone is of no immediate value, as it has no effect for several hours, but may be given after all urgent treatment has been given and reovery initiated, as it can minimize late onset or persistent symptoms. It should be given to all patients with asthma. Other measures, such as the treatment of asthma, control of hypoxia and arrhythmias and cardiovascular support, may be required depending on the clinical presentation.

An important measure, which will almost certainly reduce the incidence of fatalities from anaphylactic shock, is to ensure the patient remains in the clinic for at least 30 minutes after the injection of any drug capable of causing this type of reaction, e.g. benzyl penicillin. If this is done the patient will probably still be in the clinic when symptoms appear and immediate treatment can be given, which may be life-saving. If the patient has left the clinic before symptoms appear, treatment is unlikely to be instituted quickly enough. Furthermore, if a history of a recent drug injection is not obtained appropriate treatment may not be given. It may be of some comfort to genito-urinary physicians to know that of 94655 patients treated in STD clinics with parenteral penicillin, 52 developed anaphylaxis of varying severity and one died[60]. Most were kept in the clinic 30 minutes after the injection and this allowed early treatment and probably accounts for the low death rate. Oral penicillin is, much safer. Five cases of fatal anaphylaxis from oral penicillin had been reported up to 1971, and no cases have been reported to the Committee on Safety of Medicines.

CONCLUSION

Adverse reactions to antibiotics are common. A variety of clinical manifestations may occur from trivial rashes to fatal anaphylaxis. The mechanism of many drug reactions remains obscure, and although some are immune mediated, e.g. due to IgE or IgG antibodies, many are not truly allergic. Reactions attributed to drugs often do not recur on re-administration of the drug. In an individual, however, re-administration of the drug may cause a severe, even fatal, reaction. Drug re-administration should not be undertaken if there is a history of serious reaction, unless no other drug is available and treatment is essential. Tests for drug hypersensitivity are largely unhelpful, and sensitivity can only be established by challenge testing. This should be undertaken by experts in hospital with adequate facilities for resuscitation. Patients being treated with drugs known to cause reactions, e.g. parenteral penicillin, should be kept in the clinic for at least 30 minutes after injection, as prompt treatment of anaphylactic/anaphylactoid reactions should reduce mortality.

ACKNOWLEDGEMENTS

Dr Ewan is supported by the Medical Research Council and the Asthma Research Council. We are grateful to Ms G. Arscott, for typing the manuscript.

References

1. Ackroyd, J. F. and Rook, A. J. (1968). Allergic drug reactions. In Gell, P. G. H. and Coombs, R. R. A. (eds.). *Clinical Aspects of Immunology*, 2nd Edn. pp. 693–755. (Oxford: Blackwell Scientific)
2. Ackroyd, J. F. (1975). Immunological mechanisms in drug hypersensitivity. In Gell, P. G. H., Coombs, R. R. A. and Lachmann, P. J. (eds.). *Clinical Aspects of Immunology*, 3rd Edn. pp. 913–61. (Oxford: Blackwell Scientific)
3. Ackroyd, J. F. The diagnosis of disorders of the blood due to drug hypersensitivity caused by an immune mechanism. In Ackroyd, J. F. (ed.). *Immunological Methods*. pp. 453–513. (Oxford: Blackwell Scientific)
4. Aster, R. H. (1983). Thrombocytopenia due to enhanced platelet destruction. In Williams, W. J., Beutler, E., Erslev, A. J., Lichtman, M. A. (eds.). *Haematology*, 3rd Edn. pp. 1298–338 (McGraw Hill)
5. Shulman, N. R. (1958). Immunoreactions involving platelets. I. A steric and kinetic model for formation of a complex from a human antibody, quinidine as a haptene and platelets and for fixation of complement by the complex. *J. Exp. Med.*, **107**, 665–90
6. Smith, M. E. Reid, D. M. Jones, C. E. Jordan, J. V. Kautz, C. A. and Shulman, N. R. (1987). Binding of quinine- and quinidine-dependent drug antibodies to platelets is mediated by the Fab domain of the immunoglobulin G and is not Fc dependent. *J. Clin. Invest.*, **79**, 912–17
7. Christie, D. J. Mullen, P. C. and Aster, R. H. (1985). Fab-mediated binding of drug-dependent antibodies to platelets in quinidine- and quinine-induced thrombocytopenia. *J. Clin. Invest.*, **75**, 310–14
8. Levine, B. B. (1966). Immunologic mechanism of penicillin allergy: a haptenic model system for the study of allergic diseases in man. *N. Engl. J. Med.*, **275**, 1115–25
9. Juhlin, L. and Wide, L. (1972). IgE antibodies and penicillin allergy. In Dash, C. H. and Jones, H. E. H. (eds.). *Mechanisms in Drug Allergy: a Glaxo symposium*, pp. 139–47. (London: Churchill Livingstone)
10. Idsoe, O., Guthe, T., Willcox, R. R. and deWeck, A. L. (1968). Nature and extent of penicillin side-reactions with particular reference to fatalities from anaphylactic shock. *Bull. WHO*, **38**, 159–88
11. Myhre, J. R. (1956). Shock during penicillin therapy. *Tidskrift den Norske Laegeforening*, **76**, 256–8 (In Norwegian)
12. Harle, D. G., Baldo, B. A., Smal, M. A. and Fisher, M. M. (1987). Tests for the diagnosis of immediate hypersensitivity to drugs and identification of drug allogenic determinants. (Abstr.) *British Society for Allergy and Clinical Immunology*. Autumn meeting
13. Claas, F. H. J., van der Meer, J. W. M. and Langerak, J. (1979). Immunological effect of co-trimoxazole on platelets. *Br. Med. J.*, **2**, 898–9
14. Rose, B. (1953). In Schiller, I. W. (ed.). Allergic Reactions to Penicillin: A Panel Discussion. *J. Allergy*, **24**, 383–404
15. Driagin, G. B. (1966). Anaphylactic shock with fatal outcome following an intradermal test for sensitivity to penicillin. *Terapeuticheskii Arkhiv*, **38**, 118–19 (In Russian)
16. Dogliotti, M. (1968). An instance of fatal reaction to the penicillin scratch-test. *Dermatologica*, **136**, 489–96
17. Rosenblum, A. H. (1970). Clinical experience in testing patients with penicillin hypersensitivity. In Stewart, G. R. and McGovern, J. P. (eds.). *Penicillin Allergy: Clinical and Immunologic Aspects*. pp. 135–46. (Springfield: Charles Thomas)
18. Resnik, S. S. and Shelley, W. B. (1966). Penicilloyl polylysine skin test: anaphylaxis in absence of penicillin sensitivity. *J. Am. Med. Assoc.*, **196**, 740
19. Brown, B. C., Price, E. V. and Moore, M. B. (1964). Penicilloyl polylysine as an intradermal test of penicillin sensitivity. *J. Am. Med. Assoc.*, **189**, 599–604

20. Heaton, C. L., Posey, R. E. and Lentz, J. W. (1970). Penicilloyl polylysine skin tests in venereal disease clinics: reactions to the test antigen. In Stewart G. T. and McGovern, J. P. (eds.). *Penicillin Allergy: Clinical and Immunologic Aspects*. pp. 147–55. (Springfield: Charles Thomas)

21. Solley, G. O., Gleich, G. J. and van Dellen, R. G. (1982). Penicillin allergy: clinical experience with a battery of skin test reagents. *J. Allergy Clin. Immunol.*, **69**, 238–44

22. Adkinson, N. F., Thompson, W. L., Maddrey, W. C. and Lichtenstein, L. M. (1971). Routine use of penicillin skin testing on an inpatient service. *N. Engl. J. Med.*, **285**, 22–4

23. Kraft, D., Roth, A., Mischer, P., Pichler, H. and Ebner, H. (1977). Specific and total serum IgE measurements in the diagnosis of penicillin allergy: a long-term follow-up study. *Clin. Allergy*, **7**, 21–8

24. Rytel, M. W., Klion, F. M., Arlander, T. R. and Miller, L. F. (1963). Detection of penicillin hypersensitivity with penicilloyl polylysine. *J. Am. Med. Assoc.*, **186**, 894–8

25. Assem, E-S. K. (1981). Tests for detecting drug allergy. In Davies, D. M. (ed.). *Textbook of Adverse Drug Reactions*, 2nd Edn. Chapter 26. pp. 554–568. (Oxford: Oxford University Press)

26. Spath, P., Huber, H., Ludvan, M., Roth, A., Schwarz, S. and Zelger, J. (1979). Determinations of penicilloyl-specific IgE antibodies for the evaluation of hypersensitivity against penicillin. *Allergy*, **34**, 405–11

27. Jarisch, R., Roth, A., Boltz, A. and Sandor, I. (1981). Diagnosis of penicillin allergy by means of Phadebas RAST penicilloyl G and V and skin tests. *Clin. Allergy*, **11**, 155–60

28. Kraft, D. and Wide, L. (1976). Clinical patterns and results of radioallergosorbent test (RAST) and skin tests in penicillin allergy. *Br. J. Dermatol.*, **94**, 593–601

29. Bierlein, K. J. (1956). Repeated anaphylactic reactions in a patient highly sensitised to penicillin: a case report. *Ann. Allergy*, **14**, 35–40

30. Weinstein, L., Kaplan, K. and Chang, T. W. (1964). Treatment of infections in man with cephalothin. *J. Am. Med. Assoc.*, **189**, 829–34

31. Griffith, R. S. and Black, H. R. (1964). Cephalothin: A new antibiotic. *J. Am. Med. Assoc.*, **189**, 823–8

32. Kabins, S. A., Eisenstein, B. and Cohen, S. (1965). Anaphylactoid reaction to an initial dose of sodium cephalothin. *J. Am. Med. Assoc.*, **193**, 165–6

33. Rothschild, P. D. and Doty, D. B. (1966). Cephalothin reaction after penicillin sensitization. *J. Am. Med. Assoc.*, **196**, 372–3

34. Thoburn, R., Johnson III, J. E. and Cluff, L. E. (1966). Studies on the epidemiology of adverse drug reactions. IV. The relationship of cephalothin and penicillin allergy. *J. Am. Med. Assoc.*, **198**, 345–8

35. Batchelor, F. R., Dewdney, J. M., Weston, R. D. and Wheeler, A. W. (1966). The immunogenicity of cephalosporin derivatives and their cross-reaction with penicillin. *Immunology*, **10**, 21–33

36. Green, G. R. (1970)., Antibiotic therapy in patients with a history of penicillin allergy. In Stewart, G. T. and McGovern, J. P. (eds.). *Penicillin Allergy: Clinical and Immunologic Aspects*. pp. 162–175. (Springfield: Charles Thomas)

37. Levine, B. B. (1973). Antigenicity and cross-reactivity of penicillins and cephalosporins. *J. Infect. Dis.*, **128** (Suppl.) 364–6

38. Moellering, R. C. and Swartz, M. N. (1976). Drug therapy. The newer cephalosporins. *N. Engl. J. Med.*, **294**, 24–8

39. Committee on Safety of Medicines. (1985). *Current Problems*, (July) Number 15 (London:)

40. Jick, H. (1982). Adverse reactions to trimethoprim–sulfamethoxazole in hospitalized patients. *Rev. Infect. Dis.*, **4**, 426–8

41. Jick, S. S., Jick, H., Habakangas, J. A. S. and Dinan, B. J. (1984). Co-trimoxazole toxicity in children. *Lancet*, **2**, 631

42. Gordin, F. M., Simon, G. L., Wofsy, C. B. and Mills, J. (1984). Adverse reactions to trimethoprim sulfamethoxazole in patients with the acquired immunodeficiency syndrome. *Ann. Intern. Med.*, **100**, 495–9

43. Mitsuyasu, R., Groopman, J. and Volberding, P. (1983). Cutaneous reaction to trimethoprim sulfamethoxazole in patients with AIDS and Kaposi's sarcoma. *N. Engl. J. Med.*, **308**, 1535

44. Jaffe, H. S., Abrams, D. I., Ammann, A. J., Lewis, B. J. and Golden, J. A. (1983).

Complications of co-trimoxazole in treatment of AIDS-associated *Pneumocystis carinii* pneumonia in homosexual men. *Lancet*, 2, 1109-11

45. Winston, D. J., Lau, W. K., Gale, R. P. and Young, L. S. (1980). Trimethoprim-sulfamethoxazole for the treatment of *Pneumocystis carinii* pneumonia. *Ann. Intern. Med.*, 92, 762-9

46. Hughes, W. T., Feldman, S., Chaudhary, S. C., Ossi, M. J., Cox, F. and Sanyal, S. K. (1978). Comparison of pentamidine isethionate and trimethoprim sulfamethoxazole in the treatment of *Pneumocystis carinii* pneumonia. *J. Pediat.*, 92, 285-91

47. Kovacs, J. A., Hiemenz, J. W., Macher, A. M., *et al.*, (1984). *Pneumocystis carinii* pneumonia: a comparison between patients with the acquired immunodeficiency syndrome and patients with other immunodeficiencies. *Ann. Intern. Med.*, 100, 663-71

48. Kochen, M. M., Herrmann, C. and Goebel, F. D. (1983). Pentamidine or co-trimoxazole for *Pneumocystis carinii* pneumonia. *Lancet*, 2, 1300-1

49. Lowen, N. P., Moxham, J. and McManus, T. (1987). Reactions to azo dyes in patients with AIDS. *Br. Med. J.*, 295, 612

50. Assem, E-S. K. (1981). Drug Allergy, In Davies, D. M. (ed.). *Textbook of Adverse Drug Reactions*, 2nd Edn. chap. 25 pp. 534-53. (Oxford: Oxford Medical Publications)

51. Green, G. R., Rosenblum, A. H. and Sweet, L. C. (1977). Evaluation of penicillin hypersensitivity: value of clinical history and skin testing with penicilloyl polylysine and penicillin G. *J. Allergy Clin. Immunol.*, 60, 339-45

52. Mancini, R. E., Colombi, P. A., Galli, H. and Orcinoli, L. (1961). Effect of glucocorticoid hormones on experimentally induced allergic reactions on human skin. *J. Allergy*, 32, 471-82

53. Green, G. R., Peters, G. A. and Geraci, J. E. (1967). Treatment of bacterial endocarditis in patients with penicillin hypersensitivity. *Ann. Intern. Med.*, 67, 235-49

54. Bernstein, I. L. and Lustberg, A. (1957). Penicillin anaphylaxis occurring in a patient on steroid therapy. *Ann. Intern. Med.*, 47, 1276-9

55. Sullivan, T. J., Yecies, L. D., Shatz, G. S., Parker, C. W. and Wedner, H. J. (1982). Desensitisation of patients allergic to penicillin using orally administered β-lactam antibiotics. *J. Allergy Clin. Immunol.*, 69, 275-82

56. Sullivan, T. J. (1982). Antigen-specific desensitisation of patients allergic to penicillin. *J. Allergy Clin. Immunol.*, 69, 500-8

57. Finegold, I. (1985). Oral desensitisation to trimethoprim–sulphamethoxazole in a patient with AIDS. (Abstr. No 129) *J. Allergy Clin. Immunol.*, 75, (Suppl.) 137

58. Parker, C. W. (1975). Drug Allergy, Part III. *N. Engl. J. Med.*, 292 957-60

59. Grieco, M. H., Dubin, M. R., Robinson, J. L. and Schwartz, M. J. (1964). Penicillin hypersensitivity in patients with bacterial endocarditis. *Ann. Intern. Med.*, 60, 204-16

60. Rudolph, A. H. and Price, E. V. (1973). Penicillin reactions among patients in venereal disease clinics. A national survey. *J. Am. Med. Assoc.*, 223, 499-501

61. Lasser, E. C., Berry, C. C., Talner, L. B. *et al.* (1987). Pretreatment with corticosteroids to alleviate reactions to intravenous contrast material. *N. Engl. J. Med.*, 317, 845-9

62. Ackroyd, J. F. (1988). Corticosteroids and allergies to contrast material. *N. Engl. J. Med.*, 318, 856

NOTE ADDED IN PROOF

In the section on prophylactic steroid therapy (pg 255) reference was made to the suggestion that larger doses of steroids than those usually used might be effective in protecting patients from adverse drug reactions. The results have now been published of a large multicentre trial of the prophylatic efficacy of two doses of 32 mg of Methylprednisolone in reducing the frequency and severity of adverse reactions to intravenous radiological contrast media[61]. The trial involved 6763 patients but although the authors of the report claimed that this treatment significantly reduced the incidence of adverse reactions, this conclusion was not supported by the data presented and it can only be concluded that in this trial the administration of two doses of Methylprednisolone did not cause a significant reduction in the incidence of severe reactions[62].

12
Envoi

G. W. CSONKA

Research on sexually transmitted diseases (STD) is not a separate entity from the mainstream of medical inquiry but borrows and contributes to it, as does immunology. The great number and variety of STD has proved a powerful stimulus to immunological research and progress. Recent advances such as protective vaccination against hepatitis B is an example of the application of immunology which together with virology, has helped unravel the mechanism of AIDS, probably the most devastating infectious disease of the closing years of this century. Furthermore, immunology is perceived to be integral to the understanding and management of many STD. So far the main impact of immunology in STD has been in its diagnosis, but the prospect of vaccines becoming available in the foreseeable future for genital warts and herpes opens new ways in the prevention of other STD which pose, at present, considerable problems in this field.

However, has the modern physician in genito-urinary medicine taken up the challenge with sufficient enthusiasm, or has he missed recent opportunities by not becoming more closely involved with immunological principles and practice? The training of the specialist genito-urinary physician does not include any in-depth teaching of immunology, although it is needed to understand many of the ailments he treats. How could it become part of the continuing education? Since immunology is complex and rapidly expanding, repeated exposure to its tenets are necessary. It might with advantage form a larger component of the diploma course or board examination for the speciality of junior staff. They could also be given the chance to work for a period in a shared post between a department of immunology and genito-urinary medicine. This raises a second problem: where will immunology be practised once the genito-urinary physician is sensitized? To this end, research laboratories should become required additions for the premier GU medicine departments. There is no reason why the Oslerian revolution which has underpinned modern medicine in other fields should not also apply to genito-urinary medicine.

On the other hand, immunologists could with benefit look in some detail at the whole range of STD – there are at least 20 pathogens and 50 recognized conditions and syndromes[1] – and like all infections are characterized by an immune response, the nature of which remains, in many cases, to be elucidated. There are a number of conditions where significant involvement of immunological factors are suspected, but not yet proven, and where management is unsatisfactory, such as women with frequent or persistent unexplained candidiasis, men with relapsing non-gonococcal urethritis or recurrent genital herpes in either sex. Though these conditions may appear at first sight comparatively trivial, they cause an inordinate amount of frustration and unhappiness for the luckless patient.

One may further question whether genito-urinary physicians have taken into full account the unprecedented changes which have occurred within the past 10 years in their speciality? It would appear that a number have quietly abrogated much of their clinical role in managing an important section of their patients. It must be remembered that until the end of the 19th century, syphilology was almost wholly clinical and hospital-based and treated entirely by venereologists. The introduction of penicillin in the 1940s radically changed the attitude to management. The effective treatment of syphilis and gonorrhoea caused departments of genito-urinary medicine to evolve into out-patient clinics. The emergence of new serious diseases and the recent recognition of complexities of some of the older ones has altered our perspective yet again. In addition, the increasing need for counselling patients gives our speciality an opportunity to take stock urgently. There seem to be several options:

(1) To treat simpler forms of STD, mostly those of non-viral aetiology as out-patients, and to refer others with complicated conditions to practitioners in other disciplines.

(2) To create multipurpose departments which include the basic clinic as under (1) with added facilities to deal with HIV infection and counselling, with genital warts and cervical and other dysplasias including a colposcopy service and hepatitis B screening and vaccination. Some would wish to go further, and suggest that it would be sensible to accommodate family planning, subfertility and psychosexual counselling clinics, all of which operate by appointment, under the same roof. Neither of these options facilitate the basic research or the intensive investigations the subject requires if it is to prosper.

(3) The last option is to have in addition, in-patient accommodation to care for individuals with such conditions as severe genital herpes, pelvic inflammatory disease, Reiter's disease and most aspects of HIV infection. In practice, this would require departments of genito–urinary medicine to be located within large general hospitals preferably with research laboratories, and not, as it too often the case, left entirely isolated from the major hospital or attached to a declining, run-down hospital with limited pathological and high technology supporting facilities.

I recall that when I started my career at St Mary's Hospital, London, there was a small male and female ward serving the speciality, where syphilis in *all* manifestations was treated, as well as other patients with venereal diseases with complications needing admission. There was no question that if an acute medical emergency arose, the genito-urinary physician treated the patient, so that the speciality retained its place at the centre of internal medicine. This arrangement worked well for patients, staff and students alike. It is felt that the univesity hospitals and for those aspiring to excellence, this third option should be considered the most desirable. The teaching of students and young doctors would improve immeasurably in such an environment, reflecting the epidemiological importance of STD as numerically the most frequent cause of infection in the young throughout the world.

Imagine if you will that in addition to hepatitis B vaccine, vaccines for the prevention or treatment of HIV infection, chlamydia, gonorrhoea, genital warts and genital herpes became available. The obvious choice for their administration to achieve optimal benefit for the patient and the community would be a department of genito-urinary medicine that is well staffed and provided with comprehensive community liaison and counselling support. Under these circumstances, vaccines could be modified at the production stage, evaluated clinically and then delivered to the relevant 'high-risk' population. At the same time new rapid diagnostic tests should be routinely available within the clinics of the future – the aim being to diagnose and where possible treat the patients at their first attendance. The reason why a quick diagnosis and short concentrated treatment is particularly relevant in patients with STD, is that it improves compliance, allows a better control of the spread of infection and reduces the number of complications.

As the best possible laboratory service is essential for success, one could argue that there is a place in establishing central laboratories which might include departments of microbiology, immunology and possibly epidemiology. Such centres do exist in a very few places in the world, as within the Center of Communicable Diseases in Atlanta, Georgia in the USA or the State Serum Institute in Copenhagen which deals with all laboratory aspects of gonorrhoea and syphilis for the whole of Denmark. These centres thus have at their disposal extensive and valuable laboratory and epidemiological data and are able to monitor trends which may be of practical importance in the treatment of individual patients as well as wider aspects of public health. In a large country such as Great Britain a number of regional laboratory centres might be more appropriate. Such centres would also encourage both fundamental and applied research, and they could be expected to attract candidates of the highest calibre. This aspect may be further aided by WHO or government sponsored fellowships. However, it would only complement specialized local research to be undertaken in each individual department. Within this framework immunology of STD would have a place.

Venereologists of old, by that I mean those working between the two World Wars, had skills at their disposal, and within the limits of available knowledge were successful. Present-day physicians of genito-urinary medicine still have to retain the old clinical skills, but will have to acquire new skills including a thorough understanding of immunology. It is possible that the number, scope and complexity of some of the new techniques – e.g. colposcopy, the intelligent management of HIV infection or effective counselling for this and other STD – may create the need for some specialization within the practice of genito–urinary medicine. I would expect that such specialists would be accommodated in the existing larger clinics in Great Britain, the clinics needing only comparatively modest modification and extension.

The many small part-time clinics in this country, and elsewhere, still have a purpose and might with advantage continue in their present role. They offer good treatment for the simpler STD together with adequate tracing of patients' contacts and managing of sexual partners, but could refer the more complex case to the nearest now envisaged specialized regional centre.

Historically, the network of STD clinics was created in 1917 in Great Britain, in response to the then very taxing problem of the syphilis outbreak. In this objective they proved effective. It appears that we have now reached a watershed. Changes in the practice of genito–urinary medicine, some of which have been outlined, are urgently needed. The golden age of venereology is passed with such Nobel laureates as Ehrlich and Wagner–Jauregg. If the modern physician in genito–urinary medicine is to inherit his birthright he must adapt; the opportunities are waiting.

ACKNOWLEDGEMENT

I thank S. O'Connor for her secretarial help.

Reference

1. Antal, G. (1987). The epidemiology of sexually transmitted diseases in the tropics. In Osoba, A. O. (ed.). *Clinical Tropical Medicine and Communicable Diseases.* pp. 1–16. (London: Balliere Tindall)

Index

Printed in the United States
By Bookmasters